Advances in Mental Health and Addiction

Series Editor
Masood Zangeneh

More information about this series at http://www.springer.com/series/13393

Thalia MacMillan • Amanda Sisselman-Borgia
Editors

New Directions in Treatment, Education, and Outreach for Mental Health and Addiction

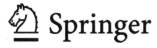 Springer

Editors
Thalia MacMillan
SUNY Empire State College
Community and Human Services
New York, NY, USA

Amanda Sisselman-Borgia
Department of Social Work
Lehman College
Bronx, NY, USA

Advances in Mental Health and Addiction
ISBN 978-3-319-72777-6   ISBN 978-3-319-72778-3   (eBook)
https://doi.org/10.1007/978-3-319-72778-3

Library of Congress Control Number: 2018931374

Printed on acid-free paper

This Springer imprint is published by Springer Nature
The registered company is Springer International Publishing AG
The registered company address is: Gewerbestrasse 11, 6330 Cham, Switzerland

Acknowledgments

From Thalia:
Thanks to my husband Andy and all of my family for all of the love, support, encouragement, and laughter.

From Amanda:
Thank you to my husband Richard Borgia, my mom Peggy Sisselman, my brother Stephen Sisselman, and my in-laws (Gail and Rich Borgia Sr., Dawn Borgia and Michelle Accardi, Michael Borgia, and Denise and Mark Pugach) for all of their consistent support and love. Thank you also to my colleagues at Lehman College, Department of Social Work, who have been very supportive of this project.

Contents

Contributors

Jill Becker Feigeles Wurzweiler School of Social Work, Yeshiva University & Lehman College/CUNY, Livingston, NJ, USA

Kevin Coffey University of Rochester – Psychiatry, SUNY Empire State College – Community and Human Services, Rochester, NY, USA

Rebecca K. Eliseo-Arras, PhD, MSW SUNY Empire State College, Division of Community and Human Services, University at Buffalo, New York, NY, USA

David A. Fullard, PhD, CRC, LMHC Empire State College/SUNY, New York, NY, USA

Rachel Henes, LMSW Freedom Institute, Hallways, New York, NY, USA

E. Gail Horton Florida Atlantic University, School of Social Work, Boca Raton, FL, USA

Naelys Luna Florida Atlantic University, School of Social Work, Boca Raton, FL, USA

Thalia MacMillan, PhD, MSW, EMT SUNY Empire State College, Community & Human Services, New York, NY, USA

Justine McGovern Lehman College, Department of Social Work, Bronx, NY, USA

Jenny Mincin, PhD, MPhil, MPA SUNY Empire State College, Human Services, Saratoga Springs, NY, USA

Jermaine J. Monk Lehman College, City University of New York, Bronx, NY, USA

Rosalind October-Edun SUNY Empire State College, Human Services, Saratoga Springs, NY, USA

Manoj Pardasani, PhD, LCSW, ACSW Graduate School of Social Service, Fordham University, New York, NY, USA

Peter J. Pociluyko SUNY Empire State College, Community & Human Services, Saratoga Springs, NY, USA

Audrey Redding-Raines, PhD, MPA, MSW Rutgers University-Newark, Newark, NJ, USA

Stephanie Sarabia Ramapo College, Department of Social Work, Mahwah, NJ, USA

Amanda Sisselman-Borgia CUNY Lehman College, Department of Social Work, Bronx, NY, USA

Jennifer Spitz SUNY Empire State College, Community & Human Services, Hartsdale, NY, USA

Brenda Williams-Gray, DSW Lehman College/CUNY, Bronx, NY, USA

A. Jordan Wright, PhD, ABAP New York University, Department of Applied Psychology, Steinhardt School of Culture, Education, and Human Development, New York, NY, USA

Part I
Diagnosis

Chapter 1
Dual Diagnosis: An Introduction

Kevin Coffey

Dual Diagnosis: An Introduction

This introductory chapter will discuss (1) the complexity associated with making a specific diagnosis when individuals have both mental illness and substance use disorder, (2) treatment associated with dual diagnosis, (3) issues of cultural competency as it pertains to this topic, and (4) overall implications for this topic for the future. There will be clinical examples throughout the chapter that will hopefully help to illustrate the information presented.

Diagnosis and Prevalence of Co-occurring Disorders

Clinicians often think of diagnosis as specific and exact. In reality, most individuals treated by mental health clinicians have a combination of diagnoses (Blazer, 2000). Individuals who experience depression often have some anxiety (Beck, 1974). Individuals who are treated for anxiety often have some issues associated with depression. In mental health clinics, many individuals present for treatment of anxiety and depression. Often when individuals are not improving in a mental health clinic, they are referred for higher levels of care, such as psychiatric inpatient and/or partial hospital. While being treated at higher levels of care, it may be discovered that individuals being treated for mental illness also experience significant issues with substance abuse. Most mental health clinics assess for substance abuse during their evaluative sessions. Some individuals will identify their use of alcohol and

K. Coffey (✉)
University of Rochester – Psychiatry, SUNY Empire State College – Community and Human Services, Rochester, NY, USA
e-mail: Kevin.coffey@esc.edu

© Springer International Publishing AG 2018   3
T. MacMillan, A. Sisselman-Borgia (eds.), *New Directions in Treatment, Education, and Outreach for Mental Health and Addiction*, Advances in Mental Health and Addiction, https://doi.org/10.1007/978-3-319-72778-3_1

drugs as a form of treatment or self-medication for their existing depression or anxiety. One in three people with depression and six out of ten people with bipolar disorder have experienced alcohol or substance use disorders (SUDs) during their lifetime (Regier et al., 1990).

Patients with anxiety disorders are more vulnerable to develop other comorbid conditions. In particular, there is a strong association between different anxiety disorders and substance use disorders. Nearly 24% of patients with anxiety disorders suffer from a comorbid substance abuse use disorder in their lifetime (Sanchez et al., 2006). According to Sanchez and colleagues (2006), 18% of individuals with anxiety disorders have comorbid diagnoses related to alcohol use, and 12% have comorbid diagnoses related to other illegal substances.

Suicidal thoughts and behaviors are higher among people with comorbid SUDs and mental health diagnoses than among the general population and those with only one type of mental health or substance misuse issue (Comer, 2014; Rosen & Amador, 1996). Depression and alcohol misuse, in particular, are common among suicide victims (Bebbington, 2004). Many individuals that present with suicidal thoughts and behavior are under the influence of alcohol or other drugs. Often these individuals cannot recall events or the precipitant of their suicidal episode the following day. Many of these individuals do not seek follow-up treatment because of shame and embarrassment (Rosen & Amador, 1996).

Treatment of Comorbid Mental Health and Substance Use Disorders

Treatment of comorbid diagnoses can be more complex to treat because of numerous artificial boundaries between agencies that treat substance abuse disorders and those that treat mental health disorders. Substance abuse treatment agencies are often governed by substance abuse regulatory agencies, whereas mental health disorders are governed by mental health treatment regulatory agencies. To be effectively treated, individuals with dual diagnoses need an operative course of treatment for each disorder. There is significant dispute and debate about which disorder needs to be treated first. Individuals who experience dual disorders are most effectively treated in an integrated treatment model, which entails treating both mental health and SUD symptoms simultaneously and in a coordinated manner (Daley & Thase, 2004).

Recovery is the process of managing addiction as well as managing symptoms of a mental illness. Recovery requires hard work, discipline, a commitment to change, and a willingness to address dual disorders. Sobriety from alcohol or other drugs is generally the first recovery task, and abstinence from substance use is the ultimate goal, as continued substance misuse can have an adverse effect on mental health and coexisting mental health diagnoses. Continued use of substances also may impact treatment for mental illness. Use of alcohol and drugs can negate the positive impact of sustained use of psychotropic medications (Daley, 2006).

Knowledge and psychological education is an important component to recovery. It will help the individual understand the etiology of their disorder which may be quite different for each individual. It will help them develop an understanding about how each disorder affects the other and how they may dovetail to prevent recovery. This learning is not just academic, but must become experiential. Individuals do not change from ideas, but from experience. This may require making significant changes in behavior and relationships (Daley & Thase, 2004).

Recovery from both mental illness and substance abuse requires individuals to develop effective support systems. They need other people to share their experiences, including problems, feelings, successes, and interests. These supports may include family both of origin and procreation, friends, professional relationships, and support groups. It is sometimes difficult for family and friends to forgive past experiences associated with addiction and mental illness. Although this is painful, individuals in recovery from mental illness and substance abuse need to accept that forgiveness is a process and may take time. Individuals accepting responsibility and accountability for transgressions to friends and family can greatly support the forgiveness process. Individuals may need to develop new supports while family and friends engage in the forgiveness process (Daley & Thase, 2004).

Early treatment for dual diagnosis involves engagement and stabilization. Stabilization may involve detoxification. Medications may be utilized in this process. In this phase of treatment, the individual also needs to except that he or she has a dual diagnosis. This phase of recovery may be influenced by levels of ambivalence. Individuals who become addicted enjoy or are comforted by their use of substances. Leaving behind addiction is a significant loss that often involves pain. Individuals during this phase of treatment also need a great deal of encouragement and support to remain in treatment (Daley & Thase, 2004).

Early recovery really focuses on how to deal with the cravings associated with substance abuse. When individuals are engaged in a life that revolves around substance misuse, there are places and friends that support this lifestyle. During this phase of treatment, individuals need to begin to change these lifestyle choices and find alternative activities that bring them job so that they can remain clean and sober. Following this early recovery stage, individuals need to build a more secure support system and make amends to others for transgressions committed during their addiction. Developing a sense of spirituality has been shown to support recovery (Daley & Thase, 2004). During later recovery, individuals explore the issues that may have brought them to misuse substances in more depth. Taking medications for coexisting mental health disorders will likely cross all the phases of treatment and recovery, but accepting that these medications might be necessary to deal with other symptoms is an important part of recovery (Daley, & Thase, 2004).

Maintenance is the final phase of treatment. This is a time for individuals to maintain earlier gains and to continue to grow and develop as a human being. Many individuals choose to stay involved in recovery long after symptoms and use of alcohol or substances have improved. Ongoing adherence to medications to treat symptoms of coexisting mental health disorders is important for successful recovery. Recovery is a difficult and complex process (Daley & Marlatt, 2006). Individuals need to make a long-term commitment to it. It will require discipline, sustained effort, and sacrifice. Individuals need to take responsibility for their own recovery and develop a solution-focused approach to recovery. Perfection should not be expected.

Individuals will need the guidance of their treatment team as well as their support system; thus family treatment may be indicated for individuals in recovery, particularly those with comorbid diagnoses (Gilbert, 2004). Family treatment may help family members contextualize the difficulties they might have experienced with the identified client/family member in treatment. Family work can also help to change dysfunctional patterns that may have contributed to the SUD for the individual and may also contribute to treatment compliance for the individual recovering from a SUD (Daley & Thase, 2004). Finally, group treatment is an important component to SUD treatment programs and development of support systems. It is especially important for dually diagnosed patients. It is critical for them to know they are not alone in their struggle to overcome their dual diagnosis. It becomes another forum for them to build trust and enhance social supports (Daley, & Thase, 2004).

Cultural Implications

Many intoxicating drugs are illegal in the United States. This means that making the drugs, buying them, or using them could result in stiff sentences that lead to jail time. Statistics suggest that people of color are arrested at rates that exceed those seen in people who are Caucasian (Daley, 1992). For example, laws written in the 1980s provided to different lengths of sentences for cocaine, depending on the form in which it was sold or used. Sentences involving crack were 100 tines harsher than sentences for powdered cocaine. These laws were revised in 2010. Unfortunately, a disparity still exists, as crack offenses are still 18 times more stringent than powder defenses. This means African-American users often have longer prison sentence than white users (Scott & Wahl, 2011).

In a sample of 179 dual diagnosis clients, there was a significantly larger proportion of African-American individuals in the drug treatment cohort than in the mental health cohort. There were differences between African-Americans and Caucasians in the type of substance use disorders found but not in the types of mental health disorders experienced by sample. African-American individuals were less likely to receive mental health treatment and Caucasian individuals were less likely than African-Americans to receive drug treatment. This is an alarming finding given the apparent racist attitudes that have recently emerged in the political arena in the United States (Ziedonis et al., 1994). Latino individuals born and raised in the United States are more likely to experience addiction than those that are raised in their native countries and emigrate here (Spiegler, Tate, Aitken, & Christian, 1989; Vega, Cannino, & Alegia 2009).

Future Ramifications

There are clear and important implications for the training of individuals in helping professions. Most training for helping professionals either focuses on mental health treatment or on treatment for substance misuse. Given the rates of dual diagnosis patients, this seems like an extremely shortsighted strategy for training. Courses pertaining to dual diagnosis treatment should be added and integrated into training programs without adversely lengthening training programs. Given the rates of SUDs and dual diagnosis, these issues and warning signs should be part of a preventive curriculum in primary and secondary education. Since numerous individuals begin their experimenting with substances as youth, these educational programs have potential to save lives. It may also help children and adolescents to understand the SUDs that they may experience in their own parents, siblings, and other family members.

References

Bebbington, P. E. (2004). The classification and epidemiology of unipolar depression. In M. Power (Ed.), *Mood disorders: A handbook of science and practice* (pp. 3–29). West Sussex, England: Wiley.

Beck, A. (1974). The development of depression: A cognitive model. In R. Friedman & M. Katz (Eds.), *The psychology of depression: Contemporary theory and research*. New York: Wiley.

Blazer, D. G. (2000). Mood disorders: Epidemiology. In B. J. Sadock & V. A. Sadock (Eds.), *Comprehensive textbook of psychiatry* (7th ed., pp. 1385–1430). Baltimore: Lippincott Williams & Wilkins.

Comer, R. (2014). *Fundamentals of abnormal psychology* (7th ed.). Worht: New York.

Daley, D. (1992). Substance abuse and offending: Clinical and social perspectives. *Current Opinions in Psychiatry, 5*, 792–798.

Daley, D. C. (2006). *Addiction and mood disorders: A guide for clients and families*. New York: Oxford Press.

Daley, D. C., & Marlatt, G. A. (2006). *Overcoming your alcohol or drug problem: Effective recovery strategies* (2nd ed.). New York: Oxford.

Daley, D. C., & Thase, M. E. (2004). *Dual disorders recovery counseling: Integrated treatment for substance use and mental health disorders* (3nd ed.). Independence, MO: Independence Press.

Gilbert, P. (2004). A biopsychosocial, integrative and evolutionary approach. In M. Power (Ed.), *Mood disorders: A handbook of science and practice* (pp. 99–142). Wiley, West Sussex, England.

Regier DA, Farmer ME, Rae DS, et al. (1990). Comorbidity of mental disorders with alcohol and other drug abuse. Results from the Epidemiologic Catchment Area (ECA) Study. *JAMA, 264*, 2511–2518.

Rosen, L. E., & Amador, X. F. (1996). *When someone you love is depressed*. New York: Free Press.

Sanchez, P., Ramiriz, D., Fernandez, L., Dominguez, M., Garrido-Torres, N., Rodriguez-Martnez, Biedma Martin, A. S., & Gonzalez-Macias, C. (2006). Anxiety disorders and substance abuse. *European Psychiatry Journal, 25*, 384–390.

Scott, M., & Wahl, O, (2011) *Substance abuse stigma and discrimination among African American abuser*. Stigma Research and Action . Accessed January 9, 2016.

Spiegler, D., Tate, D., Aitken, S., & Christian, C. (1989). *Alcohol use among U.S. ethnic minorities. Research monograph 18.* Rockville, MD: National Institute on Alcohol Abuse and Alcoholism.

Vega, W. A., Cannino, G., & Alegria, M. (2009). Prevalence and correlates of dual diagnosis in U.S. Latinos. *Drug and Alcohol Dependence, 100,* 32–38.

Ziedonis, D. M., Rayford, B. S., Bryant, K. J., & Rounsaville, B. J. (1994). Psychiatric comorbidity in white and African-American cocaine addicts seeking substance abuse treatment. *Hospital Community Psychiatry, 45*(1), 43–49.

Chapter 2
Evolution of Addiction Terminology

Peter J. Pociluyko and Thalia MacMillan

Introduction

Substance abuse has reached epic proportions with one in ten individuals reporting the use of substances (National Institute on Drug Abuse; NIDA, 2015). However, depending upon the source, estimates of substance use disorder vary widely, and our definitions within the field are constantly evolving. While differences in statistics may be a function of the population being examined, the stigma of reporting, the type of drug under study, or how use is defined, the statistics highlight that rates of use have been rising over time. There is no one portrait of a person with an addiction disorder, as addiction has the potential to span every age, gender, ethnicity, religion, and socioeconomic bracket. This chapter will provide an introductory explanation as to what defines a drug, the history of addiction, how we currently define addiction, relevant terminology, co-occurrence, and the various types of treatment. In this chapter, the terms substance abuse and addictions will be used interchangeably.

What Defines a Drug?

A drug can be defined under many different standards. The most common definition is that a drug is any substance used as a medication or another substance used for the preparation of a medication.

P. J. Pociluyko
SUNY Empire State College, Community & Human Services, Saratoga Springs, NY, USA
e-mail: Peter.Pociluyko@esc.edu

T. MacMillan (✉)
SUNY Empire State College, Community & Human Services, New York, NY, USA
e-mail: thalia.macmillan@esc.edu

© Springer International Publishing AG 2018   9
T. MacMillan, A. Sisselman-Borgia (eds.), *New Directions in Treatment,
Education, and Outreach for Mental Health and Addiction*, Advances in Mental
Health and Addiction, https://doi.org/10.1007/978-3-319-72778-3_2

In the United States per *the 1938 Food, Drug, and Cosmetic Act*, a drug is defined as (1) a substance recognized in an official pharmacopoeia or formulary; (2) a substance intended for use in the diagnosis, cure, mitigation, treatment, or prevention of disease; (3) a substance other than food intended to affect the structure or function of the body; and/or (4) a substance intended for use as a component of a medicine but not a device or a component, part, or accessory of a device (Public Law, 1938).

Drugs are typically classified into classes or groups of related drugs that have (a) similar chemical structures, (b) the same mechanism of action, and (c) a related mode of action and/or are used to treat the same disease (Mahoney & Evans, 2008). However, no single classification system can meet all needs as one drug may cross over different classifications and effect a variety of systems within the body.

Psychoactive drugs (also called psychotropics) are one class of drugs. Psychotropics are those substances that affect the function of the central nervous system by altering perceptions, thinking process, mood or consciousness, and subsequently alter behavior. These include sedative-hypnotics (depressants), stimulants, opiates (depressants with analgesic capability), anesthetics (depressants that include phencyclidine/PCP, ketamine, and nitrous oxide), and psychedelics (including consciousness expanding and ego-fragmenting effects).

Psychoactive substances typically bring about subjective changes in cognition, awareness, and mood that the user finds rewarding and pleasant. Not all of these changes may be objectively observed, but are more subjective in nature from the individual using the drug. It is important to clarify that only psychoactive drugs that affect the pleasure center in the brain (the mesolimbic dopamine system or MDS) have addictive potential. Drugs such as antidepressants, neuroleptics, lithium, mood stabilizers, and anticonvulsants do not affect the MDS and hence lack this ability. The use of most psychoactive drugs can lead to a degree of tolerance and withdrawal, which we will explain later, and is not to be equated with addiction.

Addiction: The Origin of the Term

The term addict is derived from classic Latin word "addictus" or "addico," which means to "devote or surrender to." The word addiction was derived from the classic Latin word of "addicere" meaning "to surrender, to enslave, to devote, to sentence or condemn."

Over the centuries, the word's meaning changed to mean those compelled to repeatedly act out habitual behaviors such as gluttony or having a devotion to an occupation. During the 1800s, due to a rise of the alcohol temperance and anti-opium movements, addiction was used to link to any use of alcohol, narcotics, and vices, thus taking on a negative and undesirable reference. Currently, the terms "addict" and "addiction" have highly negative, pejorative implications and are used along with street slang such as "crack head, pot head, and junkie." While many professionals argue that the term addict is demeaning, it is still commonly used in the field. Thus shifting the language to "people with an addictive disorder" or "people with addiction" would be more appropriate as it places the person first and disorder second.

Addiction: What It Is and What It Is Not? What Does Science Say?

In order to define what an addiction is, it is important to first define what addiction is not. Many of us often hear people loosely use the term. For example, "I am addicted to chocolate, to coffee, to potato chips, etc." This common usage makes the operational definition of the term poorly understood and less useful.

Addiction is often confused with physical dependence and withdrawal. The presence of tolerance and withdrawal (e.g., rebound symptoms opposite to the drug's main effects, which occur when the drug is abruptly stopped) is the criteria for physical dependence. By themselves, physical dependence and tolerance are not addiction; rather these are reversible medical conditions such that once a person is tapered off a drug, he/she is no longer tolerant or physically dependent on that drug. Tolerance and withdrawal are common conditions that can occur with the regular use of many substances including those that are not psychoactive and occur even when a drug is taken as prescribed for a moderate or prolonged period as often occurs in medical care. Tolerance and withdrawal develop because the body is repeatedly exposed to a drug; hence, it adapts to the drug presence. An analogy that can be used is the pendulum rebound effect. One will notice the pendulum will swing an equal and opposite distance from a previous position past its resting state. If released or already in motion, a pendulum will swing back and forth for a time, until it returns to a non-motion state. So, imagine if you pull a pendulum further to one side, then release it, the "rebound reaction" will be equal in distance to its prior position, and it will take longer to return to a non-motion state. Now imagine each day you pull the pendulum a little further, then let go, and do this day after day. The effects of a drug on the body and brain work in a similar manner due to biochemical changes and basic physics.

When a drug has been used often for many days or weeks and is abruptly stopped, the person will experience symptoms opposite to the actions of the drug until the body re-acclimates to the loss of the substance. The severity of this reaction is dependent upon dose, drug potency, and frequency of use. For example, a sedating drug used several times a day for many weeks, then abruptly stopped, will produce rebound symptoms of agitation, hyperexcitability, restlessness, anxiety, etc. A stimulant drug used for many consecutive days, then stopped, will be followed by symptoms of lethargy, possibly exhaustion, depressed mood, etc. Although many people with substance-related addiction will experience significant tolerance and physical dependence, as we will explain, this is not the same as addiction.

Addiction is a chronic, neurobiological disease of the brain that results from biological, psychological, and environmental factors (Savage et al., 2003). Addiction to a drug is not inherently due to the drug itself, but due to the individual's response to the drug (Erickson, 2007). Addiction to a drug indicates impaired ability to control use due to neurobiological changes in the brain circuitry resulting from the drug altering one's neurobiology (Erickson, 2011). It is characterized by specific features, including persistent episodes of impaired control over use, compulsive and repetitive use of the drug, intense cravings to use (even when there are no external stressors or pressures), and continued use despite the drug induced harm to the individual and others (American Psychiatric Association, 2013). It is not the same thing as willful, conscious excess use, or what might be called "poor judgment," nor is addiction due to a lack of willpower or lack of a moral compass regarding drug use.

Substance Use Disorder vs Substance Abuse vs Substance Misuse

With the advent of the *Diagnostic and Statistical Manual for Mental Disorders, Fifth Edition* (DSM 5), the separate classifications of substance abuse (SA) and substance dependence (SD) were merged into a single dimensional (a continuum or range) classification of substance use disorder, plus specific drug type. The advantage of this change is adding specifiers with a severity rating based upon the number of symptoms presented. This requires some clinical translation and understanding. For example, those people with two to three symptoms (mild severity) would likely be similar to those who were formerly classified under the DSM-IV criteria for the disorder of substance abuse, while those with a moderate (four to five symptoms) to a severe rating (six or more symptoms) would likely meet criteria for the former disorder of substance dependence aka substance addiction. Another important change is that the DSM 5 criteria no longer use tolerance or withdrawal as key diagnostic specifier symptoms (e.g., with or without physiological withdrawal). This change also highlighted that addiction is not defined by whether or not the individual shows evidence of withdrawal, but focuses instead on symptoms that indicate clinically significant impairment and/or distress across different areas of functioning.

An additional strength of a single classification (by combining substance abuse and substance dependence) was the elimination of the hierarchy of classification, with substance dependence being considered the more severe disorder than substance abuse. Many practitioners assumed that if an individual met criteria for substance abuse, but not dependence, then substance abuse represented a milder form of addiction (Hasin et al. 2013). Another concern noted by Hasin et al. (2013) was lower reliability and validity for diagnoses of substance abuse, often made by evidence of a single symptom; a single symptom is often assumed to mean the "milder" disorder of substance abuse. However, a single symptom such as not fulfilling one's responsibilities due to substance use is often a severe type of symptom, and hence reliability and validity based on the presence of that sole symptom for a diagnosis was problematic. Symptom presentation and resulting categorization of substance abuse versus dependence can potentially be extremely problematic as an individual could potentially meet either disorder (Grant et al., 2007; Hasin et al., 2013; Hasin, Hatzenbueler, Smith, & Grant, 2005; Hasin & Grant, 2004).

The disadvantage and counterargument against the DSM 5 criteria change is that substance abuse and substance dependence are distinct disorders and are not necessarily part of a continuum (Erickson, 2007). Furthermore, not everyone who uses a drug in excess or excessively uses on a frequent basis necessarily has impaired control, which is typically indicative of addiction (Hasin et al., 2013). As listed in DSM-IV, substance abuse implies willful, conscious, and excessive use most often related to poor judgment; therefore while it could be classified as a disorder, it was not a disease. This distinction made the disorder best addressed by education, supportive counseling, and sanctions to curb the behavior. In contrast, substance dependence per DSM-IV was equated with the onset of addiction; therefore, this was considered a disease to be treated with medication, therapy, abstinence, plus adjunctive supports such as education about the disease of addiction, exposure to mutual help/12-step groups, etc. Hence, the classification of substance abuse may still carry value when effectively understood and applied diagnostically in contrast to the new classification of substance use disorder with severity specifier.

The term substance misuse, which is commonly used in Europe, also has value as it relates to misuse or non-therapeutic use, such as taking more medication than prescribed, taking medication that one is not authorized to use, sharing medications with others, etc. The position of the US Food and Drug Administration (2015) is that the differences are one of intention. For example, when a person knows that s/he will obtain a pleasant or euphoric effect by taking a drug (such as at higher doses than prescribed) or mixing with alcohol or another drug, this is considered drug abuse because of the intent to obtain a euphoric response. However, if a person isn't able to fall asleep after taking a standard sleep aid drug, they may take an additional dose that is not authorized per prescription instructions soon thereafter, by assuming, "One was not enough, so two will work." A person may also offer his prescribed pain or headache medication to a friend who is in pain. These are considered drug misuse since these people did not follow medical instructions, but the intent was not to obtain euphoria. In effect they are treating themselves, but not following the directions of their healthcare provider.

The Concept of Enabling and Co-dependence

When used in context of addiction and substance use disorder, the term "enabling" has developed an incorrect meaning and a negative connotation. To enable is to "give (someone or something) the authority or means to do something" (e.g., to enable a student to learn and apply math concepts) or "to make someone or something able to do something by providing whatever is necessary to achieve that aim" (Cambridge Dictionary, 2017). However, within the helping professions, the term has evolved to mean an effort by others to protect or shield a person with a substance use, gambling, or mental health disorder from experiencing the natural consequences that will occur from their symptomatic behavior. This definition also can imply an intent is to help maintain the person's impairment, which is attached for some type of needs by the "enabler." This term is also used to subtly and overtly label family and friends as "sick, having a family disease, being co-dependent, etc." and often to subtly blame others for an individual's lack of recovery.

The reality is that people are naturally protective of others whom they love and care about, even though their actions often have unintended, negative consequences and can prevent the affected person from facing and overcoming the consequences of his/her actions. People who "protect others from consequences" often feel very ambivalent about their actions and the affected person. Frequently, protective people oscillate between feelings of love, concern, fear of harm, wanting to protect the affected person, feeling frustrated, annoyed, and angry that the other is not changing. More often the fear that something terrible will happen to the loved one, if no one intercedes, will tip the balance toward a protective effort that prevents consequences from occurring; thus, this creates a cycle of an unchanging status quo.

It is more useful and effective to avoid the term "enabling" and for the practitioner to reframe her/his thinking about such protective behavior and its intentions. Thinking and describing the so-called "enabling" behavior as "loving, concerned, caring, and repeated in the hope that things will improve" is a useful reframe that is also more readily accepted by the so-called enabler(s). As providers to family and friends, it is helpful to start with the eliciting questions about behavior and its outcomes: "Your concern, love, devotion, etc. for your spouse, son, daughter, etc. is noble. Is that what drives you to keep trying to protect him/her? What do you fear will happen if you do not continue what you do?" By doing so, it later allows the conversation to examine the results of such efforts, "So let's review what you have done in the past and how often you have tried. What has been the result?" The provider and individual could then discuss alternative actions and efforts without criticism or negative labeling and, equally important, without implying pathology on the part of the protective individual(s).

When there is a presence of addictive disorders in one or more family members or a significant other, it has the potential to impact others with whom the addicted person interacts. As a result, the term co-dependency developed and is commonly used in the addiction treatment literature as a parallel to substance/chemical dependence. Co-dependency refers to adverse interpersonal behaviors and implies symptoms and pathological psychological qualities about the individual. The effort to "pathologize" and medically define the construct of co-dependency began when some addiction professionals assumed they could reliably identify and define such behaviors and the alleged symptoms as a disease. This was done by creating a list of criteria for diagnosis and claiming there was existing treatment for the disease (van Wormer, 1989).

Co-dependency as a disorder is often presumed to be present among any and all members where there is a member with an addictive disorder. Proponents like

Cermak (1986), Kitchens (1991), and others suggest this is a diagnostic entity (Gierymski & Williams, 1986). The literature almost universally labels women for having this disorder. Schaef (1986) claims that the disorder has a specific onset, with a course of progression and a predictable outcome, while Beattie (1987) claimed 96% of Americans are affected by co-dependence. However, neither Schaef (1986) nor Beattie (1987) cites any scientific data or clear evidence to support this claim. The literature that does describe co-dependency often implies that this behavioral pattern is the result of childhood and leads to a tendency to engage in unhealthy relationships, often involved addicted individuals. Cermak (1986) and Kitchens (1991) both claim that co-dependency is equal to a personality disorder along the characteristics of dependent personality disorder, yet little scientific evidence exists for use of this concept. These perspectives are related to a faulty assumption that family members and/or friends of addicted individuals will always be adversely affected by the relationship. While a large portion of significant others do experience long-term consequences (e.g., develop their own addiction, a mental health disorder, become less functional), others find ways to set limits and become stronger and more functional and more resilient. The assumption that all significant others are "damaged" by the impact of addiction from a significant other has not been proven to be universal.

The application of the disease process for addiction being used to conceptualize interpersonal behaviors that is broadly labeled "co-dependency" presents many problems. Using terms that are not formally accepted as diagnostic labels reduces individual credibility and that of the addiction and mental health treatment profession. It is not a concept or classification described in recent or past DSM editions. The definition of co-dependency is so broad that it creates impossibility for measurement; hence, this is a key reason why there is scant scientific literature on this topic. The term also carries the same negative consequences that befall a misunderstanding of many diagnostic labels. Another issue is the high potential for the family member to view themselves as ill, has little or no strengths, and feeling blamed. It would be more professionally appropriate to assign existing DSM 5 classifications to family members who show evidence of symptomatic distress and reduced functioning.

Co-occurring Disorders? Dual Diagnosis? What Is the Correct Terminology?

The use of terminology of terms such as "dual diagnosis," "mentally ill and chemically addicted," and/or "substance addicted and mentally ill" is rather dated as they have inherent limitations. Unfortunately, such terms continue to be used without always understanding the implications. Dual diagnosis implies people have just two disorders. Many people with substance use disorder typically have three or more disorders, including multiple substance use disorder, one or more mental health disorders, and oftentimes HIV, hepatitis, or related disorders which also can affect judgment, behavior, thinking, or overall functioning (Regier et al., 1990).

Terms such as "mentally ill/chemically addicted" or "substance addicted and mentally ill' imply mental illness and addiction. However, mental illness (vs mental disorder) generally signifies severe disorders such as psychotic disorders, bipolar I disorder, chronic PTSD, severe personality disorders, and anxiety disorders, plus reflects significant impairment in functioning, etc. Only a smaller percentage of people with substance use disorder have severe mental illness, and most have a wide range of mild to moderate mental disorders from persistent depressive disorder, impulse control disorders, mild to moderate severe personality disorders, mild to moderate anxiety disorders, attention deficit disorder, sleep disorders, and tics, among others (SAMSHA, 2011). People often do not demonstrate all the features of addiction but instead have a few symptoms or mild specifier of substance use disorder that indicates severity akin to the former DSM -IV substance abuse diagnostic criteria.

In terms of etiology, many believe that co-occurring disorders are predominately due to self-medication that has gone awry, (i.e., the self-medication hypothesis or SMH), where substance use to curb existing mental health symptoms has gone out of control. The SMH is a theory that seems logical yet can be overly simplistic as there is often a cascade of different weighted factors involved in etiology and, as a result, has not been consistently supported by empirical research. One reason is that people with substance use and mental health disorders often confuse what they perceive as a benefit of drug use; for example, patients may say "alcohol or tobacco use helps me cope with anxiety and low mood from my mental disorder." Initial use of the drug may change over time from positive reinforcement (getting high) to negative reinforcement, for example, using the drug to counteract rebound effects such as withdrawal-induced anxiety, restlessness, agitation, or depressed mood. Hence people mistakenly believe that a drug is helping them control their primary mental health symptoms, rather than the symptoms of addiction. Practitioners also mistakenly assume the drug is being used by the patient to control primary symptoms of a mental health disorder.

Moreover, many people begin and continue the use psychoactive drugs for the same basic reasons: curiosity, desire to feel euphoric, to enhance or facilitate social interaction, temporary pain or other symptom reduction, and as self-distraction (SAMSHA, 2011). Theories that appear to have increasing support suggest differing disorders often have some common genetic and neurochemical basis, plus are further impacted by environmental stressors and negative life experiences (SAMSHA, 2011). A substance use disorder can precede the development of a mental disorder or can develop well after the onset of a mental disorder. For example, a person may develop alcohol or cannabis dependence and then develop depression, bipolar disorder, or panic disorder later, or the reverse order may occur. In either case, each disorder amplifies and negatively affects (as in aggravates) the other.

Knowing which disorder came first is generally not important for purposes of treatment. What is often helpful is identifying and describing how the disorders impact each other, as well as how the patient reacts to various symptoms. Properly assessing, identifying, and treating all disorders is essential, ideally with the same team of practitioners. A common belief from "clinical folklore" and "12-step folklore" is that once the person stops using a mood-altering substance, most or all mental health symptoms will disappear. While that does sometimes occur for people who have secondary or drug-induced mental health symptoms, often people have developed one or more primary mental disorder that requires treatment along with treatment for their substance use disorders. Among the most common co-occurring mental health disorders are depression, persistent depressive disorder (formerly dysthymia), bipolar disorder, anxiety disorders, and personality disorders.

Any discussion of co-occurring addiction and mental health disorders still sometimes raises a philosophical question of inquiry—which disorder came first. This is followed by the illusory correlation that one disorder must be causing the other disorder; hence, it leads to a hidden assumption that if the "underlying issue is treated" the other disorder will cease. The evidence accrued over the decades continues to indicate that onset of any disorder increases the risk of developing a second, third, or more disorders and should be the expectation, not the exception for people entering treatment. The practice and assumption for treating one disorder then the next in sequence is based on an outdated view of "underlying causal factors." The evidence supports that substance use and mental health disorders have multiple casual factors, and the evidence suggest that many disorders co-occur so often that common factors likely underlie many disorders. Therefore, the best practice is well-coordinated and integrative treatment of all disorders (Kelly and Daley, 2013).

Defining Recovery

Many members of 12-step fellowships believe that for people who are active in recovery, all understand and know what recovery means. For people in recovery from an addiction or a co-occurring disorder (and even for professionals) this lack of a clear definition can become more elusive. The National Council on Alcohol and Drug Dependence (2011) states "recovery is a complex and dynamic process encompassing all the positive benefits to physical, mental and social health that can happen when people with an addiction to alcohol or drugs, or their family members, get the help they need." That definition could also apply to people with co-occurring disorders.

The Substance Abuse and Mental Health Administration ([SAMHSA], 2011) attempted to create a similar definition, "Recovery from alcohol and drug problems is a process of change through which an individual achieves abstinence and improved health, wellness and quality of life," followed by attempts to identify a dozen guiding principles of recovery, such as: "There are many pathways to recovery; Recovery is self-directed and empowering; Recovery involves a personal recognition of the need for change and transformation."

In 2012, SAMHSA updated this to a Working Definition of Recovery from Mental Disorders and/or Substance Use Disorders identifying four areas:

Health: overcoming or managing one's disease(s) or symptoms—for example, abstaining from use of alcohol, illicit drugs, and non-prescribed medications if one has an addiction problem—and for everyone in recovery, making informed, healthy choices that support physical and emotional wellbeing

Home: a stable and safe place to live

Purpose: meaningful daily activities, such as a job, school, volunteerism, family caretaking, or creative endeavors, and the independence, income, and resources to participate in society

Community: relationships and social networks that provide support, friendship, love, and hope

(Source: Recovery and Recovery Support. https://www.samhsa.gov/recovery)

Individuals suffering from any serious illness generally can state they want symptom remission, improved function, and a more satisfying quality of life. The Betty Ford Center (2007) attempted to characterize this term and found it was not easily explained by a simple definition. They noted, *"recovery is not synonymous with a specific method of attaining it recovery is an acquired lifestyle, not a particular method."* Recovery is best described by key characteristics:

1. Abstinence vs sobriety. Sobriety was defined as key feature of a recovery lifestyle. According to this group sobriety is synonymous with abstinence from alcohol and all non-prescribed drugs. In contrast, the literal definition of sobriety and as implied in the traditions of 12-step programs explains that sobriety is about having self-control, balance in one's life, and doing things within moderation.
2. Medication-assisted sobriety provision that one could be considered to be "in recovery" while taking medications as prescribed. This is a shift from a commonly held belief of some traditionalist professionals and 12-step members who view any substance use, even psychiatric medication, as active drug use. If formerly dependent individuals who are taking medications for a diagnosed medical condition with a potential for abuse liability (e.g., sedatives or opiods), and the medication is taken as prescribed, then the definition of recovery is met. It also stands to reason that if addiction is viewed as a medical illness, the use of properly prescribed medications is acceptable and does not run contrary to the definition of recovery.
3. The issue whether recovery also means tobacco abstinence was not fully addressed, even though tobacco (not just nicotine) dependence is a very deadly and serious health issue and a leading cause of death for those actively using drugs and those in recovery. This is equally a concern for those with co-occurring mental health disorders, who have some of the highest tobacco use patterns of any healthcare population. Tobacco abstinence should be part of a definition or active recovery.

4. Citizenship which is described as not only cessation of individual and socially harmful behaviors, but active pro-social behaviors (being a productive citizen, living a productive life, helping others, etc.).
(Betty Ford Institute Consensus Panel, 2007)

Kaskutas et al. (2014) identified four domains of abstinence in recovery, essentials of recovery, enriched recovery, and spirituality of recovery. Recovery should be framed within specifiers as per DSM 5 by time periods along with specific outcomes and behavior results, within the frame of early, stable, and sustained sobriety. For example, early sobriety is defined as 1–12 months, sustained sobriety is 1–5 years, and stable sobriety is 5 or more years.

Finally, a practical definition that can be set to measurable standards is that recovery from a SUD or MHD is defined by continuous improvement in the life of the individual as reflected by increasing periods of abstinence, improvement in overall health, overall stability in their life areas, increasingly longer periods without or with limited symptoms, increasing ability to maintain independence, and maintenance of positive relationships with others (American Psychiatric Association, 2013). This definition would allow for patients to customize or individualize to their own cultural or spiritual needs whereby demonstrating physical, psychological, social, spiritual changes, and specific improvements in those areas. While the above definitions are descriptive, they need to more clearly address how one quantifies and operationally measures progress of recovery.

Mutual Help vs Professional Treatment

Many patients and practitioners widely refer to "self-help groups" to describe 12-step and other support groups. As a point of clarification, the term self-help is for books, not groups. The accurate term is mutual help groups. Mutual help groups and the "sponsorship" of people in recovery for substance use or mental health disorders have similarities and provide important elements for recovery. Still, sometimes patients, family members, the general public, and even some professionals sometimes confuse the different roles and functions of mutual help and professional group treatment methods.

The common elements between professional group treatment and mutual help groups include sharing personal information through open group discussion, self-recognition of having a substance use or mental health disorder, self-examination of one's behavior, learning about one's illness(es), correcting misconceptions about addiction, and learning practical steps to support recovery (Ekleberry, 2008). A key aspect is learning to ask for and seek help from others rather than "trying to go through it alone."

Mutual help groups like Alcoholics Anonymous, Dual Recovery Anonymous, Narcotics Anonymous, Double-Trouble, and others follow a mutual fellowship model based on guiding principles, practical advice from folklore, and practices passed down from successful members, and not via strict rules, professional standards, laws, and ethical standards. Twelve-step mutual help groups select their own "chairperson" from within the individual group. The group chair typically uses a "leader-centric" approach to organize the group, sets the topic of the session, selects the lead speaker for a specific meeting, and may call on others to share. Guiding principles and steps for 12-step groups are not theoretical models but follow the membership steps and traditions established by the fellowships founders. The groups and sponsors share practical ideas for recovery derived from current and past member's experiences. As a nonprofessional group, there is no accountability, no record keeping or records of attendance, no supervision of sponsors, and no standards of practice. There is no fee for services rendered and each group is self-supporting via member donations. The focus is on mutual support toward abstinence from mood-altering drugs; for Double Trouble or dual recovery groups, this also includes managing one's mental health symptoms. An abstinence from alcohol, drugs, or gambling is a foundation for recovery for people attending substance use, dual recovery, and gambling focused 12-step groups. Termination from the mutual help group is purely voluntary, and the only membership requirement is a "sincere desire" to stop drug or alcohol use or gambling behavior and/or focus on learning to manage one's mental health.

The emphasis remains on three levels of recovery—physical, psychological, and spiritual. Inherently there is a recovery related to regaining a functional social aspect of one's life. Twelve-step sponsors are like non-paid recovery coaches, serving as a personal, non-paid guide who developed his/her own stable recovery and voluntarily agrees to help support others practice the steps and principles to support recovery. Just like a coach, sponsors serve as an outside and objective observer who can point out hidden or unrecognized problems, emotional or attitudinal blind spots, and signals of pending relapse.

In contrast, professional treatment relies on scientific methods, scientific theoretical models for behavior, and research-based practices that underlie treatment. There must be professional accountability, clinical supervision, treatment plans, patient record keeping, standards of practice, and ethical standards, and it is subject to professional organization standards as well as state and/or federal laws. Addiction and mental health professionals also meet individually with patients to complete a psychosocial assessment, develop individualized treatment plans, help people explore specific issues that impede recovery, help patients develop a relapse prevention plan, and often hold sessions with family members. Professionals often help patients more deeply explore their emotions, feelings, behaviors, and maladaptive beliefs and to identify discrepancies between actions and statements. Professionals will typically (with patient-written consent) report to referral agencies, probation/parole officers, the courts, and even to family members or employers on the individual's overall progress. While there is attention to the "how" to recover, there is also emphasis on the what, when, who, and how for symptoms of a substance use or mental disorder. There is often attention to what factors have kept the person from improving or continuing to use, the reasons behind relapse, and factors that support recovery. Attention is also given as to how to address family, social, religious or spiritual, and cultural issues that can support or impede recovery.

In contrast to mutual help groups, professionally led treatment groups are led by trained professionals. Such groups can vary from an educational focus on substance use or mental health disorders to a coping skills or topic-specific group (e.g., relapse prevention, anger control) to a process-oriented group. The approach of the group leader and group task typically includes some structure, rules for interaction, start and end times, task and purpose of the group, and specific interventions to keep the group on task, helping individual members to share and discuss specific issues to gain support or feedback.

Professional group therapy must follow agency and professional standards of practice and relies on oversight from a clinical supervisor or clinical director. While educational and task groups are often leader centered (leader chooses the topic, controls the agenda, and calls on people to speak), interactional process groups are group centered, with the leader serving as a facilitator. The structure in a group allows the members to select their own topics in each session and allows the members' issues to unfold within the group over time. Members will also learn to give specific behavioral feedback to each other and to tolerate and manage conflict within the group. Therapy groups will have a written set of rules and boundaries defining acceptable behavior, purpose and goals of the group, meeting times, and specific expectations of the members, including the process for transfer out or termination from the group.

In closing, mutual help and 12-step groups are not considered professional treatment, and professional treatment is not equal to attending a mutual help group. At the same time, there is an important synergism (the principle that one plus one equals much more than two) such that an individual's recovery often progresses faster, more effectively, and more holistically when people use mutual help groups along with professional treatment. The value of both approaches should not be underestimated.

Summary

In summary, much of what we "know" about substance use, addiction, assessment, the role of family and friends, recovery, and treatment has evolved as we continue to learn more. The way that we define and classify drugs has grown to encompass function and purpose. The way that we think about addiction has both been broadened and narrowed; more specifically, we no longer view addiction as out of control drug use due to a singular cause (e.g., genetics or underlying mental disorder), but one that has multiple symptoms and represents a chronic, neurobiological disease resulting from a multitude of factors. As a result, the way that we classify and diagnose addiction has changed. In later chapters, different types of assessment will be discussed. What we know about recovery and treatment is also seen to be multifaceted and will be explored in further chapters. Knowledge, treatment, and the terminology will continue to evolve as we learn more.

References

American Psychiatric Association. (2013). *Diagnostic and statistical manual of mental disorders* (5th ed.). Washington, DC: American Psychiatric Publishers.

Beattie, M. (1987). *Co-dependent no more*. San Francisco: Harper & Row.

Betty Ford Institute Consensus Panel. (2007). What is recovery? A working definition from the Betty ford institute. *Journal of Substance Abuse Treatment, 33*, 221–228.

Cambridge Dictionary. (2017). *Dictionary*. New York: Cambridge University Press.

Erickson, C. K. (2007). *The science of addiction: From neurobiology to treatment*. New York: W.W. Norton.

Erickson, C. K. (2011). *Addiction essentials: The go to guide for clinicians and patients*. New York: W.W. Norton.

Cermak, T. L. (1986). Diagnostic criteria for codependency. *Journal of Psychoactive Drugs, 18*(1), 15–20.

Ekleberry, S. C. (2008). *Integrated treatment for co-occurring disorders: Personality disorders and addiction*. NY: Routledge.

Gierymski, T., & Williams, T. (1986). Codependency. *Journal of Psychoactive Drugs, 18*(1), 7–13.

Grant, B. F., Compton, W. M., Crowley, T. J., Hasin, D. S., Helzer, J. E., Li, T. K., et al. (2007). Errors in assessing DSM-IV substance use disorders. *Archives of General Psychiatry, 64*, 379–382.

Hasin, D. S., O'Brien, C. P., Auriacombe, M., Borges, G., Bucholz, K., Budney, A., et al. (2013). DSM-5 criteria for substance use disorders: Recommendations and rationale. *American Journal of Psychiatry, 170*(8), 834–851.

Hasin, D. S., Hatzenbueler, M., Smith, S., & Grant, B. F. (2005). Co-occurring DSM-IV drug abuse in DSM-IV drug dependence: Results from the National Epidemiologic Survey on alcohol and related conditions. *Drug & Alcohol Dependence, 80*, 117–123.

Hasin, D. S., & Grant, B. F. (2004). The co-occurrence of DSM-IV alcohol abuse in DSM-IV alcohol dependence: Results of the National Epidemiologic Survey on alcohol and related conditions on heterogeneity that differ by population subgroup. *Archives of General Psychiatry, 61*, 891–896.

Kaskutas, L. A., Borkman, T. J., Laudet, A., Ritter, L. A., Witbrodt, J., Subbaraman, M., et al. (November 2014). Elements that define recovery: The experiential perspective. *Journal of Studies on Alcohol and Drugs, 75*(6), 999–1010.

Kelly, T. M., & Daley, D. C. (2013). Integrated treatment of substance use and psychiatric disorders. *Social Work in Public Health, 28*(0), 388–406.

Kitchens, J. A. (1991). *Understanding and treating codependence*. New Jersey: Prentice Hall.

Mahoney, A., & Evans J. (2008). Comparing drug classification systems. *AMIA annual symposium proceedings*. November 6, 2008: 1039.

National Council on Alcohol and Drug Dependence. (2011). *Definition of recovery*. Retrieved from https://www.ncadd.org/people-in-recovery/recovery-definition/definition-of-recovery

National Institute on Drug Abuse. (2015). Drug Facts. Retrieved from https://www.drugabuse.gov/publications/finder/t/160/drugfacts

Public Law 75-717, 52 STAT 1040. Act of June 25, 1938. *Federal food, drug, and cosmetic act*.

Regier, D. A., Farmer, M. E., Rae, D. S., Locke, B. Z., Keith S. J., Judd, L. L., & Goodwin, F. K. (1990). Comorbidity of mental disorders with alcohol and other drug abuse. Results from the Epidemiologic Catchment Area (ECA) Study. *Journal of the American Medical Association, 264*(19), 2511–2518.

Savage, S. R., Joaranson, D. E., Covington, E. C., Schnool, S. H., Heir, H. A., & Gilson, A. M. (2003). Definitions related to medical use of opiods: Evolution towards agreement. *Journal of Pain Management., 26*, 655–667.

Schaef, A. W. (1986). *Co-dependence: Misunderstood—Mistreated*. Minneapolis: Winston Press.

Substance Abuse and Mental Health Administration. (2011). *Definitions*. Retrieved from https://www.samhsa.gov/newsroom/press-announcements/201112220800

Substance Abuse and Mental Health Administration. (2012). *Recovery and recovery support.* https://www.samhsa.gov/recovery

US Food and Drug Administration. (2015, August 30). Combating misuse and abuse of prescription drug. Available online at https://www.fda.gov/ForConsumers/ConsumerUpdates/ucm220112. htm

van Wormer, K. (1989). Co-dependency: Implications for women and therapy. *Women & Therapy, 8*(4), 51–63.

Chapter 3
Comprehensive Assessment of Substance Abuse and Addiction Risk in Adolescence

A. Jordan Wright

Assessing substance use, misuse, abuse, and problems in adolescence is a key way to help identify risk, intervene early, and potentially prevent addiction and other substance-related problems in adulthood (Buchman et al., 2013; Bukstein & Kaminer, 2015; Ehlers et al., 2007; Gillespie, Neale, & Kendler, 2009; Grant & Dawson, 1997; Grant, Stinson, & Hartford, 2001; Hingson, Heeren, & Winter, 2006; Johnson & Novak, 2009; Kendler et al., 2013; Lisdahl, Gilbart, Wright, & Shollenbarger, 2013; Morrell, Song, & Halpern-Felsher, 2011; Moss, Chen, & Yi, 2014; Swift, Coffey, Carlin, Degenhardt, & Patton, 2008; Westling, Andrews, Hampson, & Peterson, 2008). Adolescence is a particularly sensitive risk period for alcohol and other substance-related problems to begin and progress (Jordan & Anderson, 2016), with many individuals beginning problematic use during adolescence (Degenhardt et al., 2008; Johnston, O'Malley, Bachman, & Schulenberg, 2010, 2011). Thus, evaluating risks for problematic use during adolescence and future dependence and other problems is key in prevention and early intervention. While necessarily imperfect, comprehensive evaluation can be useful in identifying those adolescents at greatest risk for developing problem patterns and future substance-related disorders.

A. J. Wright (✉)
New York University, Department of Applied Psychology, Steinhardt School of Culture, Education, and Human Development, New York, NY, USA
e-mail: ajordanwright@nyu.edu

© Springer International Publishing AG 2018   25
T. MacMillan, A. Sisselman-Borgia (eds.), *New Directions in Treatment, Education, and Outreach for Mental Health and Addiction*, Advances in Mental Health and Addiction, https://doi.org/10.1007/978-3-319-72778-3_3

Levels of Assessment

In the quest to try to understand exactly what to evaluate as part of a comprehensive assessment of risk, many theoretical, empirical, and even practical issues must be taken into account. While it is often impossible to evaluate every single area enumerated in this chapter, an understanding of the potential impacts of different factors is important. When prioritizing, it is often most important and feasible to focus on individual risk and protective factors for the adolescent, which are among the most important and predictive, such as current substance use, history of substance use, and mental and behavioral health issues (Swadi, 1999). However, when given the freedom, flexibility, and resources to be more comprehensive, many other factors at different levels play a role in risk for developing substance-related problems. Families are obviously a major context in which adolescents develop, and family factors like direct modeling of problematic substance abuse, poor parental monitoring, high family conflict, poor family bonding, overly harsh disciplinary practices, and positive family attitudes regarding substance use heavily influence onset of adolescent use and progression from use to misuse to major problems (Lochman & van den Steenhoven, 2002). The other major contexts in which adolescents develop are schools, and in addition to peer and friend influence, actual school factors play a role in adolescent substance use problems. For example, a low commitment to academics, disengagement and disconnection from the school community, and actual school failure have all been identified as predictive risk factors for adolescent substance abuse (Fletcher, Bonnell, & Hargreaves, 2008; Friedman, 1983; Gottfredson, 1987; Hundleby & Mercer, 1987; Jessor, 1976; Robins, 1980; Smith & Fogg, 1978).

Neighborhood factors have also been identified as predictive risk factors for adolescent substance-related problems. Among these factors are actual physical deterioration and community disorganization, as well as adolescents disengaging from and feeling unsafe in the neighborhood community (Fagan & Deslonde, 1988; Hays, Hays, & Mulhall, 2003; Herting & Guest, 1985; Murray, 1983; Sampson, 1986; Sampson, Castellano, & Laub, 1981; Wilson & Herrnstein, 1998). Larger social and cultural factors play a significant role in problematic substance use, from concrete factors like extreme poverty, availability of substances, and laws regulating substances (Bachman, Johnston, & O'Malley, 1981; Brook, Brook, Gordon, Whiteman, & Cohen, 1990; Cook & Tauchen, 1982; Dembo, Farrow, Schmeidler, & Burgos, 1979; Gorsuch & Butler, 1976; Gottfredson, 1987; Krieg, 1982; Levy & Sheflin, 1985; Maddahian, Newcomb, & Bentler, 1988; Murray, Richards, Luepker, & Johnson, 1987; Robins & Ratcliff, 1978; Saffer & Grossman, 1987; Zucker & Harford, 1983) to more subtle influences about attitudes and expectations, including exposure to large-scale advertising campaigns (Atkin, Hocking, & Block, 1984). With so many different factors influencing risk, comprehensive evaluation can easily become unwieldy and overwhelming. However, understanding that these factors all play a part in risk can help professionals contextualize and make decisions about just how "at-risk" adolescents are.

Validity of Assessment in Adolescence

An overall assumption can be made that most adolescents who are being evaluated for substance use, misuse, abuse, or related problems will be motivated to underreport their actual use of substances. Because of stigma, legal issues, and just generally getting into trouble (with parents and others), a system has been set up to encourage adolescents to underreport. However, many studies have shown that adolescent self-report of actual use is relatively valid and in concordance with other measures, such as biological measures (Dillon, Turner, Robbins, & Szapocznik, 2005; Johnston & O'Malley, 1997; Maisto, Connors, & Allen, 1995; Winters, Stinchfield, Henly, & Schwartz, 1990). This is most true with alcohol, cigarettes, and marijuana and less true with cocaine, but only a small percentage of adolescents surveyed in schools or in clinics tend to use an extreme response bias in their reporting of actual alcohol and other drug use (Dillon, Turner, Robbins, & Szapocznik, 2005; Winters, Stinchfield, Henly, & Schwartz, 1990). In general, though, self-report of substance use remains temporally stable upon retest and generally agrees with biological measures, such as urinalysis.

Multiple methods have been shown to improve the validity of adolescent self-report of substance use. As with most evaluations, triangulation of data using multiple methods, multiple modes, and multiple reporters is always wise (Groth-Marnat & Wright, 2016; Wright, 2010). Beyond multi-method assessment, though, specific methods can increase the likelihood that self-reports are valid. Building rapport (Winters, 2003) and ensuring confidentiality (Harrell, Kapszk, Cisin, & Wirtz, 1997) have been shown to increase adolescent truthfulness on self-reports, as have using concurrent biological measures, such as saliva or urinalysis, so that adolescents know that their self-reports will be "verified" in a way (Evans, Hansen, & Mittelmark, 1977; Wish, Hoffman, & Nemes, 1997). It should be noted that even using a fake biological data collection procedure, such as the bogus pipeline technique, in which the adolescent blows into a tube and is told it will measure substance levels (even though it will not), has been shown to increase validity of self-reports (Murray, O'Connell, Schmid, & Perry, 1987).

While adolescent self-report should be closely monitored for potential validity issues, it should also be noted that parents generally tend to underreport the extent of substance use by their children (Winters, Anderson, Bengston, Stinchfield, & Latimer, 2000), and the comparison between parent and adolescent self-reports has led to extremely low agreement of diagnosis of substance use disorders (Edelbrock, Costello, Dulcan, Conover, & Kala, 1986; Weissman et al., 1987). Similarly, sibling and peer reports of adolescent substance use have been shown to have significant problems with reliability and validity (Winters, Latimer, & Stinchfield, 2002). There is no perfect measurement technique to evaluate substance abuse and risk in general for substance-related problems, but in general the more different methods and reporters that can be enlisted and used, the more confident the evaluator can be in the validity of the assessment.

The valid use of assessment measures requires evaluators to consider cultural context in their interpretation (Council of National Psychological Associations for the Advancement of Ethnic Minority Interests, 2016). Equally important are the understanding of the psychometric properties of individual instruments with diverse populations (focused on the specific cultural background of the individual being evaluated) and the potential impact of cultural factors on how the individual being assessed is responding to the individual measures. Gender, racial, ethnic, religious, sexual, and other cultural factors should be considered when interpreting scores on each individual assessment. Most major psychological measures have healthy, if not robust, empirical literature on use with diverse populations (e.g., see the multiple tests in Groth-Marnat & Wright, 2016); however, many of the more targeted and less-often used measures may not have the research available, necessitating evaluators to keep culture and its potential impact on assessment measures in the forefront of their mind throughout the process.

Assessing Substance Use and Abuse

Perhaps most intuitive, evaluating the extent and consequences of actual current substance use is one of the most important areas to assess in adolescence, as use is highly predictive of later problems. Earlier onset of actual use has been related to substance-related problems and disorders later on (Lee & DiClemente, 1985; Parrella & Filstead, 1988), and so it is important to evaluate actual substance use. However, it is important not to conflate and confuse substance use, which in some circumstances can be normative and even adaptive, with substance abuse (Martin & Winters, 1998). For example, some have found that it is early drunkenness, not early drinking, that is a predictive risk factor for other problematic outcomes (Kuntsche et al., 2013), and as substance use increases in frequency and quantity, it becomes a significantly greater risk factor (Saal, Dong, Bonci, & Malenka, 2003). However, it has been shown that when actual substance use behaviors are controlled in adolescence, there is no link between identified risk factors and problems related to substance use (dependency or consequences) in adulthood (Bukstein & Kaminer, 2015), so it is still extremely important to evaluate the level of actual current substance use.

The Center for Substance Abuse Treatment (1999) proposed a continuum of severity in substance use during adolescence, ranging from (1) abstinence to (2) experimental use, (3) early abuse, (4) abuse, and (5) dependence. A continuum of severity like this can help delineate appropriate treatments (see Treatment Planning section later in this chapter), but it should also be flexible enough to incorporate other information, circumstances, and risk factors. Newcomb and Bentler (1989) suggested an "abuse threshold" that may be different in different circumstances. For example, minimal, recreational use of alcohol may be categorized as "experimental," but the experimental use of heroin may meet the abuse threshold and trigger a more significant intervention. In any evaluation, the extent of substance use and its history should be assessed, but they should also be contextualized within the adolescent's current circumstances, as well as within her or his other risk factors and supports.

In evaluating substance use and its history, a comprehensive assessment should include evaluation of the severity of use and problems, including onset of use, onset of regular use, frequency of use, quantity of use, duration of use, and drugs of preference (Petraitis, Flay, & Miller, 1995). Further, an evaluation of *why* the adolescent is using substances and *what purpose* they serve is helpful. Substances can provide relief from anxiety or depression, enhance mood, help individuals cope with stress, have social benefits, and can be purely recreational (Christenson & Goldman, 1983; Christenson, Smith, Roehling, & Goldman, 1989; Johnson & Gurin, 1994; Petraitis, Flay, & Miller, 1995; Zucker, Kincaid, Fitzgerald, & Bingham, 1995). There is some evidence that adolescents who use substances primarily for enhancing their mood are at greater risk for developing drug dependence (Henly & Winters, 1988). It should be noted that some adolescents use alcohol or drugs for the first time in a moment of weakness or stupidity, without significant risk for further use, problematic use, or later dependence/addiction.

Screening Instruments for Assessing Substance Use and Abuse

There are many brief screening instruments to evaluate actual substance use and its history. Many of them break down specific substances and ask about onset and frequency of use in the past and frequency, duration, and amount of current use. For example, the Adolescent Alcohol and Drug Involvement Scale (AADIS; Moburg, 2003), the Rutgers Alcohol Problem Index (RAPI; White & Labouvie, 1989), the Adolescent Drinking Index (ADI; Harrell & Wirtz, 1989), the Personal Experience Screening Questionnaire (PESQ; Winters, 1992), and the Problem Oriented Screening Instrument for Teenagers (POSIT; Dembo & Anderson, 2005) all include this information. However, some instruments include a distinction between normative and problem use of substances (like the ADI), some include measures of potential for faking (like the PESQ), and many include issues related to potential psychosocial consequences of and problems related to alcohol and drug use (like the PESQ, POSIT, and RAPI). The POSIT, for example, includes general questions about problems in areas like family and peer relations, education status, social skills, delinquent behavior, and physical and mental health and as such can be used to "cover" both the substance use/abuse screening and other areas of interest. There are other much briefer inventories, but they tend not to provide nearly enough useful information.

Perhaps one of the most useful screening instruments for substance abuse is the Adolescent Substance Abuse Subtle Screening Inventory (SASSI-A2; Miller & Lazowski, 2001). It includes the information that many other screening instruments include, such as current alcohol and other drug use (labeled "face valid" alcohol and other drug use), as well as other more obvious indicators of risk, like friend and family use questions, attitudes about use, and symptoms. However, it also includes subtler indicators of risk for use; that is, items are included that respondents may not identify as directly related to substance use. In addition to accomplishing a screening for actual use, this measure adds this important component on subtle risk factors (see section in this chapter on Assessing Substance Knowledge and Expectancies).

Survey Questionnaires for Assessing Substance Use and Abuse

While screening instruments may be adequate for surface-level information or a brief understanding of what problems may likely be present or may warrant further evaluation, more in-depth questionnaires have been developed to provide much more detail about substance use, abuse, dependency, and related consequences. Some of these include the Adolescent Self-Assessment Profile (ASAP-II; Wanberg, 1992), the Chemical Dependency Assessment Profile (CDAP; Harrell, Honaker, & Davis, 1991), the Hilson Adolescent Profile (HAP; Inwald, Brobst, & Morrissey, 1987), the Juvenile Automated Substance Abuse Evaluation (JASAE; Ellis, 1987), and the Personal Experience Inventory (PEI; Winters & Henly, 1988), all of which are significantly longer (most a few hundred questions) than related screening instruments. All of these include direct questions about use of specific substances, including frequency, duration, and physical and social consequences. However, most also include in-depth measures of potential, related problem areas and of potential response bias. The ASAP-II focuses on some strength (protective) areas, such as family and peer supports, school adjustment, and mental health, while the CDAP includes measures of self-concept and interpersonal relations. The HAP includes evaluation of educational difficulties; home life problems; sexual problems; mental health problems like depression, suicidality, and anxiety; and personality correlates for substance abuse problems, such as frustration tolerance, risk-taking, assertiveness, rigidity and obsessiveness, and suspicious temperament. Each of these includes validity and response bias indicators, such as the HAP evaluating both unusual and guarded responses and the PEI including five validity indicators, including response bias to "fake good" or "fake bad." While obviously significantly longer and more cumbersome to take, these surveys can provide important information that goes beyond substance use, abuse, dependency, and consequences, aligned with the more comprehensive approach to evaluating adolescents for risk for significant later problems presented in this chapter.

Clinical Interviews for Assessing Substance Use and Abuse

Clinical interviews that evaluate substance use, abuse, and dependence can be useful, though there are both benefits and drawbacks to this methodology. Primarily, issues like rapport and perceived confidentiality can significantly affect the results of a clinical interview, especially with an adolescent (who most often does not have the privilege of confidentiality from her or his parents or guardians). Still, several clinical interviews have been developed to evaluate substance use and its history in adolescents.

Most clinical interviews are highly structured and include face valid questions about alcohol and other drug use and its history, such as the Adolescent Diagnostic Interview (ADI; Winters & Henly, 1993), the Global Appraisal of Individual Needs (GAIN; Dennis, Titus, White, Unsicker, & Hodgkins, 2003), the Composite International Diagnostic Interview Substance Abuse Module (CIDI-SAM; Cottler, 2000), the Customary Drinking and Drug Use Record (CDDR; Brown et al., 1998), the Substance Use Disorders Diagnostic Schedule (SUDDS-IV; Harrison & Hoffman, 1989), the Adolescent Drug Abuse Diagnosis (ADAD; Friedman & Utada, 1989), the Teen Severity Index (T-ASI; Kaminer, Bukstein, & Tarter, 1991), and the Adolescent Problem Severity Index (APSI; Metzger, Kushner, & McLellan, 1991). All of these include specific, structured questions about the quantity and frequency of use of different substances, and most include information about the physical and psychosocial consequences of use. They are mostly aligned quite clearly with the diagnostic criteria in the DSM (American Psychiatric Association, 2013). Some include related problem (context) areas, such as the ADI including psychosocial stressors, school functioning, and cognitive problems; the SUDDS-IV including screening for anxiety and depression; and the APSI including measures of legal and medical issues, personal relationships, and the adolescent's understanding of the reason for the interview. The Comprehensive Addiction Severity Index for Adolescents (CASI-A; Meyers, 1991) is a semi-structured interview that assesses both substance use and abuse and other related areas, such as health, mental health, relationships, educational functioning, and stressors.

Assessing Substance Knowledge and Expectancies

Beyond actual use, its history, and its purpose, evaluations focused on risk for problematic substance use and potential subsequent substance-related disorders and related problems benefit from a clear understanding of the knowledge, attitudes, and values about using substances. Lack of knowledge about the negative effects of substance use and misuse and believing it is more "normal" or normative than it is have been linked to greater risk of problem use, somewhat intuitively (Kandel et al., 1978; Krosnick & Judd, 1982; Smith & Fogg, 1978), as have positive attitudes about using substances and positive expectancies (Christenson & Goldman, 1983; Christenson, Smith, Roehling, & Goldman, 1989; Johnson & Gurin, 1994; Zucker, Kincaid, Fitzgerald, & Bingham, 1995). Specifically, positive expectancies relate to adolescents believing that they will have both positive effects from using substances, including reduction of stress and negative affect and positive social consequences, and no negative effects from using substances, including physical, health-related, and psychosocial consequences. Evaluating knowledge and values, attitudes, and expectancies about substance use can both reveal a specific risk factor and provide guidance on specific interventions that would benefit the adolescent at risk.

Screening Instruments for Assessing Substance Knowledge and Expectancies

In addition to the SASSI-A2 (Miller & Lazowski, 2001), which has a number of items related to attitudes about substances, there are specific screening tools that focus just on attitudes, values, expectancies, and knowledge about substance use. Most focus on beliefs about using alcohol and other drugs. Some, like the Alcohol (and Illegal Drugs) Decisional Balance Scale (ADBS; DiClemente, 1999) and the Perceived Benefit of Drinking Scale (PBDS; Petchers & Singer, 1987) focus on the effects, often positive, that using substances currently has on the individual, such as the individual liking her- or himself better when drinking or using drugs, being more oneself when drinking or using drugs, and using substances helping an individual relax or feel better about her- or himself. Some also include potentially negative effects, like using substances causing problems with others or others trying to avoid the individual when she or he is drinking or using drugs. The Alcohol and Drug Consequences Questionnaire (ADCQ; Cunningham, Sobell, Gavin, Sobell, & Curtis Breslin, 1997) asks specifically about what is *likely to* happen, good and bad, if the respondent stops using drugs or alcohol. This is more effective with adolescents who are known to be using substances already and can pair well with stages of change measures (discussed later in this chapter).

Survey Questionnaires for Assessing Substance Knowledge and Expectancies

When it comes to longer, more in-depth questionnaires about attitudes, values, and knowledge, there are a few psychometrically solid measures from which to choose. Professionals should strongly consider how much the depth of these measures will add to the overall understanding and decision-making process in each individual case, as some of these are quite lengthy. For example, the Alcohol Effects Questionnaire (AEQ; Fromme, Stroot, & Kaplan, 1993) consists of 40 items related to the perceived effects of heavy alcohol use (like the individual feeling more powerful, sexy, clumsy, and flushed), and the Alcohol Expectancy Questionnaire—Adolescent Form (AEQ-A; Brown, Christiansen, & Goldman, 1987) includes 100 items focused on the negative effects of using alcohol. The AEQ-A provides seven different scales that relate to what the respondent expects from using alcohol, including globally positive changes, social behavior change, improved cognitive and motor skills, sexual enhancement, cognitive and motor impairment, increased arousal, and tension reduction. Each of these may or may not ultimately be useful in the overall picture of an adolescent and her or his risk of developing problem use or addiction.

Assessing Mental and Behavioral Health

Research has revealed that having a mental or behavioral disorder is a significant risk factor for problematic substance use, predicting both the onset of use and the transition from use to problematic use of substances (Conway, Swendsen, Husky, He, & Merikangas, 2016). Specifically, individual difference and personality factors that relate to mental health, including those related to both internalizing and externalizing problems, have been found to be predictive of patterns of substance use and abuse, different motivations and reasons for using, and differential sensitivity to substance reinforcement (Armstrong & Costello, 2002; Cerda, Sagdeo, & Galea, 2008; Comeau, Stewart, & Loba, 2001; Conrod, Peterson, & Pihl, 1997; Conrod, Pihl, Stewart, & Dongier, 2000; Conrod, Pihl, & Vassileva, 1998; Cooper, Frone, Russel, & Mudar, 1995; Woicik, Stewart, Pihl, & Conrod, 2009).

Many of the risk factors for substance-related problems are also related to externalizing problems. Specifically identified in the literature have been externalizing problems like impulsivity, aggressiveness, oppositionalism, disinhibition, sensation seeking, and conduct disorder symptoms (Bjork et al., 2004; Conrod, Castellanos-Ryan, & Mackie, 2011; Conrod, Stewart, Comeau, & Maclean, 2006; Dawe, Gullo, & Loxton, 2004; Demir, Ulug, Ergun, & Erbas, 2002; Dom, D'haene, Hulstijn, & Sabbe, 2006; Kaminer, 1991; Lee, Humphreys, Flory, Liu, & Glass, 2011; O'Leary-Barrett, Mackie, Castellanos-Ryan, Al-Khudhairy, & Conrod, 2010; Pingault et al., 2013; Varma, Basu, Malhotra, Sharma, & Mattoo, 1994; Wilens et al., 2011). Specifically, the traits of disinhibition and behavior problems related to conduct and antisocial behavior have been linked to an underlying pathology of addiction proneness (Hicks, Durbin, Blonigen, Iacono, & McGue, 2012; Iacono, Malone, & McGue, 2008; Kirisci, Tarter, Ridenour, Reynolds, & Vanyukov, 2013; McGue & Iacono, 2008; Tarter et al., 2003; Vanyukov & Ridenour, 2012; Vanyukov et al., 2003). Further, a great deal of research has linked the underlying traits that place adolescents at risk for attention-deficit/hyperactivity disorder (ADHD) with those that predispose them to substance-related disorders (Dalsgaard, Mortensen, Frydenberg, & Thomsen, 2014; Groenman et al., 2013).

In addition to links with externalizing problems, substance-related problems and disorders have been linked to internalizing problems. General psychological well-being has been identified as a specific factor related to the onset of problem substance use (Petraitis, Flay, & Miller, 1995), as have general coping skills, self-esteem, and emotion regulation (Berkowitz & Begun, 2003; Botvin, 2000; Khantzian, 1997). Two traits often associated with the broad construct of neuroticism (Costa & McCrae, 1995) and negative emotionality (Harkness & McNulty, 1994) have also been found to be specifically predictive of substance abuse and substance-related problems: hopelessness and anxiety sensitivity (Conrod, Castellanos-Ryan, & Mackie, 2011; Conrod, Stewart, Comeau, & Maclean, 2006; O'Leary-Barrett et al., 2010). Between the predictive risks and the potential common underlying pathological traits of both externalizing and internalizing problems and problems related to substance use, it is essential that a comprehensive evaluation of adolescent risk for eventual addiction and other substance-related problems includes an evaluation of mental and behavioral health.

Screening Instruments for Assessing Mental and Behavioral Health

There are many instruments for screening for mental and behavioral health problems, and there are many reviews of such measures. As the scope of mental and behavioral health evaluation is vast, this chapter will limit its discussion of screening instruments (as well as interviews and survey questionnaires) to mentioning some of the more widely used measures. Perhaps one of the most widely used screening measures for mental health is the Brief Symptom Inventory (BSI; Derogatis, 1993), a very brief (53 item) inventory that yields scores on multiple mental health problems, including depression, anxiety, hostility, and paranoia, as well as global indicators of general mental health. Other widely used broad screenings include the Behavior Rating Profile (BRP-2; Brown & Hammill, 1990), the Child/Adolescent Psychiatry Screen (CAPS; Bostic, 2004), the Adolescent Symptom Inventory (ASI-4; Gadow & Sprafkin, 1998), and the Social-Emotional Dimension Scale (SEDS-2; Hutton & Roberts, 1986). Some are quite lengthy for screening measures, like the Conners Comprehensive Behavior Rating Scales (Conners CBRS; Conners, Pitkanen, & Rzepa, 2011) and the Achenbach System of Empirically Based Assessment (ASEBA; Achenbach & Rescorla, 2013). Other scales, like the Strengths and Weaknesses of ADHD Symptoms and Normal Behavior (SWAN; Swanson et al., 2001), focus primarily on one set of adolescent problems, in this case those related to attention-deficit/hyperactivity disorder (ADHD).

Survey Questionnaires for Assessing Mental and Behavioral Health

While the above brief surveys screen for overall mental health, some self-report and other report inventories that are widely used focus on a deeper investigation into mental and behavioral health issues. Measures like the Behavior Assessment System for Children (BASC-3; Reynolds, 2004) allow for multiple informers (self, parents/caregivers, and teachers) to rate and triangulate information about a variety of mental health indicators, including strengths like social skills and leadership. Other measures focus less on specific disorder-related information (though it is often included in these measures) and more on the structural makeup of personality, such as the Personality Inventory for Children (PIC-2; Lachar & Gruber, 2001) and the adolescent and preadolescent versions of some of the most widely used adult tests of personality, such as the Minnesota Multiphasic Personality Inventory-Adolescent (MMPI-A; Butcher, 1992) and Adolescent RF (MMPI-A-RF; Archer, Handel, Ben-Porath, & Tellegen, 2016), the Millon Adolescent Clinical Inventory (MACI; Millon, 1993) and Millon Pre-Adolescent Clinical Inventory (M-PACI; Millon & Tringone, 2005), and the Personality Assessment Inventory-Adolescent (PAI-A; Morey, 1999). Although significantly longer than most of the screening measures above, these instruments can provide a broader mental and behavioral health "context" for what is going on for an adolescent, helping determine a broader picture of social-emotional risks and protective factors for potential problematic substance use.

Clinical Interviews for Assessing Mental and Behavioral Health

As part of a truly comprehensive evaluation, some evaluators prefer to include structured clinical interview measures of mental and behavioral health functioning, although most often this is unnecessary unless there are specific indicators that there is likely a major mental health disorder present. For a helpful review of such diagnostic interviews, refer to Leffler, Riebel, and Hughes' (2015) article in *Assessment*. Among the more common clinical interviews are the Diagnostic Interview for Children and Adolescents (DICA-IV; Reich, 2000), the Diagnostic Interview Schedule for Children (DISC-IV; Shaffer, Fisher, Lucas, Dulcan, & Schwab-Stone, 2000), the Schedule for Affective Disorders and Schizophrenia for School-Aged Children (Kiddie-SADS; Kaufman et al., 1997), the Structured Clinical Interview for DSM-IV, Childhood Diagnoses (KID-SCID; Hien et al., 2004), the Child and Adolescent Psychiatric Assessment (CAPA; Angold & Costello, 2000), and the Global Appraisal of Individual Needs (GAIN; Dennis, Titus, White, Unsicker, & Hodgkins, 2003). Each of these is lengthy, requires specific training to administer and score, and provides fairly traditionally DSM-oriented results about diagnostic criteria.

Assessing Executive Functioning

Related to mental and behavioral health are issues of executive functioning, including impulse control, frustration tolerance, disinhibition, and general organization, planning, and future orientation. Emotional and behavioral self-control are central to executive functioning and have been found to be important predictors (and personal "contexts") of problematic substance use (Armstrong & Costello, 2002; Cerda, Sagdeo, & Galea, 2008; Khantzian, 1997) and are well considered in evaluations of ADHD, also related to substance-related disorder risk (Dalsgaard, Mortensen, Frydenberg, & Thomsen, 2014; Groenman et al., 2013). While screenings may rightfully choose not to evaluate executive functioning specifically, comprehensive evaluations should consider evaluating executive functioning (Petraitis, Flay, & Miller, 1995).

Survey Questionnaires for Assessing Executive Functioning

Executive functioning is often evaluated with performance-based cognitive measures, but there are some surveys that evaluate it. The Comprehensive Executive Function Inventory (CEFI; Naglieri & Goldstein, 2013) and the Behavior Rating Inventory of Executive Function (BRIEF; Gioia, Isquith, Guy, & Kenworthy, 2005) both include forms for teachers, parents, and self-report for adolescents. They each provide scales for different components of executive functioning, like emotional regulation and control, impulse control, planning and organizing, working memory, and self-monitoring.

Performance-Based Measures for Assessing Executive Functioning

While the survey measures discussed cover multiple areas of behavior related to executive functioning, many evaluations consider this area a cognitive or neuropsychological area of functioning, and as such use performance-based measures to approximate level of executive functioning. Multiple, quite creative measures have been developed to try to evaluate how well individuals control their own mental and behavioral processes. Measures like the Wisconsin Card Sort Test (WCST-IV; Heaton, Chelune, Curtiss, Kay, & Talley, 1993) and disk/ring transfer tasks like the Tower of Hanoi (TOH; Welsh, Pennington, & Groisser, 1991) and Tower of London (TOL; Levin et al., 1991) use techniques with specific rules that require inhibition of impulses to respond in certain ways in order to conform to the tasks. Other measures use verbal fluency, such as naming as many animals as possible within a time limit, or multi-trial word list learning, like on the California Verbal Learning Test (CVLT-II; Delis, Kramer, Kaplan, & Ober, 2000) to approximate mental control. There are several measures, including the Cognitive Assessment System (CAS2; Naglieri, Das, & Goldstein, 2014) and the Delis-Kaplan Executive Function System (D-KEFS; Delis, Kaplan, & Kramer, 2001) that combine multiple measures of different executive functions to evaluate the construct more fully.

Assessing Psychoeducational Functioning

As discussed previously, the relationship between an adolescent and school has been identified as a specific predictive factor for substance abuse and related problems (Fletcher, Bonnell, & Hargreaves, 2008; Friedman, 1983; Gottfredson, 1987; Hundleby & Mercer, 1987; Jessor, 1976; Robins, 1980; Smith & Fogg, 1978). School failure, lack of goal-directedness in academic pursuits, and low academic achievement have all been identified as specific risk factors (Petraitis, Flay, & Miller, 1995), and one potential key driving force behind the onset of school disconnection and academic difficulty is the presence of actual learning difficulties. As such, it may be important to evaluate the psychoeducational functioning of an adolescent in the course of a comprehensive evaluation for substance abuse and problem risk. Underlying and undiagnosed learning disabilities may be extremely important to address to mitigate their impact on deterioration of school connection and academic achievement, all problems in the overall picture of an adolescent at risk for developing problematic substance use. It should be noted that research has revealed multiple secondary emotional and social problems related to learning disabilities (Bender, 1987; Bryan, Burstein, & Ergul, 2004), likely exacerbated when the learning disability goes undiagnosed and unaddressed.

Survey Questionnaires for Assessing Psychoeducational Functioning

There are aspects of psychoeducational functioning that are more appropriate to assess using surveys (self-reports and other reports) and some that are more appropriate to use performance-based measures. While actual academic ability (including possible learning differences, attentional problems, etc.) are better evaluated with actual performance-based measures, aspects of students' relationships to school are better evaluated with survey questionnaires. Libbey (2004) discusses many different aspects of students' relationships to school and how to measure them, including attachment to school, positive orientation and feelings toward school, bonding, connection, engagement, satisfaction, and the general school climate as a context. One brief, widely used measure of school connectedness is the Psychological Sense of School Membership Scale (PSSM; Goodenow, 1993), which is a brief measure that evaluates (via self-report) an adolescent's feelings about school, including feeling like she or he is a part of the school community, has a sense of belonging, and feels respected in school. This measure has been found to be related to school effort, absences, tardiness, and academic performance, all of which are data collectable directly from an adolescent's school and may play an important role in understanding the context of an adolescent's risk for problematic substance use.

Performance-Based Measures for Assessing Psychoeducational Functioning

When assessing actual academic ability and functioning, performance-based measures are the standard in the field. Beyond the scope of this chapter, multiple models have emerged in the literature to diagnose learning disabilities, learning differences, attention deficits, and cognitive processing problems, including an ability-achievement discrepancy model, response to intervention, and the newer pattern of strengths and weaknesses (PSW) model (see Phipps & Beaujean, 2016 for a review of this model). For a more in-depth discussion of practical issues in the assessment of learning and psychoeducational functioning, see Taylor (2014), but in general these evaluations involve cognitive aptitude tests, academic achievement tests, and often neuropsychological measures of attention, concentration, and cognitive impulsivity.

Assessing Life Skills

In general, many different coping, problem solving, and social skills have been identified as related to adolescent substance use, abuse, and subsequent disorders and problems (Petraitis, Flay, & Miller, 1995). Much of the prevention literature focuses on broad-based interventions that teach many of these skills (e.g., Botvin et al., 2000; Griffin, Botvin, Nichols, & Doyle, 2003; Spoth, Redmond, Trudeau, & Shin, 2002; Trudeau, Spoth, Lillehoj, Redmond, & Wickrama, 2003), with great effect. As such, identifying some of these skills that may be lacking in an adolescent cannot only uncover specific risk but can also help make decisions on how exactly to intervene. It should be noted that life skills, broadly, do encompass many different areas, more than are feasible to assess, even in a comprehensive evaluation. Professionals should use their judgment to determine which are likely to be the most relevant to any given referral question.

Survey Questionnaires for Assessing Life Skills

There are some, though not many, measures used in clinical practice that cover multiple areas of life skills. For example, the Ansell-Casey Life Skills Assessment (ACLSA; Nollan, Wolf, Ansell, & Burns, 2000) has adolescents evaluate themselves on skills like maintaining healthy relationships, planning and goal-setting, using community resources, and daily living activities, among others. This measure, like many others focused on life skills, actually assesses skills theoretically necessary for independent living. Two measures of general life skills were developed specifically for their relationship to problematic substance use. The Developmental Assets Profile (DAP; Search Institute, 2005) focuses on multiple skills and assets theorized to be linked to better adjustment and subsequently lower risk for problems like substance abuse. Among these skills and assets are a commitment to learning (related to psychoeducational assessment, as discussed in this chapter), positive values, positive identity, and social competence. The Substance Use Risk Profile Scale (SURPS; Woicik, Stewart, Pihl, & Conrod, 2009) focuses on four major skills (worded in the negative as problems) identified in the literature as risk factors for substance abuse and related problems: anxiety sensitivity, impulsivity, hopelessness, and sensation seeking.

When it comes to specific life skills that are widely associated with substance abuse and related problems, an important one is adolescents' ability to cope with negative experiences and feelings. Several measures are useful for evaluating coping skills, and most provide information about both productive, adaptive methods of coping, such as problem solving, optimistically focusing on positive things, and seeking support from friends, family, and professionals, and nonproductive, maladaptive methods of coping, such as ignoring or avoiding the problem, using unhealthy tension reduction techniques like substance abuse, and worrying and blaming oneself. Two widely used measures include the Adolescent Coping Scale (ACS-2; Frydenberg & Lewis, 2012) and the Adolescent Coping Orientation for Problem Experiences Scale (A-COPE; Patterson & McCubbin, 1996).

Another specific life skill that is often strongly tied to substance abuse and dependence is problem solving. Measures have been developed to study problem solving in general, such as the Personal Problem-Solving Inventory (PPSI; Heppner & Petersen, 1982), and specific aspects of problem solving, like the Social Problem-Solving Inventory for Adolescents (SPSI-A; Frauenknecht & Black, 1995). Most often measures like these include scales of processes of problem solving as well as an evaluation of problem-solving skills and confidence.

Assessing the Family

As stated earlier, understanding (at least some of) the family context can significantly benefit a comprehensive evaluation of adolescent risk for developing problematic substance use. Factors to assess include both current and history of substance use, abuse, dependence, and treatment of both parents and siblings (Petraitis, Flay, & Miller, 1995), as well as a host of family context issues, like parental monitoring, family bonding and conflict, and harshness of disciplinary practices (Lochman & van den Steenhoven, 2002). Many times understanding specific risks within the family system can significantly change the direction of recommended interventions, shifting the focus from the adolescent her- or himself to the family as a whole.

Survey Questionnaires for Assessing the Family

While there are many different aspects of families that can be assessed as part of a comprehensive evaluation for drug and alcohol risk in adolescence and some previously discussed measures (like the SASSI-A2) include some family information, the general environment and context of the family are often important to understand, including family management, family cohesion, conflict within the family, and integration. Liddle and Rowe (1998) discussed many measures, including survey instruments and tasks to be coded by observers. Many of the scales that are most useful for these evaluations, including the Family Environment Scale (FES; Moos & Moos, 1994) and the Family Assessment Measure (FAM-III; Skinner, Steinhauer, & Santa-Barbara, 2009), cover many of these multiple areas of family functioning, while some measures cover a single area more in depth, such as the Conflict Behavior Questionnaire (CBQ; Prinz, Foster, Kent, & O'Leary, 1979), which focuses specifically on the level of distress different family members experience because of family interaction patterns. The Family Adaptability and Cohesion Scale (FACES-IV; Olson, 2010) is based on the Circumplex Model (Olson, 2011; Olson & Gorall, 2006) of family cohesion and family flexibility, each of which has a balanced, healthy middle range and extremes that are less healthy. Specifically, the extremes of family cohesion are disengagement at the low end and enmeshment at the high end, while the extremes of family flexibility are rigidity at the low end and chaos at the high end, both with balance in the middle range of the scales.

Several measures include multiple general family scales like cohesion, support, communication, and attachment, but also include scales that are specifically useful for adolescent substance abuse and related problems evaluations. For example, the Family Relations Scale (FRS; Gorman-Smith, Tolan, Zelli, & Huesmann, 1996) includes a scale about deviant beliefs that are shared within the family. The Student Survey of Risk and Protective Factors and Prevalence of Alcohol, Tobacco, and Other Drug Use (Arthur, Hawkins, Catalano, & Pollard, 1998) includes information about family norms, such as attitudes that are favorable toward alcohol and other drugs. Each of these measures offers information about family dynamics, norms, attitudes, and practices that either directly or indirectly affect adolescent problem substance use risk, further contributing information about the context in which the adolescent being evaluated is living.

Assessing Readiness for Change

While most often associated with actual disorders, especially substance-related disorders, readiness for behavior change is a useful construct for helping understand an adolescent's mindset with regard to how she or he perceives her or his own substance use (Christenson & Goldman, 1983; Christenson, Smith, Roehling, & Goldman, 1989; Groth-Marnat & Wright, 2016; Johnson & Gurin, 1994; Norcross, Krebs, & Prochaska, 2011; Zucker, Kincaid, Fitzgerald, & Bingham, 1995). Prochaska, DiClemente, and Norcross (1992) discussed how decisional balance (weighing pros and cons), self-efficacy to effect change (see section on Self-Efficacy later in this chapter), and temptation influence an individual's readiness to change her or his behaviors. The stages include precontemplation, in which an individual is not even considering changing her or his behavior; contemplation, during which the individual is thinking about changing; preparation, at which point she or he is ready to change; action, during which stage she or he is making changes to her or his behavior; and maintenance, focusing on staying on track with her or his behavior. Relapse occurs when an individual slips back into her or his old behavior pattern and starts the stages over again at precontemplation. Understanding an adolescent's stage of change can significantly affect the ultimate recommendations, as, for example, even with the same level of substance use, individuals in precontemplation will require a different intervention than those in preparation (Groth-Marnat & Wright, 2016; Norcross, Krebs, & Prochaska, 2011).

Survey Questionnaires for Assessing Readiness for Change

Several measures have been developed to evaluate the stage of change that an individual is in with regard to a specific problem, most often drug and/or alcohol abuse, but sometimes listed as "problem" in general. They are generally all self-report measures, and some measures include items that correspond to each of the five stages of change and yield scores on each (with the evaluator left to interpret often the most highly endorsed stage as the likely actual stage the individual is in), such as the Readiness to Change Questionnaire (RCQ; Rollnick, Heather, Gold, & Hall, 1992) and the University of Rhode Island Change Assessment Scale (URICA; Hasler, Klaghofer, & Buddeberg, 2002). Some use modified or truncated versions of the stage of change theory, such as the Stages of Change Readiness and Treatment Eagerness Scale (SOCRATES; Miller, 1991), which is organized into problem recognition, ambivalence about change, and taking steps, and the Problem Recognition Questionnaire (PRQ; Cady, Winters, Jordan, Solberg, & Stinchfield, 1996), which focuses on the early stages, with factors for contemplation, contemplation/preparation, and preparation. The Circumstances, Motivation, Readiness, and Suitability Scales (CMRS; DeLeon, Melnick, Kressel, & Jainchill, 1994) include potential motivations for treatment, including both external circumstances and internal motivators, readiness for treatment, and the individual's self-perceived appropriateness for treatment. While not directly linked to the stages of change model, it can certainly provide valuable information about an adolescent's current mindset related to engaging with treatment and earnestly working to change behavior.

Assessing Self-Efficacy

As part of the Transtheoretical Model of Change (which enumerates the stages of change; Prochaska, DiClemente, & Norcross, 1992), the level of efficacy an individual feels, the confidence in her or his personal ability to implement specific behaviors for a desired effect, is central to behavioral control and change and has specifically been implicated in the effectiveness of behavior change in substance abuse and substance-related disorders (Kadden & Litt, 2011). Much like some of the other factors presented in this chapter, while it may not relate directly to actual substance use behaviors, understanding an adolescent's level of self-efficacy can help inform appropriate interventions to recommend (Christenson & Goldman, 1983; Chrstenson, Smith, Roehling, & Goldman, 1989; Johnson & Gurin, 1994; Zucker, Kincaid, Fitzgerald, & Bingham, 1995). In order for an adolescent to feel confident changing her or his behavior with regard to using substances, she or he must have faith and confidence that she or he can actually succeed in changing the behavior. Therefore, within a comprehensive evaluation of an adolescent, self-efficacy is another piece of information that can significantly impact intervention recommendations.

Brief Survey Questionnaires for Assessing Self-Efficacy

As a very specific construct related to an individual being evaluated, most of the measures aimed at assessing self-efficacy are quite brief. Most of them are written in situational terms, presenting either vague or specific types of situations and asking the respondent to evaluate her or his confidence that she or he could refuse using substances in those situations. Many of the situations are categorized into social pressure situations, dealing with negative emotions, and general situations that present the opportunity to use alcohol or other drugs. Most of the measures are specific to a single substance, except for the Brief Situational Confidence Questionnaire (BCSQ; Breslin, Sobell, Sobell, & Agrawal, 2000), which presents the situations and asks about confidence to resist drinking heavily or using the individual's primary drug of choice, giving the option to the respondent.

For self-efficacy related to alcohol resistance, the Situational Confidence Questionnaire (SCQ; Graham & Ontario, 1988) and Self-Efficacy for Drinking Control Scale (SEDCS; Sitharthan & Kavanagh, 1991) focus on confidence in resisting the urge to drink heavily, while the Alcohol Abstinence Self-Efficacy Scale (AASES; DiClemente, Carbonari, Montgomery, & Hughes, 1994) and Drink Refusal Self-Efficacy Questionnaire (DRSEQ-R; Oei, Hasking, & Young, 2005) focus on confidence to abstain from drinking entirely. The Confidence Questionnaire for Smoking Behaviors (Condiotte & Lichtenstein, 1981) evaluates self-efficacy to resist relapse on cigarette smoking. For other drugs, the Drug-Taking Confidence

Questionnaire (Annis, Turner, & Sklar, 1997) evaluates confidence to resist using drugs, though it must be readministered repeatedly for each substance in question. The Drug Avoidance Self-Efficacy Scale (DASES; Martin, Wilkinson, & Poulos, 1995) evaluates the same construct, but specifically with multidrug use.

Treatment Planning

Making specific intervention recommendations from a comprehensive evaluation can be confusing, especially as more and more information can become increasingly overwhelming. Simply understanding an adolescent's pattern of substance use, in the absence of key contextual factors like the reasons for use, attitudes and expectancies about substance use, mental health history, academic functioning, and level of self-efficacy, may not be enough to determine the best course of action. It should be noted, though, that because of practical constraints, comprehensive evaluations that include every domain presented in this chapter are often not feasible. Even a basic screening, though, should include an evaluation of substance use and its history (including some information on the reasons for use), attitudes and expectancies about substance use, and mental and behavioral health. When possible, though, including more of the domains only serves to strengthen the utility of the evaluation.

As discussed previously in this chapter, the idea of an "abuse threshold" (Newcomb & Bentler, 1989) is useful in deciding what level of intervention is necessary, based solely on use. Winters, Latimer, and Stinchfield (2002) presented some situations that are extremely important when considering appropriate interventions to recommend. First, the use (even one-time use) of some classifications of substances (like heroin or crystal meth) is dangerous enough that significant treatment intervention (beyond what would be considered "prevention" by the Institute of Medicine [Mrazek & Haggerty, 1994] definition) should be considered. Similarly, regular very early use (childhood or young adolescence), prolonged use in moderate quantities, or acute use in large quantities are each risky enough to justify significant therapeutic intervention. Substance use in significantly inappropriate settings, such as during school or before driving a car, even if there are no acute negative consequences, should also meet the threshold for abuse that warrants significant therapeutic intervention, as should an unclear pattern of use that does have significant negative social or psychological consequences. Finally, they discuss a situation in which there is an absence of substance use and consequences, but there are multiple significant risk factors present, such as an externalizing disorder, family history of addiction, engagement with drug abusing peers, and positive expectancies about future use of substances. In this case, indicated prevention (Mrazek & Haggerty, 1994) may be a more appropriate recommendation for intervention.

When additional information like beliefs about how normative substance use is, stage of change, and self-efficacy is obtainable, more specific recommendations about intervention can be made. For example, an adolescent who is not currently using any substances and has minimal risks in terms of family use and dynamics, mental and behavioral health, and access to substances, but who believes that substance abuse is much more prevalent in her peer group than it actually is, would likely benefit from psychoeducational intervention about the actual rates of substance abuse for youth her age. Another adolescent who has extremely low self-efficacy, believing strongly that he does not have the capability to change his substance abuse behavior, would benefit from cognitive interventions targeting self-efficacy beliefs. Individuals in different stages of change also warrant different types of intervention (Groth-Marnat & Wright, 2016; Norcross, Krebs, & Prochaska, 2011); for example, an adolescent with problematic use in precontemplation would likely benefit from something like motivational interviewing, to propel them forward in the stages of change, whereas an adolescent with problematic use in action would benefit more from specific, concrete techniques, such as those found in dialectical behavior therapy or cognitive-behavioral therapy. The more information collected beyond actual use and its history, the more specific and targeted recommendations can be for intervention that is likely to have positive effects with that individual adolescent. More information, and thus more detail about different risk and protective factors, helps improve the likelihood of intervention being successful.

Conclusion

Evaluating substance use and abuse in adolescence may seem straightforward, requiring direct questions about onset, frequency, amount, and duration of use of different substances, but trying to make strong predictions about just how at risk an adolescent is for developing problematic use, eventual addiction and dependency, and negative life consequences is complicated. Many adolescents use substances (especially alcohol, nicotine, and marijuana), and many of them will not develop problems. Conducting comprehensive evaluations of factors and contexts known to be related to risk and potential later problems can help strengthen a professional's understanding of an adolescent's likely trajectory. Perhaps more importantly, information from a comprehensive evaluation can help the clinical decision-making process in countless ways, guiding recommendations toward what will likely be the most beneficial and protective for the adolescent being evaluated.

References

Achenbach, T., & Rescorla, L. (2013). Achenbach system of empirically based assessment. In *Encyclopedia of Autism Spectrum Disorders* (pp. 31–39). New York, NY: Springer.

American Psychiatric Association. (2013). *Diagnostic and Statistical Manual of Mental Disorders* (5th ed.). Washington, DC: American Psychiatric Publishers.

Angold, A., & Costello, E. J. (2000). The child and adolescent psychiatric assessment (CAPA). *Journal of the American Academy of Child & Adolescent Psychiatry, 39*(1), 39–48.

Annis, H., Turner, N. E., & Sklar, S. M. (1997). *Drug-Taking Confidence Questionnaire: DTCQ.* Addiction Research Foundation: Sample Pack.

Archer, R. P., Handel, R. W., Ben-Porath, Y. S., & Tellegen, A. (2016). *Minnesota Multiphasic Personality Inventory-Adolescent-Restructured Form (MMPI-A-RF): Administration, Scoring, Interpretation, and Technical Manual.* Minneapolis, MN: University of Minnesota Press.

Armstrong, T. D., & Costello, E. J. (2002). Community studies on adolescent substance use, abuse, or dependence and psychiatric comorbidity. *Journal of Consulting and Clinical Psychology, 70*(6), 1224–1239.

Arthur, M., Hawkins, J. D., Catalano, R. F., & Pollard, J. A. (1998). *Student Survey of Risk and Protective Factors and Prevalence of Alcohol, Tobacco, and Other Drug Use.* Seattle, WA: Social Development Research Group, University of Washington.

Atkin, C., Hocking, J., & Block, M. (1984). Teenage drinking: Does advertising make a difference? *Journal of Communication, 34*(2), 157–167.

Bachman, J. G., Johnston, L. D., & O'Malley, P. M. (1981). Smoking, drinking, and drug use among American high school students: Correlates and trends, 1975-1979. *American Journal of Public Health, 71*(1), 59–69.

Bender, W. N. (1987). Secondary personality and behavioral problems in adolescents with learning disabilities. *Journal of Learning Disabilities, 20*(5), 280–285.

Berkowitz, M. W., & Begun, A. L. (2003). Designing prevention programs: The developmental perspective. In Z. Sloboda & W. J. Bukoski (Eds.), *Handbook of Drug Abuse Prevention: Theory, Science, & Practice* (pp. 327–348). New York, NY: Kluwer Academic/Plenum Publishers.

Bjork, J. M., Knutson, B., Fong, G. W., Caggiano, D. M., Bennett, S. M., & Hommer, D. W. (2004). Incentive-elicited brain activation in adolescents: Similarities and differences from young adults. *Journal of Neuroscience, 24*(8), 1793–1802.

Bostic, J. Q. (2004). *Child/Adolescent Psychiatry Screen (CAPS).* Boston, MA: Massachusetts General Hospital. Retrieved from: http://www2.massgeneral.org/schoolpsychiatry/childadolescentpscychiatryscreencaps.pdf.

Botvin, G. J. (2000). Preventing drug abuse in schools: Social and competence enhancement approaches targeting individual-level etiologic factors. *Addictive Behaviors, 25*(6), 887–897.

Botvin, G. J., Griffin, K. W., Diaz, T., Scheier, L. M., Williams, C., & Epstein, J. A. (2000). Preventing illicit drug use in adolescents: Long-term follow-up data from a randomized control trial of a school population. *Addictive Behaviors, 25*(5), 769–774.

Breslin, F. C., Sobell, L. C., Sobell, M. B., & Agrawal, S. (2000). A comparison of a brief and long version of the situational confidence questionnaire. *Behaviour Research and Therapy, 38*(12), 1211–1220.

Brook, J. S., Brook, D. W., Gordon, A. S., Whiteman, M., & Cohen, P. (1990). The psychosocial etiology of adolescent drug use: A family interactional approach. *Genetic, Social, and General Psychology Monographs, 116*(2), 111–276.

Brown, L., & Hammill, D. D. (1990). *BRP-2: Behavior Rating Profile.* Austin, TX: Pro-ed.

Brown, S. A., Christiansen, B. A., & Goldman, M. S. (1987). The alcohol expectancy questionnaire: An instrument for the assessment of adolescent and adult alcohol expectancies. *Journal of Studies on Alcohol, 48*(5), 483–491.

Brown, S. A., Meyer, M. G., Lippke, L., Tapert, S. F., Stewart, D. G., & Vik, P. W. (1998). Psychometric evaluation of the customary drinking and drug use record (CDDR): A measure of adolescent alcohol and drug involvement. *Journal of Studies on Alcohol, 59*(4), 427–438.

Bryan, T., Burstein, K., & Ergul, C. (2004). The social-emotional side of learning disabilities: A science-based presentation of the state of the art. *Learning Disability Quarterly, 27*(1), 45–51.

Buchmann, A. F., Blomeyer, D., Jennen-Steinmetz, C., Schmidt, M. H., Esser, G., Banaschewski, T., & Laucht, M. (2013). Early smoking onset may promise initial pleasurable sensations and later addiction. *Addiction Biology, 18*(6), 947–954.

Bukstein, O. G., & Kaminer, Y. (2015). Adolescent substance use disorders: Transition to substance abuse, prevention, and treatment. In M. Galanter, H. D. Kleber, & K. T. Brady (Eds.), *The American Psychiatric Publishing Textbook of Substance Abuse Treatment* (5th ed., pp. 641–650). Washington, D.C.: American Psychiatric Publishing.

Butcher, J. N. (1992). *Minnesota Multiphasic Personality Inventory-Adolescent*. Minneapolis, MN: University of Minnesota Press.

Cady, M. E., Winters, K. C., Jordan, D. A., Solberg, K. B., & Stinchfield, R. D. (1996). Motivation to change as a predictor of treatment outcome for adolescent substance abusers. *Journal of Child & Adolescent Substance Abuse, 5*(1), 73–91.

Center for Substance Abuse Treatment. (1999). *Screening and Assessing Adolescents for Substance Use Disorders (Treatment Improvement Protocol Series no. 31)*. Rockville, MD: Substance Abuse and Mental Health Services Administration.

Cerdá, M., Sagdeo, A., & Galea, S. (2008). Comorbid forms of psychopathology: Key patterns and future research directions. *Epidemiologic Reviews, 30*(1), 155–177.

Christiansen, B. A., & Goldman, M. S. (1983). Alcohol-related expectancies versus demographic/background variables in the prediction of adolescent drinking. *Journal of Consulting and Clinical Psychology, 51*(2), 249–257.

Christiansen, B. A., Smith, G. T., Roehling, P. V., & Goldman, M. S. (1989). Using alcohol expectancies to predict adolescent drinking behavior after one year. *Journal of Consulting and Clinical Psychology, 57*(1), 93–99.

Comeau, N., Stewart, S. H., & Loba, P. (2001). The relations of trait anxiety, anxiety sensitivity, and sensation seeking to adolescents' motivations for alcohol, cigarette, and marijuana use. *Addictive Behaviors, 26*(6), 803–825.

Condiotte, M. M., & Lichtenstein, E. (1981). Self-efficacy and relapse in smoking cessation programs. *Journal of Consulting and Clinical Psychology, 49*(5), 648–658.

Conners, C. K., Pitkanen, J., & Rzepa, S. R. (2011). *Conners Comprehensive Behavior Rating Scale* (pp. 678–680). New York: Springer.

Conrod, P. J., Castellanos-Ryan, N., & Mackie, C. (2011). Long-term effects of a personality-targeted intervention to reduce alcohol use in adolescents. *Journal of Consulting and Clinical Psychology, 79*(3), 296–306.

Conrod, P. J., Peterson, J. B., Pihl, R. O., & Mankowski, S. (1997). Biphasic effects of alcohol on heart rate are influenced by alcoholic family history and rate of alcohol ingestion. *Alcoholism: Clinical and Experimental Research, 21*(1), 140–149.

Conrod, P. J., Pihl, R. O., Stewart, S. H., & Dongier, M. (2000). Validation of a system of classifying female substance abusers on the basis of personality and motivational risk factors for substance abuse. *Psychology of Addictive Behaviors, 14*(3), 243–256.

Conrod, P. J., Pihl, R. O., & Vassileva, J. (1998). Differential sensitivity to alcohol reinforcement in groups of men at risk for distinct alcoholism subtypes. *Alcoholism: Clinical and Experimental Research, 22*(3), 585–597.

Conrod, P. J., Stewart, S. H., Comeau, N., & Maclean, A. M. (2006). Efficacy of cognitive–behavioral interventions targeting personality risk factors for youth alcohol misuse. *Journal of Clinical Child and Adolescent Psychology, 35*(4), 550–563.

Conway, K. P., Swendsen, J., Husky, M. M., He, J. P., & Merikangas, K. R. (2016). Association of lifetime mental disorders and subsequent alcohol and illicit drug use: Results from the National Comorbidity Survey–Adolescent Supplement. *Journal of the American Academy of Child & Adolescent Psychiatry, 55*(4), 280–288.

Cook, P. J., & Tauchen, G. (1982). The effect of liquor taxes on heavy drinking. *The Bell Journal of Economics, 13*(2), 379–390.

Cooper, M. L., Frone, M. R., Russell, M., & Mudar, P. (1995). Drinking to regulate positive and negative emotions: A motivational model of alcohol use. *Journal of Personality and Social Psychology, 69*(5), 990–1005.

Costa, P. T., Jr., & McCrae, R. R. (1995). Domains and facets: Hierarchical personality assessment using the revised NEO personality inventory. *Journal of Personality Assessment, 64*(1), 21–50.

Cottler, L. B. (2000). *Composite International Diagnostic Interview—Substance Abuse Module (SAM)*. St. Louis, MO: Department of Psychiatry, Washington University School of Medicine.

Council of National Psychological Associations for the Advancement of Ethnic Minority Interests. (2016). *Testing and Assessment with Persons & Communities of Color*. Washington, DC: American Psychological Association. Retrieved from https://www.apa.org/pi/oema.

Cunningham, J. A., Sobell, L. C., Gavin, D. R., Sobell, M. B., & Curtis Breslin, F. (1997). Assessing motivation for change: Preliminary development and evaluation of a scale measuring the costs and benefits of changing alcohol or drug use. *Psychology of Addictive Behaviors, 11*(2), 107–114.

Dalsgaard, S., Mortensen, P. B., Frydenberg, M., & Thomsen, P. H. (2014). ADHD, stimulant treatment in childhood and subsequent substance abuse in adulthood—A naturalistic long-term follow-up study. *Addictive Behaviors, 39*(1), 325–328.

Naglieri, J. A., Das, J. P., & Goldstein, S. (2014). *Cognitive Assessment System-Second Edition (2nd ed.)*. Austin, TX: Pro-ed.

Dawe, S., Gullo, M. J., & Loxton, N. J. (2004). Reward drive and rash impulsiveness as dimensions of impulsivity: Implications for substance misuse. *Addictive Behaviors, 29*(7), 1389–1405.

Degenhardt, L., Chiu, W. T., Sampson, N., Kessler, R. C., Anthony, J. C., Angermeyer, M., et al. (2008). Toward a global view of alcohol, tobacco, cannabis, and cocaine use: Findings from the WHO world mental health surveys. *PLoS Medicine, 5*(7), e141.

DeLeon, G., Melnick, G., Kressel, D., & Jainchill, N. (1994). Circumstances, motivation, readiness, and suitability (the CMRS scales): Predicting retention in therapeutic community treatment. *The American Journal of Drug and Alcohol Abuse, 20*(4), 495–515.

Delis, D. C., Kaplan, E., & Kramer, J. H. (2001). *Delis-Kaplan Executive Function System (D-KEFS)*. San Antonio, TX: The Psychological Corporation.

Delis, D. C., Kramer, J. H., Kaplan, E., & Ober, B. A. (2000). *CVLT-II: California Verbal Learning Test: Adult Version*. San Antonio, TX: The Psychological Corporation.

Dembo, R., & Anderson, A. (2005). Problem-oriented screening instrument for teenagers. In T. Grisso, G. Vincent, & D. Seagrave (Eds.), *Mental Health Screening and Assessment in Juvenile Justice* (pp. 112–122). New York, NY: The Guilford Press.

Dembo, R., Farrow, D., Schmeidler, J., & Burgos, W. (1979). Testing a causal model of environmental influences on the early drug involvement of inner city junior high school youths. *The American Journal of Drug and Alcohol Abuse, 6*(3), 313–336.

Demir, B., Uluğ, B. D., Ergün, E. L., & Erbaş, B. (2002). Regional cerebral blood flow and neuropsychological functioning in early and late onset alcoholism. *Psychiatry Research: Neuroimaging, 115*(3), 115–125.

Dennis, M. L., Titus, J. C., White, M. K., Unsicker, J. I., & Hodgkins, D. (2003). *Global Appraisal of Individual Needs: Administration Guide for the GAIN and Related Measures*. Bloomington, IL: Chestnut Health Systems.

Derogatis, L. R. (1993). *Brief Symptom Inventory: BSI; Administration, Scoring, and Procedures Manual*. Minneapolis, MN: Pearson.

DiClemente, C. C. (1999). Alcohol (and illegal drugs) decisional balance scale. *Enhancing Motivation for Change in Substance Abuse Treatment. Treatment Improvement Protocol (TIP) Series, 35.*

DiClemente, C. C., Carbonari, J. P., Montgomery, R. P., & Hughes, S. O. (1994). The alcohol abstinence self-efficacy scale. *Journal of Studies on Alcohol, 55*(2), 141–148.

Dillon, F. R., Turner, C. W., Robbins, M. S., & Szapocznik, J. (2005). Concordance among biological, interview, and self-report measures of drug use among African American and Hispanic adolescents referred for drug abuse treatment. *Psychology of Addictive Behaviors: Journal of the Society of Psychologists in Addictive Behaviors, 19*(4), 404–413.

Dom, G., D'haene, P., Hulstijn, W., & Sabbe, B. G. C. C. (2006). Impulsivity in abstinent early-and late-onset alcoholics: Differences in self-report measures and a discounting task. *Addiction, 101*(1), 50–59.

Edelbrock, C., Costello, A. J., Dulcan, M. K., Conover, N. C., & Kala, R. (1986). Parent-child agreement on child psychiatric symptoms assessed via structured interview. *Journal of Child Psychology and Psychiatry, 27*(2), 181–190.

Ehlers, C. L., Phillips, E., Finnerman, G., Gilder, D., Lau, P., & Criado, J. (2007). P3 components and adolescent binge drinking in Southwest California Indians. *Neurotoxicology and Teratology, 29*(1), 153–163.

Ellis, B. R. (1987). *Juvenile Automated Substance Abuse Evaluation* (JASAE).

Evans, R. I., Hansen, W. B., & Mittelmark, M. B. (1977). Increasing the validity of self-reports of behavior in a smoking in children investigation. *Journal of Applied Psychology, 62*(4), 521–523.

Fagan, J., & Deslonde, J. (1988). *The Social Organization of Drug Use and Drug Dealing Among Urban Gangs*. New York, NY: Criminal Justice Center, John Jay College of Criminal Justice.

Fletcher, A., Bonell, C., & Hargreaves, J. (2008). School effects on young people's drug use: A systematic review of intervention and observational studies. *Journal of Adolescent Health, 42*(3), 209–220.

Frauenknecht, M., & Black, D. R. (1995). Social problem-solving inventory for adolescents (SPSI-A): Development and preliminary psychometric evaluation. *Journal of Personality Assessment, 64*(3), 522–539.

Friedman, A. S. (1983). High school drug abuse clients. In *Clinical Research Notes*. Rockville, MD: Division of Clinical Research, National Institute on Drug Abuse.

Friedman, A. S., & Utada, A. (1989). A method for diagnosing and planning the treatment of adolescent drug abusers (the adolescent drug abuse diagnosis [ADAD] instrument). *Journal of Drug Education, 19*(4), 285–312.

Fromme, K., Stroot, E. A., & Kaplan, D. (1993). Comprehensive effects of alcohol: Development and psychometric assessment of a new expectancy questionnaire. *Psychological Assessment, 5*(1), 19–26.

Frydenberg, E., & Lewis, R. (2012). *Adolescent Coping Scale: Second Edition (ACS-2)*. Australia: Australian Council for Educational Research.

Gadow, K. D., & Sprafkin, J. N. (1998). *Adolescent symptom Inventory-4*. Checkmate Plus.

Gillespie, N. A., Neale, M. C., & Kendler, K. S. (2009). Pathways to cannabis abuse: A multi-stage model from cannabis availability, cannabis initiation and progression to abuse. *Addiction, 104*, 430–438.

Gioia, G. A., Isquith, P. K., Guy, S. C., & Kenworthy, L. (2005). *Behavior Rating Inventory of Executive Function* (Second ed.). Odessa, FL: Psychological Assessment Resources.

Goodenow, C. (1993). The psychological sense of school membership among adolescents: Scale development and educational correlates. *Psychology in the Schools, 30*(1), 79–90.

Gorman-Smith, D., Tolan, P. H., Zelli, A., & Huesmann, L. R. (1996). The relation of family functioning to violence among inner-city minority youths. *Journal of Family Psychology, 10*, 115–129.

Gorsuch, R. L., & Butler, M. C. (1976). Initial drug abuse: A review of predisposing social psychological factors. *Psychological Bulletin, 83*(1), 120–137.

Gottfredson, D. C. (1987). An evaluation of an organization development approach to reducing school disorder. *Evaluation Review, 11*(6), 739–763.

Graham, J. M., & Ontario. (1988). *Situational Confidence Questionnaire (SCQ): User's Guide*. Addiction Research Foundation.

Grant, B. F., & Dawson, D. A. (1997). Age at onset of alcohol use and its association with DSM-IV alcohol abuse and dependence: Results from the National Longitudinal Alcohol Epidemiologic Survey. *Journal of Substance Abuse, 9*, 103–110.

Grant, B. F., Stinson, F. S., & Harford, T. C. (2001). Age at onset of alcohol use and DSM-IV alcohol abuse and dependence: A 12 year follow-up. *Journal of Substance Abuse, 13*, 493–504.

Griffin, K. W., Botvin, G. J., Nichols, T. R., & Doyle, M. M. (2003). Effectiveness of a universal drug abuse prevention approach for youth at high risk for substance use initiation. *Preventive Medicine, 36*(1), 1–7.

Groenman, A. P., Oosterlaan, J., Rommelse, N., Franke, B., Roeyers, H., Oades, R. D., et al. (2013). Substance use disorders in adolescents with attention deficit hyperactivity disorder: A 4-year follow-up study. *Addiction, 108*(8), 1503–1511.

Groth-Marnat, G., & Wright, A. J. (2016). *Handbook of Psychological Assessment* (6th ed.). Hoboken, NJ: Wiley.

Harkness, A. R., & McNulty, J. L. (1994). The personality psychopathology five (PSY-5): Issues from the pages of a diagnostic manual instead of a dictionary. In S. Strack & M. Lorr (Eds.), *Differentiating Normal and Abnormal Personality* (pp. 291–315). New York, NY: Springer Publishing.

Harrell, A. V., Kapsak, K. A., Cisin, I. H., & Wirtz, P. W. (1997). The validity of self-reported drug use data: The accuracy of responses on confidential self-administered answered sheets. *NIDA Research Monographs, 167*, 37–58.

Harrell, A., & Wirtz, P. W. (1989). *Adolescent Drinking Index: Professional Manual*. Odessa, FL: Psychological Assessment Resources.

Harrell, T. H., Honaker, L. M., & Davis, E. (1991). Cognitive and behavioral dimensions of dysfunction in alcohol and polydrug abusers. *Journal of Substance Abuse, 3*, 415–426.

Harrison, P. A., & Hoffmann, N. G. (1989). *SUDDS: Substance Use Disorder Diagnostic Schedule Manual*. St. Paul, MN: New Standards, Inc.

Hasler, G., Klaghofer, R., & Buddeberg, C. (2002). The University of Rhode Island Change Assessment Scale (URICA). *Psychotherapie, Psychosomatik, Medizinische Psychologie, 53*(9–10), 406–411.

Hays, S. P., Hays, C. E., & Mulhall, P. F. (2003). Community risk and protective factors and adolescent substance use. *Journal of Primary Prevention, 24*(2), 125–142.

Heaton, R. K., Chelune, G. J., Curtiss, G., Kay, G. G., & Talley, J. L. (1993). *Wisconsin Card Sorting Test*. Odessa, FL: Psychological Assessment Resources.

Henly, G. A., & Winters, K. C. (1988). Development of problem severity scales for the assessment of adolescent alcohol and drug abuse. *International Journal of the Addictions, 23*(1), 65–85.

Heppner, P. P., & Petersen, C. H. (1982). The development and implications of a personal problem-solving inventory. *Journal of Counseling Psychology, 29*(1), 66–75.

Herting, J. R., & Guest, A. M. (1985). Components of satisfaction with local areas in the metropolis. *The Sociological Quarterly, 26*(1), 99–116.

Hicks, B. M., Durbin, C. E., Blonigen, D. M., Iacono, W. G., & McGue, M. (2012). Relationship between personality change and the onset and course of alcohol dependence in young adulthood. *Addiction, 107*(3), 540–548.

Hien, D., Matzner, F., First, M. B., Spitzer, R. L., Williams, J., & Gibbon, M. (2004). *Structured Clinical Interview for DSM-IV Childhood Diagnoses (KID-SCID)*. New York, NY: Biometrics Research.

Hingson, R. W., Heeren, T., & Winter, M. R. (2006). Age at drinking onset and alcohol dependence: Age at onset, duration, and severity. *Archives of Pediatrics & Adolescent Medicine, 160*(7), 739–746.

Hundleby, J. D., & Mercer, G. W. (1987). Family and friends as social environments and their relationship to young adolescents' use of alcohol, tobacco, and marijuana. *Journal of Marriage and the Family, 49*(1), 151–164.

Hutton, J. B., & Roberts, T. G. (1986). *Social-Emotional Dimension Scale: A Measure of School Behavior*. Austin, TX: Pro-Ed.

Iacono, W. G., Malone, S. M., & McGue, M. (2008). Behavioral disinhibition and the development of early-onset addiction: Common and specific influences. *Annual Review of Clinical Psychology, 4*, 325–348.

Inwald, R., Brobst, K. E., & Morrissey, R. F. (1987). *Hilson adolescent profile: Manual*. Incorporated: Hilson Research.

Jessor, R. (1976). Predicting time of onset of marijuana use: A developmental study of high school youth. *Journal of Consulting and Clinical Psychology, 44*(1), 125–134.

Johnson, E. O., & Novak, S. P. (2009). Onset and persistence of daily smoking: The interplay of socioeconomic status, gender, and psychiatric disorders. *Drug and Alcohol Dependence, 104*, S50–S57.

Johnson, P. B., & Gurin, G. (1994). Negative affect, alcohol expectancies and alcohol-related problems. *Addiction, 89*(5), 581–586.

Johnston, L. D., & O'Malley, P. M. (1997). The recanting of earlier reported drug use by young adults. *NIDA Research Monographs, 167*, 59–80.

Johnston, L. D., O'Malley, P. M., Bachman, J. G., & Schulenberg, J. E. (2010). *Monitoring the Future National Results on Adolescent Drug Use: Overview of Key Findings, 2009 (NIH publication no. 10–7583)*. Bethesda, MD: National Institute on Drug Abuse.

Johnston, L. D., O'Malley, P. M., Bachman, J. G., & Schulenberg, J. E. (2011). *Marijuana Use Continues to Rise Among U.S. Teens, While Alcohol Use Hits Historic Lows*. Ann Arbor, MI: University of Michigan News Service.

Jordan, C. J., & Andersen, S. L. (2016). Sensitive periods of substance abuse: Early risk for the transition to dependence. *Developmental Cognitive Neuroscience*. https://doi.org/10.1016/j.dcn.2016.10.004

Kadden, R. M., & Litt, M. D. (2011). The role of self-efficacy in the treatment of substance use disorders. *Addictive Behaviors, 36*(12), 1120–1126.

Kaminer, Y. (1991). The magnitude of concurrent psychiatric disorders in hospitalized substance abusing adolescents. *Child Psychiatry and Human Development, 22*(2), 89–95.

Kaminer, Y., Bukstein, O., & Tarter, R. E. (1991). The teen-addiction severity index: Rationale and reliability. *International Journal of the Addictions, 26*(2), 219–226.

Kandel, D. B., Kessler, R. C., & Margulies, R. Z. (1978). Antecedents of adolescent initiation into stages of drug use: A developmental analysis. *Journal of Youth and Adolescence, 7*(1), 13–40.

Kaufman, J., Birmaher, B., Brent, D., Rao, U., Flynn, C., Moreci, P., et al. (1997). Schedule for affective disorders and schizophrenia for school-age children–present and lifetime version (K-SADS-PL): Initial reliability and validity data. *Journal of the American Academy of Child & Adolescent Psychiatry, 36*, 980–988.

Kendler, K. S., Gardner, C. O., Edwards, A., Hickman, M., Heron, J., Macleod, J., et al. (2013). Dimensions of parental alcohol use/problems and offspring temperament, externalizing behaviors, and alcohol use/problems. *Alcoholism: Clinical and Experimental Research, 37*(12), 2118–2127.

Khantzian, E. J. (1997). The self-medication hypothesis of substance use disorders: A reconsideration and recent applications. *Harvard Review of Psychiatry, 4*(5), 231–244.

Kirisci, L., Tarter, R. E., Ridenour, T., Reynolds, M., & Vanyukov, M. (2013). Longitudinal modeling of transmissible risk in boys who subsequently develop cannabis use disorder. *The American Journal of Drug and Alcohol Abuse, 39*(3), 180–185.

Krieg, T. L. (1982). Is raising the legal drinking age warranted? *Police Chief, 49*(HS-036 226), 32–34.

Krosnick, J. A., & Judd, C. M. (1982). Transitions in social influence at adolescence: Who induces cigarette smoking? *Developmental Psychology, 18*(3), 359–368.

Kuntsche, E., Rossow, I., Simons-Morton, B., Bogt, T. T., Kokkevi, A., & Godeau, E. (2013). Not early drinking but early drunkenness is a risk factor for problem behaviors among adolescents from 38 European and north American countries. *Alcoholism: Clinical and Experimental Research, 37*(2), 308–314.

Lachar, D., & Gruber, C. P. (2001). *Personality Inventory for Children, Second Edition (PIC-2) Standard Form and Behavioral Summary Manual*. Los Angeles, CA: Western Psychological Services.

Lee, G. P., & DiClimente, C. C. (1985). Age of onset versus duration of problem drinking on the alcohol use inventory. *Journal of Studies on Alcohol, 46*(5), 398–402.

Lee, S. S., Humphreys, K. L., Flory, K., Liu, R., & Glass, K. (2011). Prospective association of childhood attention-deficit/hyperactivity disorder (ADHD) and substance use and abuse/dependence: A meta-analytic review. *Clinical Psychology Review, 31*(3), 328–341.

Leffler, J. M., Riebel, J., & Hughes, H. M. (2015). A review of child and adolescent diagnostic interviews for clinical practitioners. *Assessment, 22*(6), 690–703.

Levin, H. S., Culhane, K. A., Hartmann, J., Evankovich, K., Mattson, A. J., Harward, H., et al. (1991). Developmental changes in performance on tests of purported frontal lobe functioning. *Developmental Neuropsychology, 7*(3), 377–395.

Levy, D., & Sheflin, N. (1985). The demand for alcoholic beverages: An aggregate time-series analysis. *Journal of Public Policy & Marketing, 4*, 47–54.

Libbey, H. P. (2004). Measuring student relationships to school: Attachment, bonding, connectedness, and engagement. *Journal of School Health, 74*(7), 274–283.

Liddle, H. A., & Rowe, C. (1998). Family measures in drug abuse prevention research. In R. S. Ashery, E. B. Robertson, & K. L. Kumpfer (Eds.), *Drug Abuse Prevention Through Family Interventions* (pp. 324–372). Washington, DC: National Institute on Drug Abuse.

Lisdahl, K. M., Gilbert, E. R., Wright, N. E., & Shollenbarger, S. (2013). Dare to delay? The impacts of adolescent alcohol and marijuana use onset on cognition, brain structure, and function. *Frontiers in Psychiatry, 4*, 25–43.

Lochman, J. E., & van den Steenhoven, A. (2002). Family-based approaches to substance abuse prevention. *Journal of Primary Prevention, 23*(1), 49–114.

Maddahian, E., Newcomb, M. D., & Bentler, P. M. (1988). Adolescent drug use and intention to use drugs: Concurrent and longitudinal analyses of four ethnic groups. *Addictive Behaviors, 13*(2), 191–195.

Maisto, S. A., Connors, G. J., & Allen, J. P. (1995). Contrasting self-report screens for alcohol problems: A review. *Alcoholism: Clinical and Experimental Research, 19*(6), 1510–1516.

Martin, C. S., & Winters, K. C. (1998). Diagnosis and assessment of alcohol use disorders among adolescents. *Alcohol Research and Health, 22*(2), 95–105.

Martin, G. W., Wilkinson, D. A., & Poulos, C. X. (1995). The drug avoidance self-efficacy scale. *Journal of Substance Abuse, 7*(2), 151–163.

McGue, M., & Iacono, W. G. (2008). The adolescent origins of substance use disorders. *International Journal of Methods in Psychiatric Research, 17*(S1), S30–S38.

Metzger, D. S., Kushner, H., & McLellan, A. T. (1991). *Adolescent Problem Severity Index Administration Manual*. Biomedical Computer Research Institute.

Meyers, K. (1991). *Comprehensive Addiction Severity Index for Adolescents*. Philadelphia, PA: Philadelphia Canter for Studies on Addiction, University of Pennsylvania VA Medical Center.

Miller, F. G., & Lazowski, L. E. (2001). *The Adolescent Substance Abuse Subtle Screening Inventory-A2 (SASSI-A2) Manual*. Springville, IN: SASSI Institute.

Miller, W. R. (1991). *The Stages of Change Readiness and Treatment Eagerness Scale*. Albuquerque, University of New Mexico: Unpublished manuscript.

Millon, T. (1993). *Millon Adolescent Clinical Inventory*. Minneapolis, MN: National Computer Systems.

Millon, T., & Tringone, R. (2005). *Millon Pre-Adolescent Clinical Inventory (M-PACI) Manual*. Minneapolis, MN: NCS Pearson.

Moberg, D. P. (2003). *Screening for Alcohol and Other Drug Problems Using the Adolescent Alcohol and Drug Involvement Scale (AADIS)*. Madison, WI: Center for Health Policy and Program Evaluation, University of Wisconsin-Madison.

Moos, R. H., & Moos, B. S. (1994). *Family Environment Scale Manual*. Palo Alto, CA: Consulting Psychologists Press.

Morey, L. C. (1999). *Personality Assessment Inventory (PAI)*. Hoboken, NJ: Wiley.

Morrell, H. E., Song, A. V., & Halpern-Felsher, B. L. (2011). Earlier age of smoking initiation may not predict heavier cigarette consumption in later adolescence. *Prevention Science, 12*(3), 247–254.

Moss, H. B., Chen, C. M., & Yi, H. Y. (2014). Early adolescent patterns of alcohol, cigarettes, and marijuana polysubstance use and young adult substance use outcomes in a nationally representative sample. *Drug and Alcohol Dependence, 136*, 51–62.

Mrazek, P. J., & Haggerty, R. J. (1994). *Reducing Risks for Mental Disorders: Frontiers for Preventive Intervention Research*. Washington, D.C.: National Academic Press.

Murray, C. A. (1983). The physical environment and community control of crime. In J. Q. Wilson (Ed.), *Crime and Public Policy* (pp. 107–122). San Francisco: Institute for Contemporary Studies.

Murray, D. M., O'Connell, C. M., Schmid, L. A., & Perry, C. L. (1987). The validity of smoking self-reports by adolescents: A reexamination of the bogus pipeline procedure. *Addictive Behaviors, 12*(1), 7–15.

Murray, D. M., Richards, P. S., Luepker, R. V., & Johnson, C. A. (1987). The prevention of cigarette smoking in children: Two-and three-year follow-up comparisons of four prevention strategies. *Journal of Behavioral Medicine, 10*(6), 595–611.

Naglieri, J. A., & Goldstein, S. (2013). *Comprehensive Executive Function Inventory*. North Tonawanda, NY: Multi-Health Systems.

Newcomb, M. D., & Bentler, P. M. (1989). Substance use and abuse among children and teenagers. *American Psychologist, 44*(2), 242–248.

Nollan, K. A., Wolf, M., Ansell, D., & Burns, J. (2000). Ready or not: Assessing youths' preparedness for independent living. *Child Welfare, 79*(2), 159.

Norcross, J. C., Krebs, P. M., & Prochaska, J. O. (2011). Stages of change. *Journal of Clinical Psychology, 67*(2), 143–154.

Oei, T. P., Hasking, P. A., & Young, R. M. (2005). Drinking refusal self-efficacy questionnaire-revised (DRSEQ-R): A new factor structure with confirmatory factor analysis. *Drug and Alcohol Dependence, 78*(3), 297–307.

O'Leary-Barrett, M., Mackie, C. J., Castellanos-Ryan, N., Al-Khudhairy, N., & Conrod, P. J. (2010). Personality-targeted interventions delay uptake of drinking and decrease risk of alcohol-related problems when delivered by teachers. *Journal of the American Academy of Child & Adolescent Psychiatry, 49*(9), 954–963.

Olson, D. (2011). FACES IV and the circumplex model: Validation study. *Journal of Marital and Family Therapy, 37*(1), 64–80.

Olson, D. H. (2010). *Faces IV Manual*. Minneapolis, MN: Life Innovations.

Olson, D. H., & Gorall, D. M. (2006). *Faces IV and the Circumplex Model*. Minneapolis, MN: Life Innovations.

Parrella, D. P., & Filstead, W. J. (1988). Definition of onset in the development of onset-based alcoholism typologies. *Journal of Studies on Alcohol, 49*(1), 85–92.

Patterson, J. M., & McCubbin, H. I. (1996). Adolescent coping orientation for problem experiences (ACOPE). In H. I. McCubbin, A. I. Thompson, & M. A. McCubbin (Eds.), *Family Assessment: Resiliency, Coping and Adaptation: Inventories for Research and Practice* (pp. 537–583). Madison, WI: University of Wisconsin-Madison, Center for Excellence in Family Studies.

Petchers, M. K., & Singer, M. I. (1987). Perceived-benefit-of-drinking scale: Approach to screening for adolescent alcohol abuse. *The Journal of Pediatrics, 110*(6), 977–981.

Petraitis, J., Flay, B. R., & Miller, T. Q. (1995). Reviewing theories of adolescent substance use: Organizing pieces in the puzzle. *Psychological Bulletin, 117*(1), 67–86.

Phipps, L., & Beaujean, A. A. (2016). Review of the pattern of strengths and weaknesses approach in specific learning disability identification. *Research and Practice in the Schools, 4*(1), 18–28.

Pingault, J. B., Côté, S. M., Galéra, C., Genolini, C., Falissard, B., Vitaro, F., & Tremblay, R. E. (2013). Childhood trajectories of inattention, hyperactivity and oppositional behaviors and prediction of substance abuse/dependence: A 15-year longitudinal population-based study. *Molecular Psychiatry, 18*(7), 806–812.

Prinz, R. J., Foster, S. L., Kent, R. N., & O'Leary, K. D. (1979). Multivariate assessment of conflict in distressed and nondistressed mother-adolescent dyads. *Journal of Applied Behavioral Analysis, 12*, 691–700.

Prochaska, J. O., DiClemente, C. C., & Norcross, J. C. (1992). In search of how people change: Applications to addictive behaviors. *American Psychologist, 47*(9), 1102–1114.

Reich, W. (2000). Diagnostic interview for children and adolescents (DICA). *Journal of the American Academy of Child & Adolescent Psychiatry, 39*(1), 59–66.

Reynolds, C. R. (2004). *Behavior Assessment System for Children*. Hoboken, NJ: Wiley.

Robins, L. N. (1980). The natural history of drug abuse. *Acta Psychiatrica Scandinavica, 62*(s284), 7–20.

Robins, L. N., & Ratcliff, K. S. (1978). Risk factors in the continuation of childhood antisocial behavior into adulthood. *International Journal of Mental Health, 7*(3–4), 96–116.

Rollnick, S., Heather, N., Gold, R., & Hall, W. (1992). Development of a short 'readiness to change' questionnaire for use in brief, opportunistic interventions among excessive drinkers. *Addiction, 87*(5), 743–754.

Saal, D., Dong, Y., Bonci, A., & Malenka, R. C. (2003). Drugs of abuse and stress trigger a common synaptic adaptation in dopamine neurons. *Neuron, 37*(4), 577–582.

Saffer, H., & Grossman, M. (1987). Beer taxes, the legal drinking age, and youth motor vehicle fatalities. *The Journal of Legal Studies, 16*(2), 351–374.

Sampson, R. J. (1986). Crime in cities: The effects of formal and informal social control. In A. J. Reiss & M. Tonry (Eds.), *Crime and Justice: An Annual Review of Research, Communities and Crime* (Vol. 8, pp. 271–311). Chicago: University of Chicago Press.

Sampson, R. J., Castellano, T. C., & Laub, J. H. (1981). *Juvenile Criminal Behavior and its Relation to Neighborhood Characteristics*. Washington, DC: Office of Juvenile Justice and Delinquency Prevention.

Search Institute. (2005). *Developmental Assets Profile Technical Manual*. Minneapolis: Author.

Shaffer, D., Fisher, P., Lucas, C. P., Dulcan, M. K., & Schwab-Stone, M. E. (2000). NIMH diagnostic interview schedule for children version IV (NIMH DISC-IV): Description, differences from previous versions, and reliability of some common diagnoses. *Journal of the American Academy of Child & Adolescent Psychiatry, 39*(1), 28–38.

Sitharthan, T., & Kavanagh, D. J. (1991). Role of self-efficacy in predicting outcomes from a programme for controlled drinking. *Drug and Alcohol Dependence, 27*(1), 87–94.

Skinner, H. A., Steinhauer, P. D., & Santa-Barbara, J. (2009). The family assessment measure. *Canadian Journal of Community Mental Health, 2*(2), 91–103.

Smith, G. M., & Fogg, C. P. (1978). Psychological predictors of early use, late use, and nonuse of marijuana among teenage students. In D. Kandel (Ed.), *Longitudinal Research on Drug Use: Empirical Findings and Methodological Issues* (pp. 101–113). Washington, DC: Halstead-Wiley.

Spoth, R. L., Redmond, C., Trudeau, L., & Shin, C. (2002). Longitudinal substance initiation outcomes for a universal preventive intervention combining family and school programs. *Psychology of Addictive Behaviors, 16*(2), 129–134.

Swadi, H. (1999). Individual risk factors for adolescent substance use. *Drug and Alcohol Dependence, 55*(3), 209–224.

Swanson, J., Deutsch, C., Cantwell, D., Posner, M., Kennedy, J., Barr, C., Moyzis, R., Schuck, S., Flodman, P., & Spence, A. (2001). Genes and attention-deficit hyperactivity disorder. *Clinical Neuroscience Research., 1*, 207–216.

Swift, W., Coffey, C., Carlin, J. B., Degenhardt, L., & Patton, G. C. (2008). Adolescent cannabis users at 24 years: Trajectories to regular weekly use and dependence in young adulthood. *Addiction, 103*(8), 1361–1370.

Tarter, R. E., Kirisci, L., Mezzich, A., Cornelius, J. R., Pajer, K., Vanyukov, M., et al. (2003). Neurobehavioral disinhibition in childhood predicts early age at onset of substance use disorder. *American Journal of Psychiatry, 160*(6), 1078–1085.

Taylor, A. E. B. (2014). *Diagnostic Assessment of Learning Disabilities in Childhood: Bridging the Gap Between Research and Practice*. Springer Science & Business Media.

Trudeau, L., Spoth, R., Lillehoj, C., Redmond, C., & Wickrama, K. A. S. (2003). Effects of a preventive intervention on adolescent substance use initiation, expectancies, and refusal intentions. *Prevention Science, 4*(2), 109–122.

Vanyukov, M. M., & Ridenour, T. A. (2012). Common liability to drug addictions: Theory, research, practice. *Drug and Alcohol Dependence, 123*(Supplement 1), S1–S2.

Vanyukov, M. M., Tarter, R. E., Kirisci, L., Kirillova, G. P., Maher, B. S., & Clark, D. B. (2003). Liability to substance use disorders: 1. Common mechanisms and manifestations. *Neuroscience & Biobehavioral Reviews, 27*(6), 507–515.

Varma, V. K., Basu, D., Malhotra, A., Sharma, A., & Mattoo, S. K. (1994). Correlates of early-and late-onset alcohol dependence. *Addictive Behaviors, 19*(6), 609–619.

Wanberg, K. W. (1992). *Adolescent Self-Assessment Profile*. Arvada, CO: Center for Alcohol/Drug Abuse Research and Evaluation.

Weissman, M. M., Wickramaratne, P., Warner, V., John, K., Prusoff, B. A., Merikangas, K. R., & Gammon, G. D. (1987). Assessing psychiatric disorders in children: Discrepancies between mothers' and children's reports. *Archives of General Psychiatry, 44*(8), 747–753.

Welsh, M. C., Pennington, B. F., & Groisser, D. B. (1991). A normative-developmental study of executive function: A window on prefrontal function in children. *Developmental Neuropsychology, 7*, 131–149.

Westling, E., Andrews, J. A., Hampson, S. E., & Peterson, M. (2008). Pubertal timing and substance use: The effects of gender, parental monitoring and deviant peers. *Journal of Adolescent Health, 42*(6), 555–563.

White, H. R., & Labouvie, E. W. (1989). Towards the assessment of adolescent problem drinking. *Journal of Studies on Alcohol, 50*(1), 30–37.

Wilens, T. E., Martelon, M., Joshi, G., Bateman, C., Fried, R., Petty, C., & Biederman, J. (2011). Does ADHD predict substance-use disorders? A 10-year follow-up study of young adults with ADHD. *Journal of the American Academy of Child & Adolescent Psychiatry, 50*(6), 543–553.

Wilson, J. Q., & Herrnstein, R. J. (1998). *Crime and Human Nature: The Definitive Study of the Causes of Crime*. New York, NY: Simon and Schuster.

Winters, K. C. (1992). Development of an adolescent alcohol and other drug abuse screening scale: Personal experience screening questionnaire. *Addictive Behaviors, 17*(5), 479–490.

Winters, K. C. (2003). Assessment of alcohol and other drug use behaviors among adolescents. In J. P. Allen & V. B. Wilson (Eds.), *Assessing Alcohol Problems: A Guide for Clinicians and Researchers* (2nd ed., pp. 101–123). Washington, DC: National Institute on Alcohol Abuse and Alcoholism.

Winters, K. C., Anderson, N., Bengston, P., Stinchfield, R. D., & Latimer, W. W. (2000). Development of a parent questionnaire for use in assessing adolescent drug abuse. *Journal of Psychoactive Drugs, 32*(1), 3–13.

Winters, K. C., & Henly, G. A. (1993). *Adolescent Diagnostic Interview (ADI): Manual*. Western Psychological Services.

Winters, K. C., & Henly, G. A. (1988). Assessing adolescents who abuse chemicals: The chemical dependency adolescent assessment project. *NIDA Research Monograph, 77*, 4–18.

Winters, K. C., Latimer, W. W., & Stinchfield, R. (2002). Clinical issues in the assessment of adolescent alcohol and other drug use. *Behaviour Research and Therapy, 40*(12), 1443–1456.

Winters, K. C., Stinchfield, R. D., Henly, G. A., & Schwartz, R. H. (1990). Validity of adolescent self-report of alcohol and other drug involvement. *International Journal of the Addictions, 25*(sup11), 1379–1395.

Wish, E. D., Hoffman, J. A., & Nemes, S. (1997). The validity of self-reports of drug use at treatment admission and at follow-up: Comparisons with urinalysis and hair assays. *NIDA Research Monograph, 167*, 200–226.

Woicik, P. A., Stewart, S. H., Pihl, R. O., & Conrod, P. J. (2009). The substance use risk profile scale: A scale measuring traits linked to reinforcement-specific substance use profiles. *Addictive Behaviors, 34*(12), 1042–1055.

Wright, A. J. (2010). *Conducting Psychological Assessment: A Guide for Practitioners*. Hoboken, NJ: Wiley.

Zucker, R. A., & Harford, T. C. (1983). National study of the demography of adolescent drinking practices in 1980. *Journal of Studies on Alcohol, 44*(6), 974–985.

Zucker, R. A., Kincaid, S. B., Fitzgerald, H. E., & Bingham, C. R. (1995). Alcohol schema acquisition in preschoolers: Differences between children of alcoholics and children of nonalcoholics. *Alcoholism: Clinical and Experimental Research, 19*(4), 1011–1017.

Chapter 4
Portrait of Addiction

Audrey Redding-Raines and Jermaine J. Monk

Introduction

Race and gender are significant factors that contribute to the diagnosis, treatment, and intervention of substance use disorders. Because of the heterogeneous characteristics of male and female African American and Hispanic individuals who use substances in a maladaptive manner, it is important to identify culturally competent systems of care for these two communities of color. Not only should culturally competent systems of care be identified, but equally as important, if not more, culturally competent systems of care that focus on co-occurring disorders should also be identified. Individuals with substance use or co-occurring disorders who are both poor and of color may experience negative, ineffective, and/or inefficient addiction treatment services, all of which can have a profound impact in the overall recovery process. According to Substance Abuse and Mental Health Services Administration [SAMHSA] (2016), "Communities of color tend to experience greater burden of mental and substance use disorders often due to poorer access to care; inappropriate care; and higher social, environmental, and economic risk factors" (p. 1). The National Institute on Drug Abuse (NIDA) has suggested that effective addiction treatment services for substance misuse should seek to not only address multidimensional aspects of an individual's addiction but should also seek to address other sociocultural factors as well (2012). Pursuant to the American Counseling Association's Code of Ethics, counselors are ethically responsible to provide culturally appropriate counseling interventions (2014). Day-Vines and colleagues (2007) further this discussion by suggesting that counselors should consider sociopolitical

---

A. Redding-Raines
Rutgers University–Newark, Newark, NJ, USA

J. J. Monk (✉)
Lehman College, City University of New York, Bronx, NY, USA
e-mail: jermaine.monk@lehman.cuny.edu

© Springer International Publishing AG 2018
T. MacMillan, A. Sisselman-Borgia (eds.), *New Directions in Treatment,
Education, and Outreach for Mental Health and Addiction*, Advances in Mental
Health and Addiction, https://doi.org/10.1007/978-3-319-72778-3_4

factors such as race and ethnic influences along with the lived experiential realities of the client. Failure to do so plays a significant role in counseling benchmarks.

The purpose of this chapter is to present and discuss gender-specific addiction treatment services for African American and Hispanic communities. This chapter seeks to examine the following: (1) risk factors associated with substance use disorders, (2) challenges with diagnosing co-occurring disorders, (3) treatment interventions found to be effective with these two referenced communities of color, and (4) proposed recommendations for future interventions. Additionally, throughout this chapter, the term African American will be used to identify men and women living in the United States whose ancestors came from Africa. This preferred term is used by the US Census Bureau, SAMHSA, and CSAT (Center for Substance Treatment, 2009). Likewise, the term Hispanic will be used to identify individuals whose ethnic background derives from Spanish-speaking countries (e.g., Spain, Puerto Rico, Cuba, and Central and South American countries) as opposed to the term Latino, which typically refers to an individual whose ethnic background derives from a Spanish-speaking country in Latin America (Loue, 2003).

Risk Factors

The advent of feminism during the 1970s not only highlighted the pervasiveness of gender inequalities, it also increased awareness about gender differences with respect to substance use disorders. Prior to this time period, standard protocols were implemented when addressing the treatment needs of men and women (Greenfield & Grella, 2009). Traditionally, white male populations dominated research studies, and these male-modeled programs became the basis for diagnosing and treating substance use disorders, regardless of gender, ethnicity, or etiologic differences (Minority Nurse Staff, 2013). As a result, treatment programs were not adequately prepared to address the gender-specific treatment needs of women (Green, 2006). Moreover, treatment programs usually looked at racial and ethnic groups as monolithic individuals having homogeneous patterns of substance use, cultures, and concerns (Loue, 2003). Understanding racial and gender risk factors as it relates to substance use disorders as well as co-occurring disorders is important and may lead to enhanced treatment methodologies and outcomes for both men and women.

Males

Men face a number of challenges in society that not only heightens their addiction, but, in some cases, emboldens its continued use (SAMHSA, 2013). Statistically, men experience higher rates for incarceration, suicide, homelessness, and morbidity and are more likely to be victims of violence (SAMHSA, 2013). These incidences are only compounded when race is added to the equation; African American and Hispanic males face even higher rates of unemployment and under-education (Barr, Farrell, Barnes, & Welte, 1993; Rodriguez, Henderson, Rowe, Burnett, Dakof & Liddle, 2007). African American and Hispanic males have higher frequencies of drug and alcohol use (Amaro, Arevelo, Gonzalez, Szapocznik, & Iguchi, 2006; Barr et al., 1993; Rodriguez et al., 2007; SAMHSA, 2013).

According to the 2011 National Survey on Drug Use and Health, men over 18 are almost twice as likely to misuse drugs or alcohol (SAMHSA, 2013, 2014). Male identity, regardless of race and ethnicity, plays a role in the decision to use substances or to seek help when a problem develops (SAMHSA, 2013). For example, behaviors such as binge drinking on college campuses or drinking heavily when turning 21 years of age is sometimes seen as part of a necessary ritual for men (SAMHSA, 2013). Further, illicit drug use, for many men, becomes associated as a rite of passage (SAMHSA, 2013).

Consequently, illicit drug and alcohol use in some cases precipitates violent and criminal behavior. Johnson, Striley, and Cottle (2006) posit, "Consumption and acquisition of drugs... tend to nurture violent and criminal activity" (p. 2064). However, African American and Hispanic males experience an increase in addiction rates, compared to males from other racial or cultural groups (Barr et al., 1993; Brocato, 2013; Rodriguez et al., 2007; SAMHSA, 2013, 2014).

African American and Hispanic males face an array of social, cultural, and systemic challenges that intensifies the decision to use illegal substances. Barr et al. (1993) contend that, for African American men, factors such as employment and socioeconomic status (SES) are huge contributors to their substance use. Systemic policies like the "war on drugs" and "zero tolerance" have created a vicious cycle of continued recidivism among African American males who are substance abusers (Sanders, 2002). Risk factors for Hispanic males include such factors as SES, employment, education, and ethnic and cultural identity; however, other contributing factors like acculturation, immigration status, and language are also important (Amaro et al., 2006).

In addition, experiencing trauma within the African American and Hispanic communities has been identified as an important risk factor associated with illicit drug and alcohol use (Johnson et al., 2006; Rodriguez et al., 2007). According to Rodriguez et al. "understanding important cultural processes more fully may provide direction... research-based interventions" (2007, p. 100). Understanding the influences of trauma on individuals is important to decreasing the incidences of substance use. Rodriguez and colleagues (2007) found that trauma was a significant determinate in their study of Hispanic youth and substance use, in particular males. The ability to develop and utilize coping skills was important to determine if a traumatic experience would result in substance use or not. Failure to engage coping skills often resulted in the use of illicit drugs and alcohol (Rodriguez et al., 2007). Similarly, Johnson et al. (2006) found that African American males had an increased risk of illicit drug use based on exposure to trauma.

Females

The prevalence of poverty and other sociocultural issues can play a role in the exacerbation of alcohol and illicit drug misuse (NIDA, 1998). These contextual factors give rise to specific risk barriers associated with the initiation of substance use and the subsequent development of substance use disorders (Center for Substance Abuse Treatment, 2009). Usually, the initiation of substance use for women begins after they have been introduced to the substance by an intimate partner. Although reasons why women initiate substances may vary, stress-related incidences, unhealthy relationships, and the effects of a partner's addiction have all been indicators of influence in the initial first use (Center for Substance Abuse Treatment, 2009). Novelty-seeking and sensation-seeking personalities have also been correlated with the initiation of illicit drug misuse (Agrawal, Gardner, Prescott, & Kendler, 2005). Agrawal and his colleagues have also suggested that anxiety disorders and major depression are linked to substance use disorders and are the most common co-occurring diagnoses (2005).

Additional contextual factors such as discriminatory acts ranging from everyday affronts to demoralizing violent actions may also be associated with the initiation of substance use and the subsequent development of substance use disorders for African American and Hispanic women (Center for Substance Abuse Treatment, 2009). Women of color can experience multiple forms of discrimination at the same time (e.g., gender and racial discrimination), which in turn can lead to profound multifaceted implications in how these women deal with life stressors and associated consequences (Krieger, 1999). Additionally, the interconnectedness of social status combined with race and ethnicity has typically resulted in increased social vulnerabilities and disadvantaged experiential realities for African American and Hispanic women (Amaro, Larson, Gampel, Richardson, Savage, & Wagler, 2005). Varying levels of discrimination based on "gender, race, ethnicity, language, culture, socioeconomic status, sexual orientation, age, and disability can affect their substance use and may affect their recovery" (Center for Substance Abuse Treatment, 2009, p. 24). Studies have shown that racial barriers exist within the counseling profession because traditional treatment models have not considered the implications of race and racism in the development of the human personality (Aponte & Johnson, 2000; Carter, 1995). Counseling pedagogy rooted in Eurocentric worldviews in conjunction with Western values only adds to the myopic understanding of difference. Norman-Major and Gooden (2012) go on to further state that:

> This lack of recognition of cultural differences often leads to development and implementation of ineffective, inefficient, and inequitable public services. Instead of serving the community as a whole or being open to all persons, programs and policies that lack of recognition of cultural difference often leave part of the public out of public service (p. 4).

Acculturation and cultural roles are also significant risk factors that can contribute to the substance use patterns of African American and Hispanic women. Studies have shown that "as new immigrants adapt to U.S. culture, they tend to drop or modify the norms of their countries of origin and adopt patterns of behavior that are more representative of the general U.S. population" (Collins & McNair, 2003, p. 2). Also, as immigrants acculturate into American society, alcohol and illicit drug use increases (Center for Substance Abuse Treatment, 2009). For ethnically diverse women who have substance use disorders, the likelihood of them developing hypertension, HIV/AIDS, HIV/hepatitis C virus co-infection, or other conditions or disorders is great. Moreover, accessibility to health care and cultural mistrust can also play a part in their decision to delay treatment (Center for Substance Abuse Treatment, 2009). Similarly, sociocultural factors coupled with substance use disorders are major contributing factors in the high prevalence of African American and Hispanic women being incarcerated, which can play a role in accessibility, length, or type of treatment available (Staton-Tindall, 2010). According to a 2003 National Institute of Corrections report, women offenders are more times than not, disproportionately women of color between the ages of 30 and 35. These women are likely to have low educational levels, limited accessibility to viable employment opportunities, have drug-related offenses, addiction problems, complex family dynamics, history of abuse and trauma, and mental and physical health problems (Staton-Tindall, 2010).

Racial inequities in the United States are largely saturated because of their aggregate and reinforcing characteristics, which are embedded in a historical structure where people of color ubiquitously and persistently experience pervasive negative differences. While there are moments of definitive exceptions within and among racial groups, the general inclinations even with fiat laws governing the promotion of racial equity are still prominent. Full implementation of both the intention and the spirit of these laws demands robust policies, norms, and cultural changes at both the micro and macro levels. The successful implementation of racial equity in American society requires the monitoring, assessing, and elimination of accumulated racial inequities that have been allowed to advance through varied forms of structural racism (Gooden, 2014).

The Dangers of the Inaccurate and Inequitable Diagnosis

When the experiential realities of communities of color are dialogued, their lived experiences are typically viewed and scrutinized from the vantage point of the White, Euro-American, middle-class. Often, this perspective tends to emphasize the pathological lifestyles of these communities and/or the continued perpetuation of false stereotypes (Sue & Sue, 2008). Laws coupled with professional standards of ethics are set in place to ensure that all citizens are equitably represented and serviced. However, despite having these measures in place, racism in conjunction with the disenfranchisement of racial and ethnic groups in the United States is part and parcel of the ingrained cultural psyche of US societal norms and institutions. Regardless of whether or not organizations are public or private, those same systematic inequalities are rooted in US institutions, and as a result, organizations, often inadvertently, function as tools of oppression, replicating and supporting the very marginalization that some are committed to undoing (Adams & Balfour, 2004).

The counseling profession has taken the necessary steps to address overt forms of racism, (e.g., old Jim Crow forms racism). However, it has not been as efficacious in addressing insidious forms of racism that have covertly contaminated the worldviews of well-intentioned counseling professionals. It has also not been as efficacious in addressing the prejudicial practices and policies that are continually perpetuated within the counseling profession (Sue, Nadal, Capodilupo, Lin, Torino, & Rivera, 2008). Gooden (2014) stated that "although the public sector has become more racially and ethnically diverse, there remains an uncomfortable, poorly articulate, and difficult to navigate divide between racial and ethnic minority group members and white public servants" (p. ix).

For counselors, an important step in achieving a culturally competent system of care is for them to become aware of their worldviews during the therapeutic relationship by acknowledging and understanding (i) those benchmarks used to surmise normality and abnormality, (ii) the underlying values and suppositions about human behavior, and (iii) the biases, prejudices, and stereotypes inherited from the socialized learned behavior of various institutions (Butler, 1994; Guba and Lincoln, 2005; Sue & Sue, 2003, 2008). Understanding the racial and cultural differences of populations at both the micro and macro levels is tantamount to being culturally competent. Developing culturally competent skill sets help to bring about cultural sensitivity, which can lead to providing targeted and tailored addiction treatment programs for both men and women (Resnicow, Soler, Braithwaite, Ahluwalia, & Butler, 2000).

Males

Addiction treatment for men requires a different approach. A SAMHSA (2013) report identifies several considerations when implementing treatment plans for men who are substance abusers. According to the report issues such as the gender of the clinician, motivation for treatment and clinical approaches are all areas of consideration when working with men (SAMHSA, 2013). The male client's comfortability and relatability with the clinician influenced their outcomes in treatment (SAMHSA, 2013). It was reported that male clients sometimes withheld some of their thoughts and feelings if the clinician was female. Male clients sometimes felt the female clinicians did not understand some of their feelings. Thus, they would refrain from sharing during counseling sessions or in groups (SAMHSA, 2013). In addition, external and internal factors exist which contribute to continued substance use. According to SAMHSA (2013) there is a high correlation between individuals who are active substance users and those who have co-occurring mental health disorders.

It is important for clinicians to take into account other possible disorders that may be affecting the substance use of men of color. When working with communities of color, ignoring sociodemographic factors exacerbates misdiagnosis and elongates implementing effective treatment plans (Erving, 2017). Johnson et al. (2006) contend that a "traumatic event exposure and illicit drug use are often co-occurring conditions…" (p. 2063). For example, Rodriguez and colleagues (2007) posit that Hispanic communities are at a higher risk for addiction if they are foreign born and an immigrant to the United States. The push for foreign-born Hispanics to acculturate to American culture is believed to diminish their native cultural values. An effort to better understand how significant "life trauma, in-familial stress and prevalence of comorbid disorders" increases the likelihood of refining existing research-based diagnosis and treatment processes (Rodriguez et al., 2007, p. 99).

African American and Hispanic males who use substances in a maladaptive manner have been linked to "marginalization, discrimination and acculturative stress" (Brocato, 2013). All too often, African American and Hispanic males have been diagnosed and treated for their substance use independent of co-occurring disorders. As mentioned previously, drug policy in the United States has targeted communities of color with a punitive approach with policies like the "war on drugs." Sanders reports, "While African Americans make up 15% of illicit drug consumers, they make up 37% of those arrested on drug offenses and 60% of felony drug offenders in state prison" (2002, p. 168). The statistics for the Hispanic community is just as startling. Brocato (2013) posits that Hispanic males account for 1 in 54 incarcerated and 1 in 27 on probation or parole. Even more disheartening "58% of Latino inmates meet the criteria for substance abuse disorder, yet only 8.6% receive treatment" (Brocato, 2013, p. 150).

Females

Values, assumptions, and beliefs have helped to shape treatment practices (Sue & Sue, 2008). The cause and effect of addiction, treatment engagement, and treatment retention of African American and Hispanic women have contributed to an overall lack of empathy about how to effectively engage these two groups of color (Wisdom, Hoffman, Rechbergre, Seim, & Owens, 2009). According to Sue and Sue (2008), current practices have restricted, stereotyped, damaged, and oppressed the culturally diverse in our society, and as a result, treatment practices continue to emphasize an ethnocentric monoculturalist perspective. An aspect of this perspective that is reflected in the therapeutic relationship has to do with the "common assumption that different cultural groups operate according to identical speech and communication conventions" (Sue & Sue, 2008, p. 173).

An effective therapeutic engagement is contingent upon sending and receiving verbal and nonverbal messages as accurately and appropriately as possible. The use of standard English in treatment delivery systems oftentimes may unfairly discriminate, and this can have devastating consequences against individuals who are multilingual (Sue & Sue, 2008). For example, the multilingual background of Hispanics can influence the counselor in misinterpreting the communicative discourse between them. Similarly, even African Americans who are from a different cultural background and use Black Language or Ebonics to articulate their lived experiential experiences may also be misinterpreted (Sue & Sue, 2008). Because Euro-American society sets such a high premium on the appropriate usage of standard English, a person of color's annotated, diverse, or poor verbal answers can lead to a blaming the victim narrative by inaccurate characteristics or motives being assessed. Moreover, communication styles associated with an individual's race, culture, ethnicity, or gender can greatly influence the one-on-one therapeutic engagement relationship (Sue & Sue, 2008). Additionally, verbal cues provide insight to conscious deceptions or unconscious biases. A counselor who has not sufficiently dealt with his or her own biases and racist attitudes may unknowingly communicate those feelings to a culturally different population (Sue & Sue, 2008).

Accessing Treatment Services

There are clinical factors that must be considered when advancing treatment models for substance use disorders. However, variables such as race and gender are just as important when implementing treatment options (Amaro et al., 2006). Even more crucial to the conversation surrounding treatment of addiction is how treatment should be implemented when there is a co-occurring mental health diagnosis present. Erving (2017) purports that co-occurring disorders must be taken into account when creating, implementing and evaluating addiction interventions.

The research on therapeutic interventions for African American and Hispanic communities is scant (Barr et al., 1993; Brocato, 2013). As such, there must be a concerted effort by practitioners to integrate effective treatment models when working with African American and Hispanic populations. Further, there must also be a recognition of the influence gender has on treatment implementation and outcomes. Amaro et al. (2006) contend that the gender disparities that exist within addiction treatment services must no longer be continually ignored. Effective and equitable treatment modalities can be utilized with the African American and Hispanic communities when professionals who work with these populations remain committed to exhibiting a high level of service and cultural competence (SAMHSA, 2014).

Males

A cultural theme engagement approach provides the best opportunity for treatment for African American and Hispanic males (Brocato, 2013; Liddle, Jackson-Gilfort, & Marvel, 2006). Two theoretical and practical models, multidimensional family therapy and the therapeutic community model, have been identified as effective when working with the identified population (Brocato, 2013; Liddle et al., 2006). It is important to note that pharmacotherapy is an emerging treatment intervention for substance abuse which has shown some promise (Amaro et al., 2006). However, issues of family and social support, race, ethnicity, and SES affect pharmacotherapy implementation (Amaro et al., 2006). Implementing a culturally responsive approach is necessary when treating African Americans and Hispanics for substance use and substance use disorders.

Implementing a culturally responsive approach is necessary when treating African American and Hispanics males for substance abuse. Currently, many substance abuse programs vary in their treatment of males with substance abuse issues. However, this chapter has identified specific substance abuse interventions as it relates to African American and Latino male treatment. The current research indicates that working with men who misuse substances require varied techniques. Factors such as gender and race are important to their treatment modality. The options for substance abuse treatment are varied and multidimensional. Substance abuse treatment consists of residential and outpatient programs. These programs provide varied approaches to treatment. Many treatment programs are more likely to receive participants from the criminal justice system (Brocato, 2013; SAMHSA, 2013). Providers who obtain their patients from the criminal justice system utilize intensive techniques for monitoring and implementing treatment (Brocato, 2013). However, interventions have failed to adequately address issues specific to African American and Hispanic male clients (Brocato, 2013; Johnson et al., 2006; SAMHSA, 2013; Sanders, 2002). It is important to mention that for both African American and Hispanic males, referrals for treatment also occur via a primary physician (Johnson et al., 2006; SAMHSA, 2013). Some providers approach treatment with Black and Hispanic male clients with a punitive or authoritative modality (Brocato, 2013; Liddle et al., 2006).

Females

According to Green (2006) "a person's gender has the potential to affect several critical junctures along the pathway to seeking substance abuse treatment.. ... The likelihood that a person's substance abuse problem will be identified appears to differ by gender in some settings" (para. 8). As the prevalence of addiction continues to grow, women-focused addiction treatment services should also incorporate and address co-occurring disorders. When addressing culturally variegated issues that women face, addiction and mental health counselors must provide appropriate and interrelated systems of care that incorporate mental health, addiction, and trauma services (Center for Substance Abuse Treatment, 2009). Implementing culturally competent treatment systems and programs that provide a continuity of care in addressing the multidimensional needs and long-term requirements of women with co-occurring disorders is essential (Center for Substance Abuse Treatment, 2005).

Pursuant to the American Counseling Association's Code of Ethics (2014), the mission of their organization is to "enhance the quality of life in society by promoting the development of professional counselors, advancing the counseling profession, and using the profession and practice of counseling to promote respect for human dignity and diversity" (p. 2). Counselors are ethically responsible to provide culturally appropriate counseling interventions, which include the counselor demonstrating the ability to consider sociocultural factors such as race and ethnic influences along with the representativeness of the client. Failure to do so plays a significant role in counseling benchmarks (Day-Vines et al., 2007).

Effective substance use prevention and treatment requires constructing gender-specific programs to engage in dialogues that address the explicit risks and consequences of substance use disorders that are oftentimes associated with women (National Drug Control Strategy, 2011). An appreciation of diversity must be central in all efforts to improve services for women. In the addiction field, the therapeutic alliance has often been cited as being the most important aspect of a client's addiction and subsequent recovery (Claunch, Marlow, Ramsey, Drymon, & Patterson, 2015). Understanding the needs and challenges of substance use and co-occurring disorders along with other sociocultural factors is a key component to accurately diagnose and provide successful treatment for women (Center for Substance Abuse Treatment, 2009).

Moving Forward: Strengths and Evidence-Based Helping Strategies

In addition to the referenced treatment strategies for African American and Hispanic male and female substance misusers, utilizing treatment strategies for African American women that focus on an Afrocentric perspective, as well as considering resiliency factors when engaging Hispanic women can enhance culturally and gender-responsive treatment programs (Center for Substance Abuse Treatment, 2009).

The traditional medical model of testing for symptoms, diagnosing the problem and prescribing the solution has slowly been eroding and is becoming irrelevant in addressing the complex, multilayered problems of substance use and co-occurring disorders (van Wormer & Davis, 2013). Discouraged by the inadequate effectiveness of problem-focused solutions, mental health and substance abuse counselors have started moving toward a strength-based approach (Hammond & Zimmerman, 2012). According to van Wormer and Davis (2013), strength-based practitioners believe that not focusing on deficits that are oftentimes obscured by misery, protective strategies, and the inability to achieve prescribed goals affords the opportunity for possibilities, resiliencies, and capabilities that can be transforming for the client. Saleebey (1992) suggests that individuals and groups "have vast, often untapped and frequently unappreciated reservoirs of physical, emotional, cognitive, interpersonal, social, and spiritual energies, resources and competencies" (p. 6). Embracing a strength-based approach that seeks to understand and develop the strengths and capabilities of African American and Hispanic substance users can facilitate in the process of addressing gender-specific addiction treatment services.

Additional treatment models referenced below have also shown promising results among African American and Hispanic substance users. Harm reduction is a set of practical strategies that facilitate the reduction of adverse consequences of alcoholism, substance use, and mental illness through the use of practical techniques that incorporate respect, trust, and a nonjudgmental attitude. This philosophy provides key elements to an effective therapeutic relationship (National Health Care for the Homeless Council, 2010). Harm reduction practitioners focus on reducing such barriers as (i) inaccessible treatment programs in the community, (ii) professional staff that may be perceived as having limited knowledge about street culture or survival rules, (iii) wait-listed for intake and treatment services, (iv) inability to pay for services, and (v) accepting abstinence as the goal of treatment that makes it difficult for individuals who are misusing alcohol or illicit drugs to get help (van Wormer & Davis, 2013). According to the National Health Care for the Homeless Council (2010), harm reduction is not:

> At odds with abstinence; instead, it includes it as one possible goal across a continuum of possibilities. Harm reduction is neither for nor against drug use. It does not seek to stop drug use, unless individuals make that their goal. Harm reduction focuses on supporting people's efforts to reduce harms created by drug use or other risky behaviors. Harm reduction neither condones nor condemns any behavior. Instead, it evaluates the consequences of behaviors and tries to reduce the harms that those behaviors pose for individuals, families and communities (p. 1).

Motivational interviewing is a communication style that uses specific techniques and strategies such as reflective listening, shared decision-making, and eliciting change talk (Resnicow & McMaster, 2012). According to Miller and Rollnick (2013), principles of motivational interviewing consists of the following: (i) it helps people recognize and do something about their present or potential problems, (ii) it is a useful tool to use with people who are disinclined to change and are uncertain about changing, (iii) it creates an openness to change, (iv) responsibility for change is left up to the individual and not the clinician, (v) strategies are more persuasive than coercive and more supportive than argumentative, and (vi) the client presents the arguments for change rather than the therapist. Implementing effectual motivational interviewing techniques, the practitioner is "able to strategically balance the need to 'comfort the afflicted' and 'afflict the comfortable'; to balance the expression of empathy with the need to build sufficient discrepancy to stimulate change" (Resnicow & McMaster, 2012, p. 1). To compliment motivational interviewing techniques, practitioners are also including motivational enhancement therapy to the therapeutic process. Motivational enhancement therapy provides personal feedback about where one stands in relation to others as a way to build motivation for change (van Wormer & Davis, 2013).

Solution-focused therapy challenges the assumptions of traditional theories of psychotherapy. The focus of the therapy shifted from problem resolution to solution development where clients were viewed as experts of their lives and what was the best course of action for them. From this perspective of redefinition, solution-focused therapy is now viewed as a client-centered and collaborative process between the counselor and the client (Simon & Berg, n.d.). Although rigorous research studies on the effectiveness of solution-focused therapy are dearth, an effort by solution-focused therapy researchers have been conducting studies to remedy this situation (van Wormer & Davis, 2013).

Cognitive-behavioral therapy reflects on the idea that maladaptive thinking and bad habits both cause problems and at the same time keeps them going. From this perspective, problems are viewed as larger-than-life versions of what was previously thought to be a good idea; however, the behavior has now become very onerous (van Wormer & Davis, 2013). Additionally, the utilization of cognitive-behavioral coping skills therapy for alcohol dependence offers another treatment option. This treatment approach is geared toward improving cognitive and behavioral skills that facilitate in changing drinking habits by integrating a combination of different methods that differ in length, modality, content, and treatment setting (Longabaugh & Morgenstern, 1999).

Overall, integration of treatment services for individuals with substance use and co-occurring disorders require development of comprehensive and collaborative tools that can better address the needs of the client. These tools consists of (i) employing a positive recovery perspective, (ii) adopting a multidimensional viewpoint, (iii) develop a phased approach to treatment, (iv) address experiential realities early on in treatment, (v) effectuate a plan of action for the client's cognitive and functional impairments, and (vi) use varied support systems to facilitate in the treatment process (SAMHSA, 2015).

Conclusion

> You never really understand a person until you consider things from his point of view -- until you climb inside of his skin and walk around in it -- Harper Lee, To Kill a Mockingbird.

This quote by Harper Lee (1960) epitomizes the underlying rationale for this chapter. Before an individual's experiential realities are understood, the individual is already put into a box and judged. Studies have shown that racism is part and parcel of the foundation and cultural psyche of US societal norms and institutions (Sue, 2010). Understanding the racial and cultural differences of populations at both the micro level and at the macro level is tantamount to being culturally competent.

Engaging in conversational discourse about race and racial issues that involve accumulated inequities dating back generations is not an indictment against Whites. It is not even intended to generate a guilty conscience, as no one living today would be directly responsible for those accumulated inequities. It does however, bear strange fruit that the legacy of those inequities are still perpetuated in many of today's institutions that Whites either own and/or control through laws, policies, and programs. To take advantage of the historical inherited privileges and assets of past generations yet refuse to address the historical discriminatory actions or inactions that have led to the accumulated inequities of people of color is morally irresponsible and perpetuates a cycle of reproducing racism upon future generations (Wise, 2012).

The ever-increasing seeds of cultural differences and cultural variations that are continually being planted in American soil warrant that public service organizations and administrators embrace varied opportunities and challenges by developing and incorporating a more inclusive culturally competent care system that rests upon a unified set of values (Diller, 2015). These values according to Diller (2015) "share the notions that being different is positive, that services must be responsive to specific cultural needs, and that they must be delivered in a way that empowers the client" (p. 18). Creating a more inclusive culturally competent care system pushes the addiction and mental health service delivery systems to the forefront by providing a culturally holistic approach that incorporates cultural sensitivity and brings about the opportunity to offer tangible and culturally responsive services.

References

Adams, G. B., & Balfour, D. L. (2004). *Unmasking administrative evil* (rev. ed.). Armonk, NY: M. E. Sharpe.

Agrawal, A., Gardner, C. O., Prescott, C. A., & Kendler, K. S. (2005). The differential impact of risk factors on illicit drug involvement in females. *Social Psychiatry and Psychiatric Epidemiology, 40*(6), 454–466.

Amaro, H., Arevalo, S., Gonzalez, G., Szapocznik, J., & Iguchi, M. Y. (2006). Needs and scientific opportunities for research on substance abuse treatment among Hispanic adults. *Drug and Alcohol Dependence, 84S*, S64–S75.

Amaro, H., Larson, M. J., Gampel, J., Richardson, E., Savage, A., & Wagler, D. (2005). Racial/ethnic differences in social vulnerability among women with co-occurring mental health and substance abuse disorders: Implications for treatment services. *Journal of Community Psychology, 33*(4), 495–511.

American Counseling Association. (2014). *American Counseling Association code of ethics.* Retrieved January 4, 2017, from http://www.counseling.org/Resources/aca-code-of-ethics.pdf.

Aponte, J. F., & Johnson, L. R. (2000). The impact of culture on intervention and treatment and ethnic populations. In J. F. Aponte & J. Wohl (Eds.), *Psychological intervention and cultural diversity* (pp. 18–39). Needham Heights, MA: Allyn & Bacon.

Barr, K. E. M., Farrell, M. P., Barnes, G. M., & Welte, J. W. (1993). Race, class and gender differences in substance abuse: Evidence of middle-class/underclass polarization among black males. *Social Problems, 40*(3), 314–327.

Brocato, J. (2013). The impact of acculturation, motivation and the therapeutic alliance on treatment retention and outcomes for the Hispanic drug involved probationers. *Journal of Ethnic Criminal Justice, 11*(3), 150–180.

Butler, S. (1994). *A conversation guide for mirrors of privilege: Making whiteness visible: Heart-to-heart conversation guide.* Word Trust Educational Services, Inc. Retrieved November 15, 2015, from www.world-trust.org.

Carter, R. T. (1995). *The influence of race and racial identity in psychotherapy: Toward a racially inclusive model.* New York, NY: Wiley.

Center for Substance Abuse Treatment. (2005, 2007, 2008, and 2011). *Substance abuse Treatment: For personas with co-occurring disorders.* Treatment improvement protocol (TIP) series 42. HHS Publication No. (SMA) 08-3992. Rockville, MD: Substance Abuse and Mental Health Services Administration.

Center for Substance Abuse Treatment. (2009). *Substance abuse treatment: Addressing the specific needs of women.* Treatment improvement protocol (TIP) series 51. HHS Publication No. (SMA) 09-4426. Rockville, MD: Substance Abuse and Mental Health Services Administration.

Claunch, K., Marlow, S., Ramsey, A., Drymon, C., & Patterson, D. A. (2015, Sept-Oct). Therapeutic alliances in substance abuse treatment. *Counselor Magazine,* 1–9. Retrieved January 15, 2017, from http://www.counselormagazine.com/detailpageoverride.aspx?pageid=1729&id=6442455832.

Collins, R. L., & McNair, L. D. (2003). *Minority women and alcohol use.* National Institute on Alcohol Abuse and Alcoholism. Retrieved July 28, 2017, from https://pubs.niaa.nih.gov/publications/arh26-4/251-2256.htm.

Day-Vines, N., Wood, S., Grothaus, T., Craigen, L., Holman, A., Dotson-Blake, K., et al. (2007). Broaching styles of race, ethnicity, and culture during the counseling process. *Journal of Counseling & Development, 85,* 401–409.

Diller, J. V. (2015, 2011, 2007). *Cultural diversity: A primer for the human services.* (5th ed.). Stamford, CT: Cengage Learning.

Erving, C. L. (2017). Physical-psychiatric comorbidity: Implications for health measurement and the Hispanic epidemiological paradox. *Journal of Social Science Research, 64,* 197–213.

Gooden, S. T. (2014). *Race and social equity: A nervous area of government.* Armonk, NY: M. E. Sharpe Inc.

Green, C. A. (2006). *Gender and use of substance abuse treatment services.* National Institute on Alcohol Abuse and Alcoholism. https://pubs.niaaa.nih.gov/publications/arh291/55-62.htm.

Greenfield, S., & Grella, C. (2009). What is "women-focused" treatment for substance use disorders? *Psychiatric Services, 60*(7), 880–882.

Guba, E. G., & Lincoln, Y. S. (2005). Paradigmatic controversies, contradictions, and emerging confluences. In N. K. Denzin & Y. S. Lincoln (Eds.), *The Sage handbook of qualitative research* (3rd ed., pp. 191–215). Thousand Oaks, CA: Sage.

Hammond, W., & Zimmerman, R. (2012). A strengths-based perspective. *Resiliency Initiatives.* Retrieved January 15, 2017, from http://resiliencyinitiatives.ca/cms/wp-content/uploads/2013/03/STRENGTH_BASED_PERSPECTIVE-Dec-10-2012.pdf.

Johnson, S. D., Striley, C., & Cottle, L. B. (2006). The association of substance abuse disorders with trauma exposure and PTSD among African American drug users. *Addictive Behaviors, 31,* 2063–2073.

Krieger, N. (1999). Embodying inequality: A review of concepts, measures, and methods for studying health consequences of discrimination. *International Journal of Health Services, 29*(2), 395–352.

Lee, H. (1960). *To kill a mockingbird.* New York, NY: Grand Central Publishing.

Liddle, H. A., Jackson-Gilfort, A., & Marvel, F. A. (2006). An empirically supported and culturally specific engagement and intervention strategy for African American adolescent males. *American Journal of Orthopsychiatry, 75*(2), 215–225.

Longabaugh, R., & Morgenstern, J. (1999). Cognitive-behavioral coping-skills therapy for alcohol dependence: Current status and future directions. *Alcohol Research & Health, 23*(2), 78–85.

Loue, S. (2003). *Diversity issues in substance abuse treatment and research.* New York, NY: Kluwer/Plenum Publishers.

Miller, W. R., & Rollnick, S. (2013). *Motivational interviewing: Helping people change.* New York, NY: Guilford Press.

Minority Nurse Staff. (2013). African Americans, substance abuse and spirituality. *Minority Nurse.* Retrieved January 15, 2017, from http://minoritynurse.com/african-americans-substance-abuse-and-spirituality.

National Drug Control Strategy (2011). Washington, DC. From obamawhitehouse.archives.gov.

National Health Care for the Homeless Council. (2010). *Harm reduction: Preparing people for change.* Retrieved January 7, 2015, from http://www.nhchc.org/wp-content/uploads/2011/09/harmreductionFS_Apr10.pdf.

National Institute on Drug Abuse (NIDA). (1998, 1995). *Drug use among racial/ethnic minorities.* NIH Publication No. 98-3888. Bethesda, MD.

National Institute on Drug Abuse (NIDA). (2012). *Principles of drug addiction treatment: A research-based guide* (3rd ed.). Retrieved January 8, 2017, from https://www.drugabuse.gov/publications/principles-drug-addiction-treatment-research-based-guide-third-edition.

Newmann, J. P., & Sallmann, J. (2004). Women, trauma histories, and co-occurring disorders: Assessing the scope of the problem. *Social Service Review, 78*(3), 466–498.

Norman-Major, K. A., & Gooden, S. T. (2012). Cultural competency and public administration. In K. A. Norman-Major & S. T. Gooden (Eds.), *Cultural competency for public administrators* (pp. 3–16). New York, NY: M. E. Sharpe.

Resnicow, K., & McMaster, F. (2012). Motivational interviewing: Moving from why to how with autonomy support. *International Journal of Behavioral Nutrition and Physical Activity.* Retrieved December 15, 2016, from http://www.ijbnpa.org/content/9/1/19.

Resnicow, K., Soler, R., Braithwaite, R. L., Ahluwalia, J. S., & Butler, J. (2000). Cultural sensitivity in substance use prevention. *Journal of Community Psychology, 28*(3), 271–290.

Rodriguiez, R. A., Henderson, C. E., Rowe, C. L., Burnett, K. F., Dakof, G. A., & Liddle, H. A. (2007). Acculturation and drug use among dually diagnosed Hispanic adolescents. *Journal of Ethnicity in Substance Abuse, 6*(2), 97–113.

Saleebey, D. (1992). Introduction: Power in the people. In D. Saleebey (Ed.), *The strengths perspective in social work practice.* New York, NY: Longman.

Sanders, M. (2002). The response of African American communities to addiction: An opportunity for treatment providers. *Alcoholism Treatment Quarterly, 20*(¾), 167–174.

Simon, J. K., & Berg, K. (n.d.). *Solution-focused brief therapy with long-term problems.* Retrieved January 8, 2017, from http://www.0to10.net/sflong.pdf.

Staton-Tindall, M. (2010). *Female offender drug use and related issues.* Retrieved January 8, 2017, from https://www.nij.gov/topics/drugs/markets/adam/Documents/staton-paper.pdf?Redirected=true.

Substance Abuse and Mental Health Services Administration (SAMHSA). (2013). *Addressing the specific behavioral health needs of men. Treatment improvement protocol (TIP) series 56.* HHS Publication No. (SMA) 13-4736. Rockville, MD.

Substance Abuse and Mental Health Services Administration (SAMHSA). (2015). *Quick guide for clinicians: Substance abuse treatment for persons with co-occurring disorders (TIP) series 42.* Rockville, MD.

Substance Abuse and Mental Health Services Administration (SAMHSA). (2016). *Racial and ethnic minority populations.* Retrieved August 28, 2017, from http://www.samhsa.gov/specific-populations/racial-ethnic-minority.

Substance Abuse and Mental Health Services Administration (SAMHSA), Center for Behavioral Health Statistics and Quality. (2014, April 3). *The TEDS report: Gender differences in primary substance abuse across age groups.* Rockville, MD.

Sue, D. W. (2010). *Microaggressions in everyday life: Race, gender, and sexual orientation.* Hoboken, NJ: Wiley.

Sue, D. W., Nadal, K. L., Capodilupo, C. M., Lin, A. I., Torino, G. C., & Rivera, D. P. (2008). Racial microaggressions against black Americans: Implications for counseling. *Journal of Counseling & Development,* Summer, *86,* 330–338.

Sue, D. W., & Sue, D. (2008). *Counseling the culturally diverse: Theory and practice* (5th ed.). Hoboken, NJ: Wiley.

van Wormer, K., & Davis, D. R. (2013). *Addiction treatment: Strengths perspective* (3rd ed.). Belmont, CA: Brooks/Cole Cengage Learning.

Wisdom, J. P., Hoffman, K., Rechbergre, E., Seim, K., & Owens, B. (2009). Women-focused treatment agencies and process improvement: Strategies to increase client engagement. *Women & Therapy, 32,* 69–87.

Wise, T. (2012). *Dear white America: Letter to a new minority.* San Francisco, CA: City Lights Books.

Chapter 5
The Relationship Between Attachment and Addiction

Kevin Coffey

This chapter will initially postulate a potential relationship between addiction and attachment style. The chapter will then present attachment theory and review attachment styles. The implications of treating individuals with addiction from an attachment perspective will be explored. Clinical examples from practice will be utilized to illuminate theory.

Addiction and Its Relationship to Attachment

Addiction is increasingly experienced by many individuals in our society. The growing numbers of individuals addicted to psychoactive substances cannot be explained by any one dimension or etiology. There is no single cause for addiction. These problems can stem from a number of biological, psychological, social, or environmental factors that vary from one person to the next. It is biologically impossible for humans to self-regulate their affect for any extended period of time without the support of other humans (Flores, 2004). There is growing evidence that prolonged use of drugs and alcohol alters brain functioning and erodes psychic structures. The individual will lose social skills throughout the course of their addiction (Parson & Farr, 1981). As humans, we are pack animals, in need of other humans to help us to self-regulate. Increasingly, those suffering from addiction are utilizing psychoactive substances to assist with self–regulation. Hence, one view of addiction is that it is an attachment disorder.

K. Coffey (✉)
University of Rochester – Psychiatry, SUNY Empire State College – Community and Human Services, Rochester, NY, USA
e-mail: Kevin.coffey@esc.edu

© Springer International Publishing AG 2018   73
T. MacMillan, A. Sisselman-Borgia (eds.), *New Directions in Treatment, Education, and Outreach for Mental Health and Addiction*, Advances in Mental Health and Addiction, https://doi.org/10.1007/978-3-319-72778-3_5

In my early career, I was sure that I could help teenagers with conduct disorders transform their lives. It took me some time to realize that attachment style was critical to mental health and this important process was set early in life. Healthy attachment starts early in the life of an infant with his/her caregivers through bonding. There is mounting evidence that correlates attachment style to substance abuse, emotional distress, and interpersonal problems in adults (Davidson & Ireland, 2009; Doumas, Blasey, & Mitchell, 2006; Molnar, Sadava, Courville, & Perrier, 2010; Throrberg & Lyvers, 2010).

Attachment Theory

The theory of attachment was originally developed by John Bowlby (1979), who was attempting to understand the intensity experienced by infants who had been separated from their parents. Bowlby (1979) observed that infants went to extraordinary lengths to prevent separation from caregivers or to reconnect with them. Popular psychodynamic theory prior to Bowlby's work held that these efforts were primitive coping mechanisms to prevent hurt (Klein, 1948). Drawing on ethological theory, Bowlby proposed that these attachment behaviors, such as crying and searching, were adaptive responses to separation from a primary attachment figure. Since infants cannot care for themselves, they are completely dependent on caregivers for their needs to be met. Bowlby theorized that through natural selection, over time an attachment behavior system was designed to regulate proximity to an attachment figure. Attachment theory according to Bowlby indicates an infant feels content and secure if a caregiver is nearby and responsive. Further, if a caregiver is absent or unresponsive, the infant feels anxious and insecure. Although Bowlby believed this was the essence of the attachment behavioral system, he did recognize there was individual difference in how individuals negotiate proximity to caregivers.

Ainsworth (1969) began to examine infant-parent separation. Her research led to a more formal understanding of individual difference in the attachment behavioral system. Ainsworth and her students developed a technique called the strange situation. This was a laboratory exercise where 1-year-olds and their caregivers were brought to the laboratory. Eventually, the caregivers and their child were separated. Over 60% of the individuals studied responded as Bowlby postulated. They were anxious and upset when the parent left the room. When the parent returned to the room, they readily calmed and sought comfort from the caregiver. Ainsworth indicated that these youth had secure attachment. A second reaction was noted in about 20% of her study. These infants were upset by the separation from the caregiver, but when reunited with the caregiver they were not comforted. These children appeared to experience ambivalence between wanting to be soothed and wanting to punish the parent for the absence. These youth were labeled anxious resistant. The third pattern of attachment identified by Ainsworth and her colleagues is called avoidant. These youth were not distressed by the separation nor did they seek reunification with the caregiver upon return to the room. These youth did not focus on the caregiver and comprised about 20% of the sample studied by Ainsworth and her colleagues.

Attachment theory provided scientific authority to the study of relationships between caregivers and their children. Although human development specialists have always placed significant import to early childhood experiences, influencing adult psychology, it took attachment theory to identify the import of early attachments. Intimate and long-lasting relationships are essential to a meaningful life. Capacity to form these relationships has their etiology in early life attachments. Difficulty overcoming ineffective attachment styles (Ainsworth, 1969) can leave certain individuals vulnerable to addictive compulsion as compensatory behavior.

Ainsworth's research focused on how parental responses to children, or the lack of response, impacted secure and insecure attachment style. Securely attached children were not necessarily the infants who were taken up the most into their mother's arms most frequently or held the longest. Rather, the securely attached children had mothers who would consistently pick them up and hug them when they wanted to be picked up and hugged and put them down when they were ready to be put down. When they were hungry, their mothers fed them. If they began to tire, their mother would sense it and put them in their bassinet.

Hazen and Shaver (1987) extended attachment theory to adult relationships. They noted there were similarities between how children interact with caregivers and how adults interact with romantic partners. Adults use these relationships for support and to shield against the calamities of life. It was noted that there are significant differences between the relationship of children and caregivers and that of two adults. The similarity is in the core principles of attachment theory which apply to both relationships. Attachment experiences are required for brain development. When an infant is born, they are unable to seek out attachment experiences to help developing synapses in the brain. Stimulating interactions between caregivers lead to the further development of these synapses. When these important relational experiences do not occur for the infant, the brain begins to prune synapses that have not been stimulated. This is ending the potential of that brain synapse for the remainder of the child's life. Attachment theorists have honed in on the limbic system as the core mediator of attachment. This part of the brain has function over emotional regulation and emotional memory (Ekman, 1992).

There is a false separation between biology and psychology that is gradually changing. Scientific research has recently demonstrated the following principles:

1. Attachment can alter gene expression.
2. Attachment and psychotherapy can alter brain chemistry.
3. Learning-based experiences alter neuronal connectivity.
4. Potentiation requires activation, which alters the strength and autonomous patterns of brain functioning.
5. Synaptic strength is an experience-dependent phenomenon.
6. Talking in a meaningful way, paying attention, and attachment alter brain's biochemistry and lead to changes in synaptic transmission, strength, and numbers of synapses (Kandel, 2000).

There is increasing data on how early loss and trauma influence the developing brains of infants. Many youth who are raised in orphanages develop reactive attachment disorder.

Many individuals who do not have secure attachment develop personality disorders. Individuals without secure attachment can develop multiple substance use issues. It is not atypical to see an individual who cuts for self-soothing, who is addicted to drugs or alcohol, or who may also experience eating disorder issues in clinical practice. Many individuals who lack secure attachment experience feelings of chronic emptiness.

What Should Attachment Teach Us About Substance Abuse Treatment?

Chemical dependency treatment has changed a great deal over the last 20–30 years. In the past it could be rigid and judgmental. Prior to motivational interviewing, the substance abuse treatment field was harsh and robustly judgmental regarding relapse. Clients were often discharged from care because of relapse, and this experience was often quite shameful. This had the potential to further reinforce a client's already shaky attachment style and leave these individuals in the care of primary care physicians or mental health professionals who may have lacked training in substance abuse. This experience often put clients further into relapse mode and moved them increasingly away from healthy attachment.

Effective change strategies begin with genuine exposure to other people. A powerful attachment experience can alter a person's nervous system as well as changing brain chemistry. Exposure to healthy attachment helps the individual learn and develop new rules and boundaries for relationship. This leads to a radical change in implicit memory. It can be argued that powerful attachment experiences can alter old patterns of relatedness and help an individual forge new patterns of relatedness. Effective psychotherapy has to utilize the underpinnings of attachment in order to work. An important factor to keep in focus during psychotherapy is it alters brain neurobiology. Hence, when an individual is working toward changing his or her life, they are also altering their neurophysiology (Flores, 2004). Good therapy is not just a casual conversation. It is a powerful mutual experience of attachment that is helping both client and therapist to self-regulate. Although the experience is intended to help the person seeking help, it will also have powerful changing effects on the therapist. It is also altering the neurobiology of the therapist (Flores, 2004).

Early treatment of individuals addicted to drugs and alcohol is a complex task. The individual needs to give up the drug they have become attached to. An individual has to hold the belief that their life is better without the drug. This is a complex premise for an individual to grasp early in sobriety. You cannot present a logical argument to the individual to convince them that their life will be better by being clean and abstinent. Sadly, when an individual becomes clean and abstinent, they struggle with regulating their emotions. They have relied on substances to mediate emotions for them. In addition, their life catches up with them. Relationships that may have been damaged as well as professional responsibilities or legal issues they have not attended to often lead to mounting stress. The first 3 months of sobriety is a very painful time. The presence of significant and powerful attachment figures at this time is the incentive for individuals to do this painful and difficult work.

Early recovery work can be greatly aided by understanding by the therapist of motivational interviewing (Millner & Rollnick, 2002) and the transtheoretical change model (Prochaska & DiClemente, 1992). Therapists come to understand that most individuals are not ready to do everything to ensure their successful sobriety. All of us have varied motivation to make change in our lives. Motivational interviewing strategies will help. What helps some initiate sobriety is quite different than what helps in sustaining sobriety. A client must learn to create mutually supported attached relationships and to utilize their emotions as a guide. Emotions are critical data informing us about our experiences.

Individuals in recovery often have difficulty experiencing pleasure. Their substance use had become their own only source of pleasure. Encouraging new and different pleasurable activities including new ways to attach to others becomes critical skills later in treatment. During the final phase of treatment, the therapist becomes a transformational object, a source of continual interactive relationships that provide the environmental backdrop for the old self to transform into the new self. In other words, the person who is addicted must develop new and different ways of relating (Shane, Shane, & Gales, 1997).

In summary, the following principles from attachment theory should impact and inform substance abuse treatment strategies:

1. Humans need other humans to self-regulate. Human beings cannot self-regulate on their own.
2. Attachment is a primary human drive.
3. Secure attachment liberates. The stronger the earliest attachment experience, the less a person will require excessive sources of external affect regulation.
4. Those who develop insecure attachment are more vulnerable to external sources of self-regulation.
5. Prolonged substance abuse produces changes in a person's brain.
6. Healthy forms of affect regulation must be developed, or an individual remains vulnerable to addiction.
7. Early treatment requires removal of the source of addiction.
8. Individuals need to develop a new sense of themselves through the attachment experience in treatment (Flores, 1997; 2004).

In this next section of this chapter, I will discuss the importance of group treatment for providing attachment experiences for individuals recovering from addiction.

Clinical Examples

A male in his 40s had been a long haul truck driver for many years driving all over the USA while severely intoxicated. When he was born, his mother had a 1-year-old son and her husband was dying of cancer. His mother often joked with him that she had three people in diapers when he was born. His mother was working at being a good mother, but she likely did not possess the psychological energy to meet his developmental needs. Although married with two children as an adult, this man had a limited relationship with his wife and children. He reported never feeling at home with his family. Oddly, the only strong connections he could identify were to beer and a special grill at his home. The early unfortunate experiences he had with his mother apparently influenced his attachment style and clearly impacted his capacity for a meaningful life.

A young woman born to a substance misusing mother and an older sister were removed from their biological mother when the young woman was 2 years old. They were adopted by a well-meaning intact family, but the new adopted family could not manage this young woman and she was placed in a residential treatment center until she was 18 years old. This woman was discharged from the residential treatment center into the adult outpatient treatment world. This patient had extreme difficulty with attachment. Her life had no boundaries and was full of chaos. She spread these difficulties to each situation she encountered. She had a personality that led many individuals to attempt to rescue her, yet these rescue attempts usually resulted in increased chaos. Sadly, this woman is now almost 40 and still has difficulty with organizing her life.

A Caucasian man in his 50s experienced depression and alcoholism, with an anxious/insecure attachment style. He had a difficult relationship with his wife and had few friends. He did work but did not report it to be very satisfying. He described going to a bar in a group and indicated that he liked that the bartender would remember what he drank. He discussed how this made him feel cared about by the bartender. He reported that by the second drink he was able to connect with the other individuals at the bar. In that moment, he felt connected to those individuals. The use of alcohol was blurring his perceptions of the experience, but nonetheless he would feel temporally attached. This is an experience that individuals with insecure attachment crave.

A young man who seemed to have it all together on the surface was good looking and athletic and already earned an MBA with a well-paying job as an auditor. Oddly, he had no sense or understanding about the appropriate rules and boundaries in life. He was a second child whose parents did not have enough energy for him, and he had an older brother who he perceived as his parent's favorite. This young man had been quite successful by imitating others, but had no clue about what was behind the behavior. He unfortunately did not take much joy from his successes. Therapeutic intervention was a powerful attachment experience that validated his experiences growing up. It also helped him reduce anxiety and begin to understand rules and boundaries in relationships.

References

Ainsworth, M. D. S. (1969). Object relations, dependency and attachment: A theoretical review of the mother-infant relationship. *Child Development, 40*, 969–1025.

Bowlby, J. (1979). *The making and breaking of affectional bonds.* London, UK/New York, NY: Routledge.

Davidson, S., & Ireland, C. A. (2009). Substance misuse: The relationship between attachment style, personality traits coping in drug and non-drug uses. *Drugs and Alcohol Today, 9*(3), 22–27.

Doumas, D. M., Blasey, C. M., & Mitchell, S. (2006). Adult attachment, emotional distress, and interpersonal problems in alcohol and drug dependency treatment. *Alcoholism Treatment Quarterly, 24*(4), 41–54.

Ekman, P. (1992). An argument for basic emotions. *Cognition and Emotion, 6*(3/40), 169–200.

Flores, P. (1997). *Group psychotherapy with addictive populations: An integration of 12-step and psychodynamic theory.* Binghamton, NY: Haworth Press.

Flores, P. (2004). *Addiction as an attachment disorder.* Lanham, MD: Rowman & Littlefield.

Hazan, C., & Shaver, P. R. (1987). Attachment as an organizational framework for research on close relationships. *Psychological Inquiry, 5*, 1–22.

Kandel, E. (2000). *Principles of neural science* (4th ed.). New York, NY: McGraw-Hill.

Klein, M. (1948). *Contributions to psycho-analysis 1921–1945.* London, UK: Hargrove.

Millner, W. R., & Rollnick, S. (2002). *Motivational interviewing: Preparing people for change* (2nd ed.). New York, NY: Guilford Press.

Molnar, D. S., Sadava, S. W., Courville, N. H., & Perrier, C. P. (2010). Attachment, motivation, and alcohol: Testing a dual-path model of high- risk drinking and adverse consequences in transitional clinical and student samples. *Canadian Journal of Behavioral Sciences, 42*(1), 1–13.

Parson, O. A., & Farr, S. P. (1981). The neuropsychology of alcohol & drug use. In S. B. Felsokov & T. J. Boll (Eds.), *Handbook of clinical neuropsychology* (pp. 320–365). New York, NY: Wilcy.

Prochaska, J. O., & DiClemente, C. C. (1992). Stages of change in the modification of problem behavior. In M. Hersen, R. R. Eisler, & P. M. Miller (Eds.), *Progress in behavior modification* (Vol. 28, pp. 184–214). Sycamore, IL: Sycamore Press.

Shane, M., Shane, E., & Gales, M. (1997). *Intimate attachments: Toward a new self psychology.* New York, NY: Guilford Press.

Throrberg, F., & Lyvers, M. (2010). Attachment, fear, of intimacy and differentiation of among clients in substance treatment facilities. *Addictive Behaviors, 31*(4), 732–737.

Chapter 6
Addiction and Self-Injury

Rebecca K. Eliseo-Arras

Introduction

Self-injury encompasses both non-suicidal self-injury (NSSI) and other forms of self-harming behaviors such as eating disorders, alcohol and drug abuse, suicide, and more severe forms of self-mutilation (Nock, Joiner, Gordon, Lloyd-Richardson, & Prinstein, 2006; Purington & Whitlock, 2004). It is a serious issue of public health and mental health importance. Non-suicidal self-injury (NSSI) involves the intentional infliction of bodily harm without suicidal intent that causes damage to body tissue (Moller, Tait, & Byrne, 2013; Nock, 2010). It is often done for the purposes of emotion regulation and is a maladaptive coping mechanism (Alfonso & Kaur, 2012; Roger, Flynn, Borrill, & Fox, 2009). While initially seen as a behavior specific to adolescent females, more recent research has determined that the behavior spans all age groups, genders, and racial/ethnic backgrounds (Nock, 2010). What is similar across those who engage in maladaptive coping behaviors is the motive: to quell negative emotions (Nock, 2010).

In individuals who have either comorbid or co-occurring self-harming behaviors, it may be evident which behavior occurred first (e.g., eating disorder that preceded NSSI), whereas in others the trajectory is not as clear. Recent research is attempting to uncover ways to determine which behavior occurred first, why this information is important, and why individuals trade one maladaptive behavior for another. Armed with this information, researchers and practitioners may be able to create and test more precise and appropriate treatment manuals.

R. K. Eliseo-Arras (✉)
SUNY Empire State College, Division of Community and Human Services,
University at Buffalo, New York, NY, USA
e-mail: Rebecca.Eliseo-Arras@esc.edu

© Springer International Publishing AG 2018   81
T. MacMillan, A. Sisselman-Borgia (eds.), *New Directions in Treatment,*
Education, and Outreach for Mental Health and Addiction, Advances in Mental
Health and Addiction, https://doi.org/10.1007/978-3-319-72778-3_6

Research cites prevalence rates of NSSI at 4% in the general US population (Briere & Gil, 1998). Adolescents are at an increased risk with prevalence rates as high as 14–17% (Klonsky & Olino, 2008). Intervening early and providing appropriate interventions for adolescents is extremely salient and may also decrease healthcare costs since less individuals will need to be seen in an emergency room for deep cuts or infections (Hawton & Sinclair, 2003).

Chapter Outline

This chapter will begin by discussing the origins of self-injury, the definition of NSSI, and the various terminologies that exist in the literature, will discuss the "typical" self-injurer, and will explore the ways that NSSI and other addictions overlap and co-occur. Current rates of NSSI in clinical, community, and school settings will also be discussed along with rates specific to different populations. Methods of self-injury will also be explored along with the developmental trajectory of NSSI and other self-harming behaviors. Comorbidity of self-injury with other mental health issues such as childhood abuse, sexual assault, and eating disorders will be discussed followed by talk of comorbidity of self-injury and addictions. The theoretical framework for NSSI will be explored, specifically focusing on the four-factor functional model (Nock & Prinstein, 2004). Issues of cultural diversity and competence related to addiction and self-injury will be explored next followed by a thorough discussion of practical skills related to diagnosis, practice, or education which include information on various relevant interventions such as cognitive behavioral therapy, dialectical behavior therapy, and motivational interviewing. This chapter will conclude with implications for future practice, research, and education with thoughts regarding motivational interviewing as an intervention for NSSI, clinicians' reactions to disclosure of NSSI and why that is important, and NSSI as an addiction and the steps needed to explore this avenue of research.

Origins of Self-Injury

The first mention of self-injury was in Menninger's (1938) book *Man Against Himself*, in which he felt that self-injury was purposeful and had meaning to the individual. Menninger was also one of the first to create a classification system for self-injury. This new system contained dimensions of the extent and form of the "psychological dysfunction that was caused by the self-injury, the meaning of the self-injury in a cultural context, and the intrapsychic determinants of the behavior" (Yates, 2004, p. 37). Much like current sentiments of NSSI, he felt that self-injury was more about healing oneself and eliminating negative feelings the person may be experiencing rather than suicidal intent.

Non-suicidal Self-Injury: Definition and Terminology

The definition and terminology of non-suicidal self-injury has evolved in the literature. One of the first mentions of self-injury in diagnostic manuals occurred with the third edition to the DSM in 1981 as a symptom to borderline personality disorder (BPD); however, recent research has shown that self-injury exists outside the BPD diagnosis. Terms such as deliberate self-harm (DSH; Gratz, 2001), deliberate self-injury (Klonsky, 2007b), and self-injurious behavior (SIB; Claes, Vandereycken, & Vertommen, 2001) were used in the literature, but many of the previous terms failed to fully address the core features of NSSI, i.e., the act of self-injury does not carry with it suicidal intentions, an act that causes damage to bodily tissues, and the act itself falls outside the realm of what is considered "normal" behavior within society. In addition, the previous terminology itself (e.g., deliberate self-harm, self-injurious behavior) did not convey that this is an act without suicidal intentions. These features are the major tenets of the definition outlined by the International Society for the Study of Self-Injury (ISSS) and will be used throughout this chapter. The ISSS defines NSSI as "the deliberate, self-inflicted destruction of body tissue without suicidal intent and for purposes not socially sanctioned" (www.itriples.org). "Not socially sanctioned" in the definition allows for exclusion of body piercing and tattooing. By definition, NSSI is not suicide although some earlier research and articles do not separate suicide and NSSI (e.g., Welch, 2001). This can create problems when trying to ascertain prevalence rates if other behaviors are lumped into this definition (Muehlenkamp, 2005). However, it should be noted that due to the relative immaturity of this field of study, there is a dearth of studies that explicitly use the term NSSI and the definition stated by the ISSS.

Distinction needs to be made between NSSI and self-harm. NSSI involves the actual destruction of bodily tissue, i.e., cutting, burning, intense scratching to draw blood, interfering with wound healing, and "erasing" of the skin (i.e., taking an eraser to the skin and rubbing it repeatedly and profusely). Self-harm, on the other hand, involves bodily harm, but the methods of harm are different. Suicide attempts can also be classified as a self-harm behavior. While a suicide attempt may in fact involve cutting the skin (e.g., as in slitting the wrists), suicide attempts are placed in the self-harm category separate from NSSI because NSSI involves no suicide ideation, which is the key distinction between these two behaviors. Further, while an individual may not have the awareness or the intention, chronic, progressive use of drugs and alcohol does cause damage to the body over time. Alcohol abuse can lead to cirrhosis of the liver, liver damage, damage to the brain, as well as memory loss following chronic, heavy abuse (US Department of Health & Human Services, 2004). Drug abuse can damage the kidneys, liver, and stomach and can lead to other complications such as heart failure or seizures (www.drugabuse.gov). However, these effects are long term and the methods of harm are not the same as with NSSI.

Eating disorders could also be classified as a self-harming behavior. Both anorexia nervosa (AN) and bulimia nervosa (BN) lead to damage within the body if the individual does not seek treatment and can lead to death as well (Rome &

Ammerman, 2003). Significant metabolic changes are also present with eating disorders, and organ and internal tissue damage is likely (for a review of medical complications caused by eating disorders, see Rome & Ammerman, 2003). Overall, all of these behaviors lead to one conclusion: individuals are harming themselves.

The "Typical" Self-Injurer

Knowing that NSSI and other forms of self-harming behavior such as addictions often co-occur, the next question to address is which individuals would be at a higher risk for engaging in self-injury. Early NSSI literature painted the picture of the "typical" self-injurer as being an adolescent Caucasian female, of middle to upper socioeconomic status, single, of moderate to high intelligence, and may have a history of previous self-injury (Shaw, 2002; Suyemoto & MacDonald, 1995). Only recently has research on NSSI shifted toward including males (Laye-Gindhu & Schonert-Reichl, 2005), giving the impression that men were not engaging in this behavior. Some research has found that females engage in NSSI more often than males (Laye-Gindhu & Schonert-Reichl, 2005; Whitlock, Eckenrode, & Silverman, 2006), while others have found little to no difference in rates of NSSI between males and females (e.g., Gratz, Conrad, & Roemer, 2002). This ratio is most pronounced in early adolescence with females eight times more likely to engage in NSSI than males with decreasing discrepancies as individuals mature and age (Hooley, 2008).

Rates of NSSI

Rates of NSSI vary across populations, perhaps due to the lack of a clear definition and terminology as well as differences in methodology. Within inpatient settings, 61% of individuals report engaging in self-injury (DiClemente, Ponton, & Hartley, 1991), while rates among community samples range from 8.6% (Andover, Pepper, & Gibb, 2007) to 44% (Hasking, Momeni, Swannell, & Chia, 2008). This number may seem to be rather high and is higher than rates of depression in the general population; however, NSSI does not always occur with depression. Some research has suggested that NSSI co-occurs with anxiety (Chartrand, Sareen, Toews, & Bolton, 2012; Nock et al., 2006) and eating disorders (Muehlenkamp, Claes, Smits, Peat, & Vandereycken, 2011) so this could perhaps point to these higher rates of NSSI seen in the literature.

Furthermore, Whitlock and Knox (2007) note that the rates of NSSI among adolescents and young adults are especially concerning. Among college samples, rates range from 12% (Favazza, DeRosear, & Conterio, 1989) to 35% (Gratz, 2001). Within a high school setting, the range is much smaller ranging from 14% (Ross & Heath, 2002) to approximately 16% (Muehlenkamp & Gutierrez, 2004) of students reporting that they engage in self-injury. However, Ross and Heath (2002) note in their survey study of high school students that around 21% reported they engaged in self-injury on at least one occasion, which may not necessarily indicate that it is being used as a coping mechanism but perhaps an indication of an attempt prompted by peer pressure and experimentation. Lifetime prevalence rates of NSSI among adolescents are especially concerning given that 56% of those in early adolescence report a history of NSSI (Hilt, Cha, & Nolen-Hoeksema, 2008).

Adolescence and early adulthood is also around the same developmental time-point that other self-harming behaviors tend to develop, such as alcohol abuse, drug use, and eating disorders (Chassin, Pitts, DeLucia, & Todd, 1999; D'Amico et al., 2002; Kponee, Siegel, & Jernigan, 2014). The influence of family history of alcohol abuse along with family environment may also put adolescents and young adults at an increased risk for alcohol abuse and other addictive behaviors (Brown, Tate, Vik, Haas, & Aarons, 1999).

Male Self-Injury

Studies have shown that self-injury is not limited to females, with males showing an increase in rates of self-injury (Taylor, 2003). More work in this area needs to be conducted. The research that does include males has looked at sex differences in relation to types of NSSI methods. For females, the main method is cutting, but for males the main method is burning (Claes et al., 2007; Laye-Gindhu & Schonert-Reichl, 2005). Taylor (2003) mentions that the methods of NSSI that males engage in may not fit within the typical definitions noted in the literature. In a study comparing males and females both with and without a history of NSSI, males with a history of NSSI did differ from those who did not have a history of NSSI in terms of body surveillance (i.e., the extent to which an individual is concerned about how what they are wearing makes them appear to others) (Nelson & Muehlenkamp, 2012).

Methods of NSSI

Individuals who engage in NSSI may often have a specific method for how they injure themselves. Methods of self-injury include cutting or burning of the skin as well as picking at healing wounds or intense scratching. Individuals who engage in cutting most often report using knives (Fortune, 2006), scissors, shards of glass, or other sharp instruments to cut themselves. For those who engage in burning, they often use lit cigarettes, heat up metal objects to then apply to the skin, or profusely rub an eraser on the skin to cause a burn (Klonsky, 2007a, b).

Developmental Trajectory of NSSI and Other Self-Harming Behaviors

The typical age of onset of NSSI is during the adolescent years, and this developmental period is a stage of significant cognitive and emotional development. There is increasing pressure on an adolescent from multiple sources, including parents and peers, for the individual to fit in with their peers and gain acceptance within certain crowds, to obtain good grades to get into college while either working a part-time job or participating in multiple extracurricular activities, combined with the various struggles of going through puberty, can place a significant amount of stress on an adolescent (Patterson & McCubbin, 1987). Coping mechanisms are also just beginning to develop during this developmental period, and it is at this point when confronted with a difficult situation that an adolescent can opt for various coping options (Patterson & McCubbin, 1987). Adolescents cope with these struggles in various ways, some of which are more adaptive than others. For a subset of adolescents, however, the stress and pressure can be overwhelming, and without positive coping mechanisms in place, these individuals may turn to NSSI for relief. Often, these coping strategies will survive through adulthood.

Other maladaptive coping mechanisms may also develop during this time frame as previously argued. Alcohol abuse and drug abuse typically appear during this developmental period (Christiansen et al., 2008), often as a result of peer pressure or influence (Goodman, Peterson-Badali, & Henderson, 2011; Kiesner, Poulin, & Dishion, 2010), but could also be the result of cumulative stress in an adolescent's environment (Eliseo-Arras, 2016). Sibling influence is often important, and recent research has confirmed that there is a positive relationship between older sibling use and younger sibling use and that this relationship may be transmitted via shared social networks (Whiteman, Jensen, Mustillo, & Maggs, 2016).

While most individuals begin engaging in NSSI during adolescence, some research has found that others start this behavior between the ages of 17 and 24 (Heath, Toste, Nedecheva, & Charlebois, 2008; Whitlock et al., 2006). Young adults who self-injured also engaged in more avoidant coping, more likely to use alcohol, and had more psychopathology than those who did not engage in NSSI (Hasking et al., 2008). Research has also shown that among young adults (both men and women) who experienced intimate partner violence (IPV), the experience of IPV was a predictor of self-injurious behaviors (Levesque, Lafontaine, Bureau, Cloutier, & Dandurand, 2010).

Comorbidity of Self-Injury with Other Mental Health Issues

NSSI has also been found to be occurring along with other disorders. Studies have shown a link between self-injury and eating disorders (Paul, Schroeter, Dahme, & Nutzinger, 2002), substance abuse (Haw, Hawton, Casey, Bale, & Shepherd, 2005), substance dependence (Harned, Najavits, & Weiss, 2006), and post-traumatic stress disorder (PTSD) (Weierich & Nock, 2008). Nock and Mendes (2008) showed that individuals who engage in self-injury have poorer coping strategies and difficulty with problem solving skills when faced with a stressful event. Other research has pointed to impulsiveness among those who self-injure (Herpertz, Sass, & Favazza, 1997) and peer victimization as reinforcement for self-injury (Hilt et al., 2008). However, more work needs to be conducted in terms of motivations, underlying factors for self-injury, and the role of peer influences.

Childhood Abuse

There are numerous studies that have examined the link between childhood sexual abuse (CSA) and NSSI (e.g., Gladstone et al., 2004; Muehlenkamp, 2005; Svirko & Hawton, 2007). Yates (2004) found that when using retrospective reports, up to 79% of individuals who engage in self-injury also reported a history of child abuse or neglect. When examining a group of women with depression, those who also had a history of CSA were more likely to have attempted suicide or engaged in self-harm than those women who did not have a history of CSA (Gladstone et al., 2004). Male undergraduates with a history of childhood physical abuse (CPA) who also had greater emotion dysregulation were more likely to engage in self-harming behavior than those without a history of CPA (Gratz & Chapman, 2007). Those who engage in NSSI with a history of CSA experience significant difficulties with emotion regulation and in their daily lives than those without a history of CSA or NSSI (Muehlenkamp, Kerr, Bradley, & Larsen, 2010). However, it should be noted that not all individuals who have experienced CSA will later engage in NSSI (Klonsky & Muehlenkamp, 2007).

Sexual Assault and Trauma

Research has shown that there is a link between self-injury and trauma, as well as self-injury and sexual assault. Individuals who were victims of sexual abuse may be at higher risk for engaging in NSSI than those who experienced other types of abuse (Weierich & Nock, 2008). This was found in a community sample as well (Romans, Martin, Anderson, Herbison, & Mullen, 1995). Other researchers have confirmed a possible correlation between self-injury and sexual abuse (Suyemoto & MacDonald, 1995; Warm, Murray, & Fox, 2003; Yates, 2004). Whitlock and Knox (2007) noted that individuals who reported a history of self-injury as well as previous suicide attempts were more likely to also have higher rates of sexual and emotional abuse histories than those without previous combined self-injurious behaviors and suicide attempts.

Eating Disorders

There is also a connection between self-injury and eating disorders (Muehlenkamp, 2005; Paul et al., 2002). Of those who have engaged in both NSSI and previous suicide attempts, they were more likely to have disordered eating behaviors than those without both NSSI and suicide attempts (Whitlock & Knox, 2007). Ross, Heath, and Toste (2009) found that those who engaged in NSSI also reported more negative feelings regarding their body shape and size and had higher rates of eating pathology than those who did not engage in NSSI. Favazza et al. (1989) as well as Ross et al. (2009) argue that eating disorders such as anorexia nervosa (AN) and bulimia nervosa (BN) should be included among self-injurious behaviors.

Comorbidity of Self-Injury and Addiction

Klonsky and Muehlenkamp (2007) note that both NSSI and substance abuse inflict harm on the body, as previously argued, and some individuals who self-injure are also likely to abuse substances. Haw et al. (2005) found in their study of alcohol dependence and excessive drinking among those who engage in deliberate self-harm (DSH) that the prevalence of males and females who engaged in DSH increased during the 13 years of the study. Moreover, rates of male drinkers and diagnoses of alcohol-related disorders tended to be higher than females during this period, although for the female participants rates of alcohol-related problems increased as well just not at the same rates as males. In addition, excessive consumption of alcohol occurred 6 h after a DSH act for females but not for males. It should be noted, however, that this study was conducted in the United Kingdom, where the comprehensive term of DSH is used and includes both self-injury with and without suicidal intent (Haw et al., 2007).

Theoretical Framework

Much of the theoretical work to examine NSSI thus far has been in the development of theoretical models to describe the various aspects, features, and comorbidities with other mental health disorders. Many of the studies examining theoretical models have looked at and tested multiple models rather than providing a consensus for a specific model. However, it may be that one model may not fit each person, and thus multiple models may be needed to describe the motivations for each individual. The field may benefit from a comprehensive model that includes all the motivations, comorbidities, and end results.

The act of NSSI is deliberate and self-inflicted; however, the motivations behind the act are varied. Some theoretical models suggest that NSSI is used for emotion regulation to reduce negative emotions (Kamphuis, Ruyling, & Reijntjes, 2007). Self-injury may be employed to quell internal feelings of anger, anxiety, or deep emotional pain (Suyemoto, 1998). Research by Kamphuis et al. (2007) supported the emotion regulation hypothesis in a sample of 106 female inpatients. Results indicated that participants experienced a buildup of negative emotions prior to the act of self-injury and that these emotions were released via self-injury. However, these results should be interpreted with caution, as there was a lack of a true control group within this study and the use of small inpatient sample size limits generalizability.

Another model that has received empirical support is the four-factor functional model (Nock & Prinstein, 2004, 2005). This model states that there are four domains, which NSSI encompasses, specifically, automatic positive reinforcement, automatic negative reinforcement, social negative reinforcement, and social positive reinforcement (Nock & Prinstein, 2005). These domains operate on dichotomous planes; positive reinforcement, negative reinforcement, social contingencies, and automatic/internal contingencies. More explicitly, this model suggests that the function of self-injury for the individual depends on whether it is negatively or positively reinforced and if it is related to intrapersonal or interpersonal events (Nock, 2010). Automatic negative reinforcement involves an attempt to thwart unwanted emotions or thoughts using self-injury whereas automatic positive reinforcement refers to the attempt to generate feelings so that the individual feels something (Nock & Prinstein, 2004, 2005). Social negative reinforcement states that self-injury is used to break away from demands in an individual's daily life, while social positive reinforcement explains the use of self-injury to gain social attention (Nock & Prinstein, 2004, 2005). In a follow-up study by the same authors (Nock & Prinstein, 2005), the purpose was to not only test the model but also to look at the contextual features that occur prior to an act of self-injury. Interestingly, the authors found that the less time a person spent contemplating committing an act of self-injury, the less pain they felt. Moreover, if an individual belabored over if they should self-injure or not and if they also had a friend who engaged in the behavior, the more likely they were to feel pain. This could possibly point to a dissociation factor if the individual is not feeling as much pain. Perhaps the act of contemplating NSSI short-circuits this dissociative feature enabling the individual to feel more pain. This is an avenue worthy of future exploration.

Addiction and Self-Injury and Issues of Cultural Diversity and Competence

The act of NSSI is not a new phenomenon. In various cultures throughout history, individuals have caused harm to themselves by cutting, burning, or scratching flesh as part of a religious ceremony or as an act of self-expression (Favazza & Favazza, 1987). However, the motives behind this new "wave" of NSSI are different.

Researchers point to emotion regulation as a possible factor that drives an individual to intentionally injure themselves (e.g., Williams & Hasking, 2010). Others state that it is buildup of tension that leads a person to engage in NSSI (Yearwood & Bosnick, 2012). In addition, there may be co-occurring mental health disorders, such as depression, anxiety, obsessive-compulsive disorder, eating disorders, as well as a trauma history that underlie the motivation for engaging in NSSI, and the existence of co-occurring disorders places the individual at a higher risk for later developmental concerns (Lofthouse, Muehlenkamp, & Adler, 2008). Further still, as previously mentioned, some individuals develop an "addiction" to this behavior once they discover that this act provides them relief from the negative emotions they are experiencing.

As previously stated, NSSI was thought to exist only among adolescent Caucasian females. Recent research has dispelled this previous misconception and has found that NSSI behaviors exist among the elderly (e.g., Li & Conwell, (2010), the LGBTQ population (e.g., House, Van Horn, Coppeans, & Stepleman, 2011), and the minority ethnic groups (e.g., Bhui, McKenzie, & Rasul (2007). More often than not, the underlying catalyst to a NSSI or other maladaptive coping event such as drug or alcohol abuse is a traumatic event (Klonsky & Moyer, 2008). Seeing these negative coping mechanisms from a trauma-informed care (TIC) lens as well as operating within a culturally competent framework can begin the healing process. Treatments aimed at reducing stigma of addictions and NSSI-related behavior while operating from an evidence-based TIC perspective are necessary for alleviating these behaviors.

Practical Skills Related to Diagnosis, Practice, or Education

Interventions

The two most common interventions for NSSI are cognitive behavioral therapy (CBT) and dialectical behavior therapy (DBT). These interventions have been used mostly in inpatient settings with some limited research conducted in community settings. Another promising intervention is motivational interviewing (MI), which has mostly been used in the substance abuse field. These interventions will be discussed below via intervention studies and strengths, and weaknesses of these studies will be noted. It should be noted that many of the studies cited do not use the term NSSI or the definition cited previously. Also, due to the comorbidity of NSSI with other mental health diagnoses (e.g., borderline personality disorder, depression, anorexia nervosa, bulimia nervosa, post-traumatic stress disorder), some of the intervention studies noted do address both NSSI and another diagnosis. However, due to the dearth amount of intervention studies conducted using the abovementioned definition by the ISSS, all intervention studies found in the literature will be discussed.

Cognitive Behavioral Therapy CBT has been shown to be effective in treating self-injury. CBT is a goal oriented, brief, direct, and time-limited intervention that can be used both in a group or individual setting (Williams, 1984). The focus of this intervention is on the present rather than past behaviors. This intervention helps individuals learn new cognitive and behavioral skills for dealing with self-harming thoughts and behaviors (Slee, Garnefski, van der Leeden, Arensman, & Spinhoven, 2008). During treatment, the counselor works with the client to identify how their thoughts, feelings, and behaviors perpetuate their self-injury (Slee et al., 2008). The end goal is to change their maladaptive behaviors into behaviors that are less harmful. Clients are given homework to reinforce what they learned during the session (Williams, 1984). Studies using CBT as an intervention for self-harming behavior have found that in conjunction with the client's normal treatment (i.e., pharmacotherapy, psychotherapy, or inpatient treatment) was more effective at treating self-harming behavior than stand-alone treatment as usual (Slee et al., 2008). Additionally, manual-assisted CBT (MACT) in comparison with treatment as usual (TAU) had lower rates of suicidal ideation, although low sample size of this study ($n = 34$) prohibits generalizability of these results (Evans et al., 1999). However, the results of these forms of CBT treatment show promise with this behavior.

Dialectical Behavior Therapy Dialectical behavior therapy (DBT; Linehan, 1993), a form of CBT, is a time-limited structured intervention that is most often used for treating individuals with borderline personality disorder (BPD). Developed by Marsha Linehan for use with women who were diagnosed with borderline personality disorder (BPD; Linehan, 1993), DBT has been shown to work with individuals who have emotion regulation problems, and given that some individuals who engage in NSSI also have problems with emotion regulation, this intervention is promising for this group (Klonsky, 2007a). One of the hallmark features of BPD is self-harming behavior, particularly cutting, and therefore many researchers and practitioners have reported using this treatment for their clients who engage in NSSI with successful results (e.g., Chapman, Derbidge, Cooney, Hong, & Linehan, 2009). Traditional inpatient DBT can last up to a year in length; however, there are some recent studies that are looking at the effectiveness of shorter, outpatient treatments (e.g., Miller, Rathus, & Linehan, 2007) (Nock, Teper, & Hollander, 2007). DBT helps the client reduce their self-injurious behavior by teaching them new coping skills (Muehlenkamp, 2006), which consists of both group and individual sessions and focuses on goal setting and replacing the self-harming behavior with other, healthier behaviors (Favazza, 1998). Like other interventions, DBT does not work for every individual with NSSI. This may be because self-injuring behavior, while oftentimes the presenting problem, is not the main issue of concern. Regardless, at this point in time, DBT is considered the "gold standard" for treatment of NSSI (Miller & Smith, 2008, p. 179).

Research on DBT for individuals who engage in NSSI in the absence of a diagnosis of BPD is limited. This intervention has been shown in clinical studies (Linehan et al., 2006 as cited in Nock et al., 2007; Muehlenkamp, 2006 as cited in Nock et al., 2007) to be effective at reducing self-injurious behavior and has also shown promise in adolescent populations (Nock et al., 2007). Although research on DBT for individuals who self-injure and have the diagnosis of BPD has yielded positive results, the major flaws with these studies is that they do not single out self-injury so findings on the effectiveness of DBT for self-injury are difficult to ascertain (Trepal & Wester, 2007). However, DBT has shown to be effective in both adult and adolescent populations (Nock et al., 2007).

Motivational Interviewing MI has shown success with individuals who are addicted to alcohol and other drugs such as cocaine (Stotts, Schmitz, Rhoades, & Grabowski, 2001). Developed by Miller and Rollnick (1991, 2002), MI is a counseling intervention that is client-driven and seeks to bring about change in the client's behaviors by helping them solve their ambivalence and promote change (Rubak, Sandbaek, Lauritzen, & Christiansen, 2005). It also guides the client through the process of change via the transtheoretical model (Prochaska & DiClemente, 1984) and its stages of change: precontemplation, contemplation, preparation, action, and maintenance. MI is useful in helping the client recognize on their own that there is a current problem and how this problem is having an impact on their lives (Rubak et al., 2005). MI has also been shown to be effective for use in the treatment of anxiety disorders (Slagle & Gray, 2007), sexual addictions (Del Giudice & Kutinsky, 2007), and smoking cessation (Thyrian et al., 2007).

From a developmental standpoint, MI is more appropriate for adolescents who are resistant to changing their behavior as well as resistant to instructions from others. Boyle (2007) has indicated that interviewing adolescents can be very difficult since adolescents are at different developmental stages and what they are willing to discuss varies. Also, adolescents may turn to their friends for support (Boyle, 2007), especially if their group of friends also engages in self-injury.

There is also evidence of a "contagion" factor within middle and high schools as well as in psychiatric settings (Berman & Wallace, 2007; Helibron & Prinstein, 2008; Hooley, 2008; Kamen, 2009). Some research has shown that when an individual with a history of NSSI is in a closed environment, others may begin to engage in the behavior that may not have a history of NSSI (Helibron & Prinstein, 2008). Muehlenkamp, Hoff, Licht, Azure, and Hasenzahl (2008) found empirical support for a social learning aspect of NSSI in which conformity to engage in NSSI among a group of individuals takes place regardless of gender. In fact, Muehlenkamp et al. (2008) found support for an association between an individual being exposed to NSSI and subsequent higher rates of NSSI among those who had been exposed to NSSI from those in their peer group. A subculture of "cutters" may develop within this closed environment, and new and accepted identities as a "cutter" are fostered within the group (Adler & Adler, 2008). Muehlenkamp et al. (2008) argue that perhaps the "spread" of NSSI is similar to what occurred in the 1980s among those with anorexia nervosa in that the media helped to fuel the contagion.

Implications for Future Practice, Research, and Education

There are numerous avenues for future research in regard to NSSI. One of those avenues should explore the benefits of MI with individuals who engage in self-injury, especially adolescents. Moreover, additional research should be conducted in community settings, especially schools, to ascertain exact prevalence rates in this setting. More research is needed to determine what best practice is for adolescents engaging in self-injury since this is the population most vulnerable to self-injury. Research should also be conducted on various ethnic and racial backgrounds since most of the research conducted has been on Caucasian populations. Finally, future research should explore cultural implications to ascertain whether this plays a factor in whether an individual develops this behavior or not.

Knowledge of NSSI is imperative for any social worker or mental health professional working with adolescents or young adults. Understanding how maladaptive coping mechanisms such as NSSI and addictions can often overlap is salient. In addition, knowing how to respond appropriately when an individual discloses is also critical. Trepal and Wester (2007) conducted a mail survey of mental health professionals to assess how many individuals they see that self injure and what treatments they use when working with these clients. They mailed out 1000 surveys and received a very low response rate of 9% (81 surveys returned; however 7 were dropped since they noted they were educators or students and the authors were only seeking data from mental health professionals). Out of the final sample of surveys, 81% of the mental health professionals surveyed stated that they have/had clients that engage(d) in self-injury. When asked about the intervention(s) used to treat these individuals, the most cited intervention was cognitive behavioral therapy with 40.5% of the counselors reporting its use; DBT was the next most frequently cited at 17.6%, while MI was only used by 1.4% of the counselors (Trepal & Wester, 2007). One possible reason for the low percentage of MI could be due to the lack of empirical support of this intervention with this population. As previously discussed, MI is a newer intervention for NSSI, so the groundwork on this intervention with this population has yet to be laid. A major limitation with this study is the low number of responses. Perhaps if the research team had done some follow-up on the surveys, if contact information was available, the response to the surveys would have been higher.

Clinician's Reactions to Disclosure

Individuals who engage in NSSI can be met with frustration from clinicians about their self-injury and the disclosure of their behavior. One reason for this is either a lack of experience or knowledge or not having encountered an individual who self-injures. Shaw (2002) notes in her qualitative study of women who self-injure that clinicians view individuals who engage in this behavior and refer to this population as "treatment resistant" (Shaw, 2002, p. 200). If they are also engaging in other forms of maladaptive behaviors (such as alcohol use), then treatment of these behaviors becomes a bit murky, and the clinician and the client must work on determining which behavior to treat first.

Not all individuals who self-injure need intervention or treatment as some individuals cease the behavior as they mature (Muehlenkamp, 2005). However, others do not stop engaging in self-injury and may need treatment to cease the behavior. This latter group is the one that needs the most attention from researchers and clinicians. Research should also consider what makes these two groups different so that clinicians can better treat individuals who self-injure early on.

Mental health providers need to understand why the behavior is utilized in the first place while not insisting that the client cease the behavior since this can be detrimental to treatment (Ferentz, 2002; Suyemoto & MacDonald, 1995; Warm et al., 2003). Instead, helping clients find a better coping strategy should be a focus of treatment (Haines & Williams, 1997). Research has shown that individuals who engage in self-injury have poor coping abilities across the board (Evans, 2000; Haines & Williams, 1997), so aiding them in finding a better coping strategy that will help them in all aspects of their life would be useful.

Research has shown that there are some addictive qualities to self-injury (Nixon, Cloutier, & Aggarwal, 2002; Turner, 2002; Victor, Glenn, & Klonsky, 2012). The act of cutting or burning causes a temporary euphoric "high" for the individual due to endorphins rushing to the affected area of the cut or burn. The individual then feels better and can return to a previous state of calm that occurred prior to the building up of the overwhelming feelings (Turner, 2002). This euphoric state and the relief that one feels after the act of self-injury can become addictive for some people, and they will return to this behavior when they experience overwhelming or stressful emotions (Nixon et al., 2002). In addition, for some individuals, seeing blood after an injury can reinforce the behavior, as this serves to calm them and make them feel better (Glenn & Klonsky, 2010).

This current work, albeit a smaller and newer area of the literature, has looked at NSSI within an addictions framework (Turner, 2002) or has examined potential addictive features of NSSI (Nixon et al., 2002). Hyman's (1999) book discussing her qualitative study found that some of participants view their self-injury as an addiction. Moreover, these participants mentioned that they first had an addiction to drugs or alcohol and then switched to self-injury suggesting a substitution of maladaptive coping mechanisms. Other studies discuss the various features of NSSI that fit within the addictions framework without empirical support (e.g., Turner, 2002). However, no research to date has specifically tested the theory that someone could be addicted to NSSI except for work by Victor et al. (2012), which compares craving within substance use and within NSSI. Victor et al. (2012) also concluded that craving for NSSI was enacted when an individual was dealing with negative emotions, providing further evidence that NSSI is used to quell negative feelings. While there is some literature on the endogenous opioids and their effects on the body after cutting (Sher & Stanley, 2008; Stanley et al., 2009) some of which has been used to support the addictive aspect of NSSI, there is not enough literature to date to support the biological processes that occur in cravings or changes in brain structures due to NSSI.

There exists the possibility that NSSI could meet the DSM criteria of addiction as there are many aspects of it that may overlap. Withdrawal from addictions involving substance or alcohol abuse can vary by substance; however, most of the symptoms include agitation, shaking, sweating, confusion, anxiety, and panic (Miller & Kipnis, 2006). While there has been no empirical evidence of withdrawal from self-injury (Faye, 1995), it stands to reason that if an individual is accustomed to the feelings they experience from self-injuring and the behavior ceases, they may feel anxiety, agitation, and panic since they are no longer engaging in the behavior that allows them to endure intense, negative emotions. The Cornell Research Program on Self-Injurious Behavior in Adolescents and Young Adults has suggested that since self-injury activates the endogenous opioid system, repeated activation of this system (i.e., repetitive self-injury) could produce a significant withdrawal response that may serve to perpetuate future NSSI (www.crpsib.com/whatissi.asp). The most relevant withdrawal model for this study would be the negative reinforcement model of addiction. This model suggests that individuals continue to engage in substance abuse to avoid the negative and often difficult symptoms associated with substance abuse withdrawal. Additionally, studies have shown that individuals who engage in self-injury report feeling numb during and immediately after the act of self-injury (Sutton, 2004). In addition, some individuals report feeling little to no pain during the action, which also points to dissociation (Favazza, 1992; Muehlenkamp, 2005). This numbing effect is a form of dissociation and can become problematic for a person over time. It is also within this numbing effect that we may find aspects of addiction, so future exploration into dissociation along with other aspects related to addiction is warranted. Additional areas of exploration should examine the withdrawal, tolerance, and preoccupation aspects of addiction as it relates to NSSI, which are the other three remaining DSM-IV diagnostic criteria for addiction.

Conclusion

The potential overlap or co-occurrence of NSSI and other maladaptive coping mechanisms such as drug or alcohol addictions among adolescents and young adults is an emerging area of research, one that needs further exploration. Interventions that are normed on adults may not always be appropriate for adolescents given the difference in developmental stages. Examining how NSSI could potentially be considered an addiction may answer many questions about why individuals resort to maladaptive coping mechanisms when encountering stressful, negative, or overwhelming emotions.

References

Adler, P. A., & Adler, P. (2008). Self-injury. In C. M. Renzetti & J. L. Edleson (Eds.), *Encyclopedia of interpersonal violence*. (Vol. 2). Thousand Oaks, CA: Sage Publications.

Alfonso, M. L., & Kaur, R. (2012). Self-injury among early adolescents: Identifying segments protected and at risk. *Journal of School Health, 82*(12), 537–547.

Andover, M. S., Pepper, C. M., & Gibb, B. E. (2007). Self-mutilation and coping strategies in a college sample. *Suicide & Life-Threatening Behavior, 37*, 238–243.

Berman, J., & Wallace, P. H. (2007). *Cutting and the pedagogy of self-disclosure*. Amherst, MA: The University of Massachusetts Press.

Bhui, K., McKenzie, K., & Rasul, F. (2007). Rates, risk factors & methods of self harm among minority ethnic groups in the UK: A systematic review. *BMC Public Health, 7*(336), 1–14.

Boyle, C. (2007). The challenge of interviewing adolescents: Which psychotherapeutic approaches are useful in educational psychology? *Educational and Child Psychology, 24*(1), 36–45.

Briere, J., & Gil, E. (1998). Self-mutilation in clinical and general population samples: Prevalence, correlates, and functions. *American Journal of Orthopsychiatry, 68*, 609–620.

Brown, S. A., Tate, S. R., Vik, P. W., Haas, A. L., & Aarons, G. A. (1999). Modeling of alcohol use mediates the effect of family history of alcoholism on adolescent alcohol expectancies. *Experimental and Clinical Psychopharmacology, 7*(1), 20–27.

Chapman, A. L., Derbidge, C. M., Cooney, E., Hong, P. Y., & Linehan, M. M. (2009). Temperament as a prospective predictor of self-injury among patients with borderline personality disorder. *Journal of Personality Disorders, 23*(2), 122–140.

Chartrand, H., Sareen, J., Toews, M., & Bolton, J. M. (2012). Suicide attempts versus nonsuicidal self-injury among individuals with anxiety disorders in a nationally representative sample. *Depression and Anxiety, 29*, 172–179.

Chassin, L., Pitts, S., DeLucia, C., & Todd, M. (1999). A longitudinal study of children of alcoholics: Predicting young adult substance use disorders, anxiety, and depression. *Journal of Abnormal Psychology, 108*(1), 106–119.

Christiansen, B. A., Smith, G. T., Roehling, P. V., Goldman, M. S., Crano, W. D., Siegel, J. T., et al. (2008). Using alcohol expectancies to predict adolescent drinking behavior after one year. *Journal of Consulting and Clinical Psychology, 57*(1), 93–99.

Claes, L., Vandereycken, W., & Vertommen, H. (2001). Self-injurious behaviors in eating-disordered patients. *Eating Behaviors, 2*, 263–272.

Claes, L., Vandereycken, W., & Vertommen, H. (2007). Self-injury in female versus male psychiatric patients: A comparison of characteristics, psychopathology and aggression regulation. *Personality and Individual Differences, 42*, 611–621.

D'Amico, E. J., Barnett, N. P., Monti, P. M., Colby, S. M., Spirito, A., & Rohsenow, D. J. (2002). Does alcohol use mediate the association between alcohol evaluations and alcohol-related problems in adolescents? *Psychology of Addictive Behaviors, 16*(2), 157–160.

Del Giudice, M. J., & Kutinsky, J. (2007). Applying motivational interviewing to the treatment of sexual compulsivity and addiction. *Sexual Addiction and Compulsivity: The Journal of Treatment and Prevention, 14*(4), 303–319.

DiClemente, R. J., Ponton, L. E., & Hartley, D. (1991). Prevalence and correlates of cutting behavior: Risk for HIV transmission. *Journal of the American Academy of Child and Adolescent Psychiatry, 135*, 735–739.

Eliseo-Arras, R. (2016). *Maternal mental health and alcohol use and the impact on daughter's mental health, communication, and risky sexual behavior in a dyadic longitudinal community sample* (Order No. 10127748). Available from Dissertations & Theses @ SUNY Buffalo. (1798476685). Retrieved from http://search.proquest.com.gate.lib.buffalo.edu/docview/17984 76685?accountid=14169.

Evans, J. (2000). Interventions to reduce repetition of deliberate self-harm. *International Review of Psychiatry, 12*, 44–47.

Evans, K., Tyrer, P., Catalan, J., Schmidt, U., Davidson, K., Dent, J., et al. (1999). Manual-assisted cognitive-behavioral therapy (MACT): A randomized controlled trial of a brief intervention with bibliotherapy in the treatment of recurrent deliberate self-harm. *Psychological Medicine, 29*, 19–25.

Favazza, A. R. (1992). Repetitive self-mutilation. *Psychiatric Annals, 22*, 60–63.

Favazza, A. R. (1998). The coming of age of self-mutilation. *The Journal of Nervous and Mental Disease, 186*(5), 259–268.

Favazza, A. R., DeRosear, L., & Conterio, K. (1989). Self-mutilation and eating disorders. *Suicide and Life-threatening Behavior, 19*, 113–127.

Favazza, A. R., & Favazza, B. (1987). *Bodies under siege: Self-mutilation in culture and psychiatry*. Baltimore: The Johns Hopkins University Press.

Ferentz, L. (2002). Case studies: When treating self-harming clients, therapists must first get past their own anxiety. *Psychotherapy Networker, 26*(5), 69–78.

Fortune, S. (2006). An examination of cutting and other methods of DSH among children and adolescents presenting to an outpatient psychiatric clinic in New Zealand. *Clinical Child Psychology and Psychiatry, 11*(3), 407–416.

Faye, P. (1995). Addictive characteristics of the behavior of self-mutilation. *Journal of Psychosocial Nursing and Mental Health Services, 33*(6), 36–39.

Gladstone, G. L., Parker, G. B., Mitchell, P. B., Malhi, G. S., Wilhelm, K., & Austin, M.-P. (2004). Implications of childhood trauma for depressed women: An analysis of pathways from childhood sexual abuse to deliberate self-harm and revictimization. *American Journal of Psychiatry, 161*, 1417–1425.

Glenn, C. H., & Klonsky, E. D. (2010). The role of seeing blood in non-suicidal self-injury. *Journal of Clinical Psychology, 66*(4), 466–473.

Goodman, I., Peterson-Badali, M., & Henderson, J. (2011). Understanding motivation for substance use treatment: The role of social pressure during the transition to adulthood. *Addictive Behaviors, 36*(6), 660–668.

Gratz, K. L. (2001). Measurement of deliberate self-harm: Preliminary data on the deliberate self-harm inventory. *Journal of Psychopathology and Behavioral Assessment, 23*(4), 253–263.

Gratz, K. L., & Chapman, A. L. (2007). The role of emotional responding and childhood maltreatment in the development and maintenance of deliberate self-harm among male undergraduates. *Psychology of Men & Masculinity, 8*(1), 1–14.

Gratz, K. L., Conrad, S. D., & Roemer, L. (2002). Risk factors for deliberate self-harm among college students. *American Journal of Orthopsychiatry, 72*, 128–140.

Haines, J., & Williams, C. L. (1997). Coping and problem solving of self-mutilators. *Journal of Clinical Psychology, 53*(2), 177–186.

Harned, M. S., Najavits, L. M., & Weiss, R. D. (2006). Self-harm and suicidal behavior in women with comorbid PTSD and substance dependence. *The American Journal of Addictions, 15*, 392–395.

Hasking, P. A., Momeni, R., Swannell, S., & Chia, S. (2008). The nature and extent of non-suicidal self-injury in a non-clinical sample of young adults. *Archives of Suicide Research, 12*, 208–218.

Haw, C., Bergen, H., Casey, D., & Hawton, K. (2007). Repetition of deliberate self-harm: A study of the characteristics and subsequent deaths in patients presenting to a general hospital according to extent of repetition. *Suicide and Life-threatening Behavior, 37*(4), 379–396.

Haw, C., Hawton, K., Casey, D., Bale, E., & Shepherd, A. (2005). Alcohol dependence, excessive drinking and deliberate self-harm. *Social Psychiatry and Psychiatric Epidemiology, 40*(12), 964–971.

Hawton, K., & Sinclair, J. (2003). The challenge of evaluating the effectiveness of treatments for deliberate self-harm. *Psychological Medicine, 33*, 955–958.

Heath, N. L., Toste, J. R., Nedecheva, T., & Charlebois, A. (2008). An examination of nonsuicidal self-injury among college students. *Journal of Mental Health Counseling, 30*(2), 137–156.

Herpertz, S., Sass, H., & Favazza, A. (1997). Impulsivity in self-mutilative behavior: Psychometric and biological findings. *Journal of Psychiatric Research, 31*(4), 451–465.

Hilt, L. M., Cha, C. B., & Nolen-Hoeksema, S. (2008). Nonsuicidal self-injury in young adolescent girls: Moderators of the distress-function relationship. *Journal of Consulting and Clinical Psychology, 76*(1), 63–71.

Hooley, J. M. (2008). Self-harming behavior: Introduction to the special series on non-suicidal self-injury and suicide. *Applied and Preventive Psychology, 12*, 155–158.

House, A. S., Van Horn, E., Coppeans, C., & Stepleman, L. M. (2011). Interpersonal trauma and discriminatory events as predictors of suicidal and nonsuicidal self-injury in gay, lesbian, bisexual, and transgender persons. *Traumatology, 17*(2), 75–85.

Hyman, J. W. (1999). *Women living with self-injury*. Philadelphia: Temple University Press.

Helibron, N., & Prinstein, M. J. (2008). Peer influence and adolescent nonsuicidal self-injury: A theoretical review of mechanisms and moderators. *Applied and Preventive Psychology, 12*, 169–177.

Kamen, D. G. (2009). How can we stop our children from hurting themselves? Stages of change, motivational interviewing, and exposure therapy applications for non-suicidal self-injury in children and adolescents. *International Journal of Behavioral Consultation and Therapy, 5*(1), 106–123.

Kamphuis, J. H., Ruyling, S. B., & Reijntjes, A. H. (2007). Testing the emotion regulation hypothesis among self-injuring females. *The Journal of Nervous and Mental Disease, 195*(11), 912–918.

Kiesner, J., Poulin, F., & Dishion, T. J. (2010). Adolescent substance use with friends: Moderating and mediating effects of parental monitoring and peer activity contexts. *Merrill-Palmer Quarterly, 56*(4), 529–556.

Klonsky, E. D. (2007a). Non-suicidal self-injury: An introduction. *Journal of Clinical Psychology: In Session, 63*, 1039–1043.

Klonsky, E. D. (2007b). The functions of deliberate self-injury: A review of the evidence. *Clinical Psychology Review, 27*, 226–239.

Klonsky, E. D., & Moyer, A. (2008). Childhood sexual abuse and non-suicidal self-injury: A meta-analysis. *The British Journal of Psychiatry, 192*, 166–170.

Klonsky, E. D., & Muehlenkamp, J. J. (2007). Self-injury: A research review for the practitioner. *Journal of Clinical Psychology: In Session, 63*, 1045–1056.

Klonsky, E. D., & Olino, T. M. (2008). Identifying clinically distinct subgroups of self-injurers among young adults: A latent class analysis. *Journal of Consulting and Clinical Psychology, 76*(1), 22–27.

Kponee, K. Z., Siegel, M., & Jernigan, D. H. (2014). The use of caffeinated alcoholic beverages among underage drinkers: Results of a national survey. *Addictive Behaviors, 39*(1), 253–258.

Laye-Gindhu, A., & Schonert-Reichl, K. A. (2005). Nonsuicidal self-harm among community adolescents: Understanding the "whats"and "whys" of self-harm. *Journal of Youth and Adolescence, 34*, 447–457.

Levesque, C., Lafontaine, M.-F., Bureau, J.-F., Cloutier, P., & Dandurand, C. (2010). The influence of romantic attachment and intimate partner violence on non-suicidal self-injury in young adults. *Journal of Youth and Adolescence, 39*, 474–483.

Li, L. W., & Conwell, Y. (2010). Pain and self-injury ideation in elderly men and women receiving home care. *Journal of the American Geriatrics Society, 58*(11), 2160–2165.

Linehan, M. M. (1993). *Cognitive-behavioral treatment of borderline personality disorder*. New York: The Guilford Press.

Lofthouse, N., Muehlenkamp, J. J., & Adler, R. (2008). Nonsuicidal self-injury and co-occurrence. In M. K. Nixon & N. L. Heath (Eds.), *Self-injury in youth* (pp. 59–78). New York: Routledge.

Linehan, M. M., Comtois, K. A., Murray, A. M., Brown, M. Z., Gallop, R. J., Heard, H. L., Korslund, K. E., Tutek, D. A., Reynolds, S. K., & Lindenboim, N. (2006). Two-year randomized controlled trial and follow-up of dialectical behavior therapy vs therapy by experts for suicidal behaviors and borderline personality disorder. *Archives of General Psychiatry, 63*(7), 757–766.

Miller, A. L., Rathus, J. H., & Linehan, M. M. (2007). *Dialectical behavior therapy with suicidal adolescents*. New York: Guilford Press.

Miller, A. L., & Smith, H. L. (2008). Adolescent non-suicidal self-injurious behavior: The latest epidemic to assess and treat. *Applied and Preventive Psychology, 12*, 178–188.

Miller, N. S., & Kipnis, S. S. (2006). *Detoxification and substance abuse treatment (TIP 45)*. Rockville, MD: Substance Abuse and Mental Health Services Administration.

Miller, W. R., & Rollnick, S. (1991). *Motivational interviewing: Preparing people to change addictive behavior*. New York: Guilford Press.

Miller, W. R., & Rollnick, S. (2002). *Motivational interviewing: Preparing people for change* (2nd ed.). New York: Guilford Press.

Moller, C. I., Tait, R. J., & Byrne, D. G. (2013). Deliberate self-harm, substance use, and negative affect in nonclinical samples: A systematic review. *Substance Abuse, 34*(2), 188–207.

Muehlenkamp, J. J. (2005). Self-injurious behavior as a separate clinical syndrome. *American Journal of Orthopsychiatry, 75*(2), 324–333.

Muehlenkamp, J. J. (2006). Empirically supported treatments and general therapy guidelines for non-suicidal self-injury. *Journal of Mental Health Counseling, 28*(2), 166–185.

Muehlenkamp, J. J., Claes, L., Smits, D., Peat, C. M., & Vandereycken, W. (2011). Non-suicidal self-injury in eating disordered patients: A test of a conceptual model. *Psychiatry Research, 188*, 102–108.

Muehlenkamp, J. J., & Gutierrez, P. M. (2004). An investigation of differences between self-injurious behavior and suicide attempts in a sample of adolescents. *Suicide and Life-Threatening Behavior, 34*, 12–23.

Muehlenkamp, J. J., Hoff, E. R., Licht, J.-G., Azure, J. A., & Hasenzahl, S. J. (2008). Rates of non-suicidal self-injury: A cross-sectional analysis of exposure. *Current Psychology, 27*, 234–241.

Muehlenkamp, J. J., Kerr, P. L., Bradley, A. R., & Larsen, M. A. (2010). Abuse subtypes and non-suicidal self-injury: Preliminary evidence of complex emotion regulation patterns. *Journal of Nervous and Mental Disease, 198*, 258–263.

Menninger, K. A. (1938). *Man against himself*. Oxford, England: Harcourt, Brace.

Nelson, A., & Muehlenkamp, J. J. (2012). Body attitudes and objectification in non-suicidal self-injury: Comparing males and females. *Archives of Suicide Research, 16*(1), 1–12.

Nixon, M. K., Cloutier, P. F., & Aggarwal, S. (2002). Affect regulation and addictive aspects of repetitive self-injury in hospitalized adolescents. *Journal of the Academy of Child and Adolescent Psychiatry, 41*(11), 1333–1341.

Nock, M. K. (2010). Self-injury. *Annual Review of Clinical Psychology, 6*, 339–363.

Nock, M. K., Joiner, T. E., Jr., Gordon, K. H., Lloyd-Richardson, E., & Prinstein, M. J. (2006). Non-suicidal self-injury among adolescents: Diagnostic correlates and relation to suicide attempts. *Psychiatry Research, 144*, 65–72.

Nock, M. K., & Prinstein, M. J. (2004). A functional approach to the assessment of self-mutilative behavior. *Journal of Consulting and Clinical Psychology, 72*(5), 885–890.

Nock, M. K., & Prinstein, M. J. (2005). Contextual features and behavioral functions of self-mutilation among adolescents. *Journal of Abnormal Psychology, 114*(1), 140–146.

Nock, M. K., Teper, R., & Hollander, M. (2007). Psychological treatment of self-injury among adolescents. *Journal of Clinical Psychology: In Session, 63*(11), 1081–1089.

Nock, M. K., Wedig, M. M., Holmberg, E. B., & Hooley, J. M. (2008). The emotion reactivity scale: Development, evaluation, and relation to self-injurious thoughts and behaviors. *Behavior Therapy, 39*, 107–116.

Patterson, J. M., & McCubbin, H. I. (1987). Adolescent coping style and behaviors: Conceptualization and measurement. *Journal of Adolescence, 10*(2), 163–186.

Paul, T., Schroeter, K., Dahme, B., & Nutzinger, D. O. (2002). Self-injurious behavior in women with eating disorders. *American Journal of Psychiatry, 159*(3), 408–411.

Prochaska, I. O., & DiClemente, C. C. (1984). *The transtheoretical approach*. Homewood, IL: Dorsey Press.

Purington, A., & Whitlock, J. L. (2004). *Self-injury fact sheet: Research facts and findings.* Retrieved from: http://selfinjury.bctr.cornell.edu/publications/2004_1.pdf.

Roger, D., Flynn, M., Borrill, J., & Fox, P. (2009). Students who self-harm: Coping style, rumination and alexithymia. *Counselling Psychology Quarterly, 22*(4), 361–372.

Romans, S. E., Martin, J. L., Anderson, J. C., Herbison, P. G., & Mullen, P. E. (1995). Sexual abuse in childhood and deliberate self-harm. *The American Journal of Psychiatry, 152*(9), 1336–1342.

Rome, E. S., & Ammerman, S. (2003). Medical complications of eating disorders: An update. *Journal of Adolescent Health, 33*, 418–426. https://doi.org/10.1016/j.jadohealth.2003.07.002.

Ross, S., & Heath, N. L. (2002). A study of the frequency of self-mutilation in a community sample of adolescents. *Journal of Youth and Adolescence, 31*(1), 67–77.

Ross, S., Heath, N. L., & Toste, J. R. (2009). Non-suicidal self-injury and eating pathology in high school students. *American Journal of Orthopsychiatry, 79*(1), 83–92.

Rubak, S., Sandbaek, A., Lauritzen, T., & Christiansen, B. (2005). Motivational interviewing: A systematic review and meta-analysis. *British Journal of General Practice, 55*, 305–312.

Shaw, S. N. (2002). Shifting conversations on girls' and women's self-injury: An analysis of the clinical literature in historical context. *Feminism & Psychology, 12*(2), 191–219.

Sher, L., & Stanley, B. H. (2008). The role of endogenous opioids in the pathophysiology of self-injurious and suicidal behavior. *Archives of Suicide Research, 12*(4), 299–308.

Slagle, D. M., & Gray, M. J. (2007). The utility of motivational interviewing as an adjunct to exposure therapy in the treatment of anxiety disorders. *Professional Psychology, 38*(4), 329–337.

Slee, N., Garnefski, N., van der Leeden, R., Arensman, E., & Spinhoven, P. (2008). Cognitive-behavioral intervention for self-harm: Randomized controlled trial. *The British Journal of Psychiatry, 192*, 202–211.

Stanley, B., Sher, L., Wilson, S., Ekman, R., Huang, Y.-Y., & Mann, J. J. (2009). Non-suicidal self-injurious behavior, endogenous opioids and monoamine neurotransmitters. *Journal of Affective Disorders, 124*(1), 134–140, in press.

Stotts, A. L., Schmitz, J. M., Rhoades, H. M., & Grabowski, J. (2001). Motivational interviewing with cocaine-dependent patients: A pilot study. *Journal of Consulting and Clinical Psychology, 69*(5), 858–862.

Sutton, J. (2004). Understanding dissociation and its relationship to self-injury and childhood trauma. *Counselling and Psychotherapy Journal, 15*(3), 24–27.

Suyemoto, K. L. (1998). The functions of self-mutilation. *Clinical Psychology Review, 18*(5), 531–554.

Suyemoto, K. L., & Macdonald, M. L. (1995). Self-cutting in female adolescents. *Psychotherapy, 32*(1), 162–171.

Svirko, E., & Hawton, K. (2007). Self-injurious behavior and eating disorders: The extent and nature of the association. *Suicide and Life-Threatening Behavior, 37*(4), 409–421.

Taylor, B. (2003). Exploring the perspectives of men who self-harm. *Learning in Health and Social Care, 2*(2), 83–91.

Thyrian, J. R., Freyer-Adam, J., Hannover, W., Roske, K., Mentzel, F., Kufeld, C., et al. (2007). Adherence to the principles of motivational interviewing, clients' characteristics and behavior outcome in a smoking cessation and relapse prevention trial in women postpartum. *Addictive Behaviors, 32*, 2297–2303.

Trepal, H. C., & Wester, K. L. (2007). Self-injurious behaviors, diagnoses, and treatment methods: What mental health professionals are reporting. *Journal of Mental Health Counseling, 29*(4), 363–375.

Turner, V. J. (2002). *Secret scars: Uncovering and understanding the addiction to self-injury.* Center City, MN: Hazelden.

U.S. Department of Health & Human Services. (2004). Alcohol's damaging effects on the brain. *Alcohol Alert, 63*, 1–7.

Victor, S. E., Glenn, C. R., & Klonsky, E. D. (2012). Is non-suicidal self-injury an "addiction"? A comparison of craving in substance use and non-suicidal self-injury. *Psychiatry Research, 197*, 73–77.

Warm, A., Murray, C., & Fox, J. (2003). Why do people self-harm? *Psychology, Health & Medicine, 8*(1), 71–79.

Weierich, M. R., & Nock, M. K. (2008). Posttraumatic stress symptoms mediate the relation between childhood sexual abuse and nonsuicidal self-injury. *Journal of Consulting and Clinical Psychology, 76*(1), 39–44.

Welch, S. S. (2001). A review of the literature on the epidemiology of parasuicide in the general population. *Psychiatric Services, 52*(3), 368–375.

Whiteman, S. D., Jensen, A. C., Mustillo, S. A., & Maggs, J. L. (2016). Understanding sibling influence on adolescents' alcohol use: Social and cognitive pathways. *Addictive Behaviors, 53*, 1–6.

Whitlock, J. L., Eckenrode, J., & Silverman, D. (2006). Self-injurious behaviors in a college population. *Pediatrics, 117*, 1939–1948.

Whitlock, J. L., & Knox, K. (2007). The relationship between suicide and self-injury in a young adult population. *Archives of Pediatrics and Adolescent Medicine, 161*(7), 634–640.

Williams, F., & Hasking, P. (2010). Emotion regulation, coping and alcohol use as moderators in the relationship between non-suicidal self-injury and psychological distress. *Prevention Science, 11*, 33–41.

Williams, J. M. G. (1984). Cognitive-behavior therapy for depression: Problems and perspectives. *British Journal of Psychiatry, 145*, 254–262.

Yates, T. M. (2004). The developmental psychopathology of self-injurious behavior: Compensatory regulation in posttraumatic adaptation. *Clinical Psychology Review, 24*, 35–74.

Yearwood, E. L., & Bosnick, E. (2012). Deliberate self-harm: Nonsuicidal self-injury and suicide in children and adolescents. In E. L. Yearwood, G. S. Pearson, & J. A. Newland (Eds.), *Child and adolescent behavioral health: A resource for advanced practice psychiatric and primary care practitioners in nursing* (pp. 187–203). Oxford, UK: Wiley-Blackwell.

Chapter 7
Comorbid Trauma and Substance Use Disorders

Amanda Sisselman-Borgia

Introduction

The treatment of substance use disorders (SUDs) goes hand in hand with understanding the health and mental health histories of our clients. Trauma histories and PTSD diagnoses are often found to exist comorbidly with substance use disorders, but are not always treated simultaneously. Treatment must consider the whole person, inclusive of physical and mental health symptoms and diagnoses. Treatment and professional training for SUDs does not always focus on the integration of trauma-informed care into the recovery process.

This chapter will focus on and define trauma in the context of a medical model of substance use disorders to understand best practices for treatment of comorbid substance use and trauma reactions/symptoms. Issues and skills related to cultural competence in this area will be discussed, as well as suggestions for evidence-based practices and screening protocols. Please note that the term substance use disorder will be used in place of substance abuse in order to be consistent with the newest terminology adapted by the *Diagnostic and Statistical Manual of Mental Disorders*, 5th edition (DSM-V) (American Psychological Association, 2014). The word addiction may be used interchangeably as well, as this is still a commonly used term in the literature.

A. Sisselman-Borgia (✉)
CUNY Lehman College, Department of Social Work, Bronx, NY, USA
e-mail: Amanda.sisselman@lehman.cuny.edu

© Springer International Publishing AG 2018   103
T. MacMillan, A. Sisselman-Borgia (eds.), *New Directions in Treatment,
Education, and Outreach for Mental Health and Addiction*, Advances in Mental
Health and Addiction, https://doi.org/10.1007/978-3-319-72778-3_7

The Inevitable Connection Between Trauma and Substance Abuse

Trauma, as defined in the DSM-V, involves experiencing or witnessing death, serious injury, and/or sexual violence as actual or threatened events within one of four contexts: directly experienced, witnessed, learned happened to a loved one, or repeated extreme exposure to details (such as in the case of first responders). In order to be diagnosed with post-traumatic stress disorder (PTSD), the DSM-V specifies that individuals must have had one of those experiences within one of the aforementioned contexts, experience some form of memories or flashbacks, some form of avoidance of the traumatic memories, and negative alterations in mood or numbing symptoms, such as amnesia surrounding traumatic events.

Substance users are more likely than general population to have PTSD symptoms. The rates are double that of general population among women (Najavits, Weiss, & Shaw, 1997). Trauma, specifically childhood trauma, is a big risk factor for substance use disorders in both men and women (Carlson & Dalenberg, 2000; Cosden, Larsen, Donahue, & Nylund-Gibson, 2015; Giordano et al., 2016). One study of individuals in treatment for substance use found that 85% of their participants experienced at least one traumatic event within their lifetime (Giordano et al., 2016). Individuals with a history of child abuse are ten times more likely to have a co-occurring mental health disorder, including PTSD (Banducci, Hoffman, Lejuez, & Koenen, 2014). Similarly, the presence of substance use disorders is also a risk factor for subsequent or further traumatic experiences. Having a family history of drug or alcohol misuse is associated with childhood maltreatment and trauma, which may lead to drug use later in life (Taplin, Saddichha, Li, & Krausz, 2014).

In his most recent book, *The Body Keeps the Score: Brain, Mind, and Body in the Healing of Trauma*, Bessel Van der Kolk (2015) asserts that those who have been traumatized are unable to tolerate memories of the traumatic event, so they often use drugs or alcohol to block out difficult memories. It is important to identify the types of traumas associated with substance abuse, whether it be child abuse, domestic violence, witnessing community violence, or experiencing or witnessing a serious accident (human or natural). Living in poverty exacerbates all of the abovementioned traumas, rendering the symptoms or reactions more severe. The more severe the trauma, the more likely a diagnosis of serious persistent mental illness; this includes PTSD associated with substance use disorders (Subica, Claypoole, & Wylie, 2012). A large study of over 4000 adolescents by Acierno et al. (2000) found that adolescents with histories of abuse or who had witnessed violence were at higher risk for substance abuse. Similarly, those who had PTSD symptoms were also at higher risk for substance abuse. Also, Caucasians were at higher risk than African Americans for substance abuse under these conditions (Acierno et al., 2000).

In addition to childhood trauma and abuse, experiencing interpersonal violence puts women at higher risk for SUDs (Weaver, Gilbert, El-Bassel, Resnick, & Noursi, 2015). Weaver et al. (2015) found that an average of 9% of women with domestic violence histories have SUD diagnoses. Domestic violence (DV) is also correlated with histories of child abuse and maltreatment, suggesting a complex portrait of risk factors for substance misuse for women who have survived DV. Substances may be used as a form of self-medication and as a coping mechanism to deal with such trauma as DV, as well as childhood abuse and witnessing community violence. Both the cognitive and physical symptoms of trauma reaction and PTSD diagnosis can lead to SUDs as individuals try to find ways to reduce symptoms and manage their emotions. For this reason, Ford and Russo (2006) recommend trauma-focused treatment that focuses on self-regulation of emotions and reactions, as this can help to alleviate symptoms and reduce relapse.

Individuals with longtime trauma histories are more likely to have difficulties with impulse control and emotion regulation, both of which are associated with SUDs (Weiss, Tull, Anestis, & Gratz, 2013). Similarly, studies have found better abstinence rates, fewer associated depressive symptoms, and fewer trauma symptoms in women who were in trauma-informed integrated treatment settings or groups versus those who were in usual care settings (Amaro, Chernoff, Brown, Arévalo, & Gatz, 2007; Amaro, Dai et al., 2007; Covington, Burke, Keaton, & Norcott, 2008; Morrissey et al., 2005). Interestingly, trauma integrated care also demonstrated better outcomes for ethnically diverse groups of women (Amaro, Chernoff et al., 2007; Amaro, Dai et al., 2007; Covington et al., 2008). Amaro, Chernoff et al. (2007) and Amaro, Dai et al. (2007) found that comorbid trauma and mental health symptoms were not predictive of retention issues in treatment, but that longer stays in the treatment process predicted symptom reduction. Interestingly, one recent study found that clients with a higher number of traumatic experiences reported increased satisfaction with treatment and trauma screening procedures (Sanford, Donahue, & Cosden, 2014).

Cultural Competence and Responsiveness

Cultural competence and responsiveness is of utmost importance in the context of comorbid trauma and SUDs. Understanding the dynamics and prevalence of comorbid trauma and SUDs in diverse communities is essential in order to be appropriately responsive. There are still heavy stigmas associated with seeking mental health and substance use treatment within many communities; thus education is paramount. A large study of 30,000 individuals in the USA demonstrated that ethnic minority groups were less likely to seek treatment for childhood trauma and abuse, as well as war-related trauma, even though they may be more likely to experience symptoms (Roberts, Gilman, Breslau, Breslau, & Koenen, 2011). Historical trauma often intersects with abuse histories and community violence, sometimes magnifying trauma symptoms among individuals of color. This can also make coping with trauma more difficult and lead to more SUDs as self-medication and coping mechanisms. This was particularly true among urban Native American adolescents and use of alcohol and illicit substances (Wiechelt, Gryczynski, Johnson, & Caldwell,

2012). Interestingly, a comparative study showed that the longer an adolescent lived in the USA and the further into the acculturation process they were, the higher the likelihood that they would use substances. This also held true when examined in samples utilizing Muslim and Christian adolescents (Badr, Taha, & Dee, 2014).

Use of brief treatment approaches that are designed to reach people in primary care settings might be most effective for people of color, as stigmas around mental health treatment and SUD treatment are particularly prevalent in communities of color (Blume, 2016). A meta-analysis of intervention studies found that interventions that were adapted to better understand cultural context had better outcomes and were four times more effective than those that did not take cultural context into account (Griner & Smith, 2006). However, while providing ethnic or racial matches for counselor/client in cases of SUD/trauma treatment might prove helpful for some, it was not associated with better treatment outcomes for African American individuals, regardless of gender, while it was more effective for Caucasians (Ruglass et al., 2014).

Cultural competence and responsiveness must also include individuals who identify as LGBTQ, as studies show that those who identify as sexual minority are more likely to experience multiple trauma victimizations and comorbid SUDs (Hughes, McCabe, Wilsnack, West, & Boyd, 2010). Multiple experiences of trauma victimization lead to higher likelihood of the development of SUDs. Encouraging gay-straight alliances (GSAs) in high schools might provide an antidote to bullying and create a less hostile environment for LGBTQ teens. Heck et al. (2014) found that LGBTQ teens who attended a school with a GSA were less likely to use cocaine and other illicit drugs, as well as prescription meds than teens whose schools did not have the GSA.

Practice with Individuals Who Have Comorbid Trauma and Substance Use Disorders

CBT and narrative therapies are two different, but effective ways to treat comorbid trauma symptoms and substance use disorders (Ford and Russo, 2006). It is imperative to develop concrete cognitive behavioral coping skills to understand and manage impulses and handle memories/flashbacks. However, telling one's narrative or story about substance abuse in the context of the trauma history and deciding how one will rewrite their story and move on with a more functional life that includes abstinence is another way to make a life shift. Ford and Russo (2006) provide a good review of both of these modalities in this context while describing their Trauma Adaptive Recovery Group Education and Therapy (TARGET) intervention for treating substance use in the context of trauma. A review of intervention studies examined different instruments used to screen for trauma and demonstrated both the association between trauma and SUD, as well as the importance for trauma screening in the SUD context (Weaver et al., 2015).

Family work is often an essential part of treatment for SUDs, whether the identified client is an adolescent or an adult. Many times the trauma relates to family histories or the trauma reactions greatly impact family members. Reviews of the literature reveal that family-based interventions are effective in treating adolescent SUDs (Kumpfer, 2014). The Strengthening Families Program has been found to be one of the most successful programs used to provide skills training to the entire family (Kumpfer, Xie, & O'Driscoll, 2012). Another study found that mothers of color impacted by the child welfare system had been disproportionately plagued by SUDs and trauma within their families (Stephens & Aparicio, 2017). Family history and the legacies that these histories leave behind have powerful impacts on the clients we serve.

In review, the following treatment suggestions might be helpful:

- Conduct trauma symptom screening prior to treatment to get a baseline.
- Provide trauma-informed environment training to all staff and employees to foster safe space for treatment and recovery that includes "trauma-informed" principles (Substance Abuse and Mental Health Services Administration [SAMHSA], 2014).
- Provision of integrated MH/trauma services is most effective, especially for women of color with trauma histories.
- Use of cognitive behavioral therapy to assist clients in managing nightmares and flashbacks and being able to function in daily life/interactions in combination with narrative and supportive psychodynamic therapy to understand attachment issues and reasons for certain reactions and behaviors (i.e., substance use as self-medicating, impulse control issues related to substance use and trauma, etc.).
- Family treatment models are effective in working with adolescents with SUDs.
- Screening for family histories of trauma is important for adolescents and adults dealing with SUDs.

Conclusion and Future Directions

It is clear that trauma and SUDs go hand in hand, creating difficult circumstances for clients and their families. Research is being done to learn more about these associations, but future research must focus more on the disproportionate number of individuals of color and individuals in poverty that suffer from comorbid trauma and SUDs. The impact on families is enormous, creating vicious cycles that repeat themselves over the generations. Research must also focus on new ways that SUD interventions can successfully integrate trauma care and screening into the work.

References

Acierno, R., Kilpatrick, D. G., Resnick, H., Saunders, B., De Arellano, M., & Best, C. (2000). Assault, PTSD, family substance use, and depression as risk factors for cigarette use in youth: Findings from the National Survey of adolescents. *Journal of Traumatic Stress, 13*(3), 381–396.

Amaro, H., Chernoff, M., Brown, V., Arévalo, S., & Gatz, M. (2007). Does integrated trauma informed substance abuse treatment increase treatment retention? *Journal of Community Psychology, 35*(7), 845–862.

Amaro, H., Dai, J., Arévalo, S., Acevedo, A., Matsumoto, A., Nieves, R., & Prado, G. (2007). Effects of integrated trauma treatment on outcomes in a racially/ethnically diverse sample of women in urban community-based substance abuse treatment. *Journal of Urban Health, 84*(4), 508–522.

American Psychiatric Association. (2014). American Psychiatric Association. DSM-5. APA DSM, 5.

Badr, L. K., Taha, A., & Dee, V. (2014). Substance abuse in Middle Eastern adolescents living in two different countries: Spiritual, cultural, family and personal factors. *Journal of Religion and Health, 53*(4), 1060–1074.

Banducci, A. N., Hoffman, E., Lejuez, C. W., & Koenen, K. C. (2014). The relationship between child abuse and negative outcomes among substance users: Psychopathology, health, and comorbidities. *Addictive Behaviors, 39*(10), 1522–1527.

Blume, A. W. (2016). Advances in substance abuse prevention and treatment interventions among racial, ethnic, and sexual minority populations. *Alcohol Research: Current Reviews, 38*(1), 47.

Carlson, E. B., & Dalenberg, C. J. (2000). A conceptual framework for the impact of traumatic experiences. *Trauma, Violence, & Abuse, 1*(1), 4–28.

Cosden, M., Larsen, J. L., Donahue, M. T., & Nylund-Gibson, K. (2015). Trauma symptoms for men and women in substance abuse treatment: A latent transition analysis. *Journal of Substance Abuse Treatment, 50*, 18–25.

Covington, S. S., Burke, C., Keaton, S., & Norcott, C. (2008). Evaluation of a trauma-informed and gender-responsive intervention for women in drug treatment. *Journal of Psychoactive Drugs, 40*(sup5), 387–398.

Ford, J. D., & Russo, E. (2006). Trauma-focused, present-centered, emotional self-regulation approach to integrated treatment for posttraumatic stress and addiction: Trauma adaptive recovery group education and therapy (TARGET). *American Journal of Psychotherapy, 60*(4), 335–355.

Giordano, A. L., Prosek, E. A., Stamman, J., Callahan, M. M., Loseu, S., Bevly, C. M., et al. (2016). Addressing trauma in substance abuse treatment. *Journal of Alcohol and Drug Education, 60*(2), 55.

Griner, D., & Smith, T. B. (2006). Culturally adapted mental health intervention: A meta-analytic review. *Psychotherapy: Theory,Research,Practice, Training, 43*, 531–548.

Heck, N. C., Livingston, N. A., Flentje, A., Oost, K., Stewart, B. T., & Cochran, B. N. (2014). Reducing risk for illicit drug use and prescription drug misuse: High school gay-straight alliances and lesbian, gay, bisexual, and transgender youth. *Addictive Behaviors, 39*(4), 824–828.

Hughes, T., McCabe, S. E., Wilsnack, S. C., West, B. T., & Boyd, C. J. (2010). Victimization and substance use disorders in a national sample of heterosexual and sexual minority women and men. *Addiction, 105*(12), 2130–2140.

Kumpfer, K. L. (2014). Family-based interventions for the prevention of substance abuse and other impulse control disorders in girls. *ISRN Addiction, 2014*, 23.

Kumpfer, K. L., Xie, J., & O'Driscoll, R. (2012, April). Effectiveness of a culturally adapted strengthening families program 12–16 years for high-risk Irish families. In *Child & Youth Care Forum* (41, 2, pp. 173–195). New York: Springer Publishing.

Morrissey, J. P., Jackson, E. W., Ellis, A. R., Amaro, H., Brown, V. B., & Najavits, L. M. (2005). Twelve-month outcomes of trauma-informed interventions for women with co-occurring disorders. *Psychiatric Services, 56*(10), 1213–1222.

Najavits, L. M., Weiss, R. D., & Shaw, S. R. (1997). The link between substance abuse and post-traumatic stress disorder in women. *The American Journal on Addictions, 6*(4), 273–283.

Roberts, A. L., Gilman, S. E., Breslau, J., Breslau, N., & Koenen, K. C. (2011). Race/ethnic differences in exposure to traumatic events, development of post-traumatic stress disorder, and treatment-seeking for post-traumatic stress disorder in the United States. *Psychological Medicine, 41*(1), 71–83.

Ruglass, L. M., Hien, D. A., Hu, M. C., Campbell, A. N., Caldeira, N. A., Miele, G. M., & Chang, D. F. (2014). Racial/ethnic match and treatment outcomes for women with PTSD and substance use disorders receiving community-based treatment. *Community Mental Health Journal, 50*(7), 811–822.

Sanford, A., Donahue, M., & Cosden, M. (2014). Consumer perceptions of trauma assessment and intervention in substance abuse treatment. *Journal of Substance Abuse Treatment, 47*(3), 233–238.

Stephens, T., & Aparicio, E. M. (2017). "It's just broken branches": Child welfare-affected mothers' dual experiences of insecurity and striving for resilience in the aftermath of complex trauma and familial substance abuse. *Children and Youth Services Review, 73*, 248–256.

Subica, A. M., Claypoole, K. H., & Wylie, A. M. (2012). PTSD'S mediation of the relationships between trauma, depression, substance abuse, mental health, and physical health in individuals with severe mental illness: Evaluating a comprehensive model. *Schizophrenia Research, 136*(1), 104–109.

Substance Abuse and Mental Health Services Administration. (2014). *SAMHSA's concept of trauma and guidance for a trauma informed approach. HHS publication no. (SMA) 14–4884.* Rockville, MD: Substance Abuse and Mental Health Services Administration.

Taplin, C., Saddichha, S., Li, K., & Krausz, M. R. (2014). Family history of alcohol and drug abuse, childhood trauma, and age of first drug injection. *Substance Use & Misuse, 49*(10), 1311–1316.

Van der Kolk, B. A. (2015). The body keeps the score: Brain, mind, and body in the healing of trauma. Penguin Books.

Weaver, T. L., Gilbert, L., El-Bassel, N., Resnick, H. S., & Noursi, S. (2015). Identifying and intervening with substance-using women exposed to intimate partner violence: Phenomenology, comorbidities, and integrated approaches within primary care and other agency settings. *Journal of Women's Health, 24*(1), 51–56.

Weiss, N. H., Tull, M. T., Anestis, M. D., & Gratz, K. L. (2013). The relative and unique contributions of emotion dysregulation and impulsivity to posttraumatic stress disorder among substance dependent inpatients. *Drug and Alcohol Dependence, 128*(1), 45–51.

Wiechelt, S. A., Gryczynski, J., Johnson, J. L., & Caldwell, D. (2012). Historical trauma among urban American Indians: Impact on substance abuse and family cohesion. *Journal of Loss and Trauma, 17*(4), 319–336.

Chapter 8
Substance Abuse Among Older Adults: Context, Assessment, and Treatment

Justine McGovern and Stephanie Sarabia

Introduction

Through the lens of a case study, this chapter explores substance misuse among older adults in the context of changing global demographics and social work practice. From 2006 to 2050, the proportion of people age 60 and over is projected to increase from 11% to 22% of the global population (World Health Organization [WHO], 2016). The number of people over age 65 in the USA is projected to double from 2000 to 2040 (Administration on Aging [AoA], 2014). With increasing numbers of older adults living longer worldwide, the time has come for helping professionals and social service providers to prepare for meeting diverse needs of growing numbers of older clients, as well as for addressing evolving challenges to systems and societies struggling to meet those needs with few resources.

To this end, the chapter identifies trends in service provision that affect outcomes for older adults. Further, it provides a theoretical framework through which to deepen understanding of substance issues affecting older adults and introduces assessment and treatment approaches to better meet client needs. In addition, the chapter articulates implications for social work education, practice, and research. Specifically, it calls for increasing awareness about substance misuse affecting older adults, developing standards of practice that reflect cultural competence about late life, and implementing strategies to expand the workforce in gerontology and geriatric fields of practice.

J. McGovern (✉)
Lehman College, Department of Social Work, Bronx, NY, USA
e-mail: Justine.McGovern@Lehman.CUNY.edu

S. Sarabia
Ramapo College, Department of Social Work, Mahwah, NJ, USA

© Springer International Publishing AG 2018   111
T. MacMillan, A. Sisselman-Borgia (eds.), *New Directions in Treatment,
Education, and Outreach for Mental Health and Addiction*, Advances in Mental
Health and Addiction, https://doi.org/10.1007/978-3-319-72778-3_8

While some issues affecting older adults, such as health care, housing, and retirement, have gained a degree of prominence in social work research and practice, others remain underrepresented in the literature and in service provision (AoA, 2014). Largely invisible in scholarship and practice, substance misuse among older adults is increasingly suspected by helping professionals facing affected clients. Those who report their suspicions have, heretofore, felt underprepared in terms of how to recognize, assess, and treat clients affected by substance misuse (McGovern, 2016).

Significant knowledge gaps persist. For example, little is known about how substance misuse affects older adults over the long term, when misuse arises in later life in combination with other health issues, or how substances interact at nonregulated levels. Moreover, there is little research addressing the interaction of conditions, such as the long-term effects of trauma or malnutrition and substance misuse (McInnis-Dittrich, 2016). While the Office of Alcohol and Substance Abuse Services (OASAS) and Substance Abuse and Mental Health Services Administration (SAMHSA) are beginning to include information on older adult substance misuse, the lack of a dedicated focus on the issue contributes to a lack of evidence-based practice approaches to treating substance misuse and training opportunities for helping professionals (OASAS, 2016; SAMHSA, 2016).

Substance Misuse Among Older Adults: Context

Substance misuse is a significant and growing issue affecting older adults in the USA. Alcohol continues to outrank illicit drug use among adults over 65, but prescription drugs, especially painkillers such as opioids, are the fastest growing misused substances among older adults (SAMSHA, 2016). In the USA, the number of adults over 50 who are thought to have a substance use issue is expected to double to 5.7 million by 2020 (Wu & Blazer, 2011). While 6% of these persons have a diagnosable condition, many more exceed established healthy levels of the substance of choice, usually alcohol, without meeting criteria for alcoholism or drug addiction (SAMHSA, 2016b).

Many factors combine to put older adults at risk for substance misuse. These include genetics, socioeconomic factors, lived experiences, and health habits. Moreover, lack of social support such as family, friends, and community resources can worsen the effects of chronic illness and injury, the rates of which are higher among older adults than younger adults, causing higher rates of depression and anxiety as well. This can prompt overreliance on medications (McInnis-Dittrich, 2014). In addition, less education; poor health habits such as sleeplessness and oversleeping, overeating and undereating, as well as poor nutrition; and lack of access to medical care intersect with class, race, gender, ethnicity, sexual orientation, and gender identity to influence substance use across the life span (McInnis-Dittrich, 2016).

Although often gradual, the aging process itself can produce changes that put older adults at risk for developing problem substance use. As the body ages, its capacity to process alcohol and other drugs becomes less efficient. Due to decreased lean muscle mass and a slower digestive system, substances remain in the body longer resulting in higher levels of intoxication (Benshoff, Harrawood, & Koch, 2003; Shibusawa & Sarabia, 2015). This process is even more pronounced for aging women for whom gender-based disparities in tolerance increase over time (Kerr-Correa, Igami, Hiroce, & Tucci, 2007).

Beyond age, life stage also plays a part in substance use patterns among older adults (McInnis-Dittrich, 2014). Social changes common to later life can promote use of alcohol and mood-altering drugs. Aging is accompanied by multiple losses: loss of work with retirement; family roles as parenting decreases and family hierarchies are upended; loss of spouse, family, and friends due to death; physical capacity; and independence with the onset of physical and cognitive limitations. These compounded losses can contribute to increased rates of depression and anxiety, which can exacerbate underlying mental health issues. There is mounting evidence of a relationship between substance misuse and mental health issues among older adults (Nunes & Levin, 2004; Satre, Sterling, Mackin, & Weisner, 2011). National surveys estimate that 25% of adults over 65 meet the criteria for a mental health issue, such as depression or anxiety disorder, in the USA (SAMHSA, 2016b). Since co-occurring mental health and substance use disorders complicate the treatment of both disorders, it is essential to screen older adults for both to effectively provide treatment (Satre et al., 2011).

Relying on alcohol or prescription drugs to manage feelings associated with these losses is particularly apparent among women (Farkas, 2014). Gender is the greatest risk for substance abuse among older adults. Women are at greater risk for substance abuse as compared to men of the same age, especially women living on their own (Shibusawa & Sarabia, 2015). Several factors contribute to this disparity. Women have more body fat, less muscle mass, and a slower metabolism than men, which affects their processing of alcohol. In addition, women's bodies not only contain less water to dilute alcohol, but also alcohol remains in their bodies longer and at higher levels, with negative effects, referred to as the telescoping effect. Significantly, women advance more quickly into addiction and develop cirrhosis more quickly than men (Pape & Sarabia, 2014).

Early- and Late-Onset Alcohol Misuse

Most older adults suffering the ill-effects of alcohol use fall into one of two categories, those who are long-term users and those who started misusing alcohol later in life. Referred to as early-onset alcohol abusers, two-thirds of older adults with alcohol-related issues started drinking in their younger years. Long-term usage of high doses of alcohol puts older adults at risk for comorbid diagnoses, often requiring treatment that requires prescription medications, further complicating matters (NIAAA, 2016). Combining alcohol with complex medication prescriptions can cause additional problems, such as increasing rates of falls and delirium (McInnis-Dittrich, 2016).

Beyond physical ailments, alcohol abuse is associated with social issues, such as isolation and rejection by family members, unemployment and poor retirement preparation, and homelessness or poor living conditions. Further, older adults with early onset who have been drinking more than the recommended amounts for most of a lifetime account for two-thirds of older drinkers and are at greater risk for psycho-emotional issues, such as depression and enduring memory problems (Bogunovic, 2012). Prognosis for these individuals reflects the interaction of substances, poor physical health, and psycho-emotional vulnerability and is not good (McInnis-Dittrich, 2016). Studies suggest that the majority of older adults are also managing a chronic illness, which is more difficult to do if one is consuming alcohol (Center for Substance Abuse Treatment [CSAT], 1998).

In contrast, prognosis for persons abusing alcohol suddenly in later life is better, for several reasons. Often precipitated by a traumatic event, for example, death of a spouse, retirement, injury or health problems, or loneliness, late-onset alcohol misuse often presents without the long-term physical, social, and psycho-emotional effects and comorbid diagnoses that affect early-onset users. Moreover, late-onset alcohol abusers often benefit from stronger support systems and better overall health than persons who have been abusing alcohol for many years (McInnis-Dittrich, 2016).

Illicit Drug Use and Dependence

Persons abusing illicit drugs do not tend to live as long as those who do not, falsely suggesting that illicit drug use and dependence is not an issue among older adults. However, it is the definition of "old" that needs to be adjusted for this population. Due to ravages on the physical being and to social and emotional life, mortality rates for drug users are high (Reardon, 2012). Rates of hospital admission for drug use among mid-life adults have been rising since 1998. In contrast, alcohol-related admissions among the same demographic have remained the same (Reardon, 2012).

Born between 1946 and 1964, baby boomers have had a significant impact on many factors affecting quality of life for older adults, including recreational drug use. Specifically, social acceptance of recreational drug use reflects baby boomer advocacy and experiences many shared during the 1960s and 1970s. Among adults aged 50+, rates of marijuana and cocaine usage have doubled since the 1990s (McInnis-Dittrich, 2016).

Abuse and Misuse of Prescription Drugs

Where prescription medications are concerned, misuse refers to underuse, overuse, erratic use, and abuse, defined as nontherapeutic medication use, as well as medications that are misprescribed (Kalapatapu & Sullivan, 2010). Access to medications is easier, and prescription of medications is more common now than ever, which contributes to medication misuse. Amounts of prescription drug purchases by adults over 65 have increased to $15 billion a year, four times more than among younger populations. Moreover, symptoms of medication misuse are often difficult to separate from those of common conditions affecting older adults. Common symptoms include listlessness, confusion, depression or mania, cognitive issues such as memory loss, frequent falls, and more (McInnis-Dittrich, 2016).

There are many causes of medication misuse beyond prescription issues and drug interaction problems. Poor eyesight that impairs reading, memory issues that affect tracking dosages, irregular sleeping habits that cause confusion, and many more factors that affect older adults disproportionately can interfere with medication use (McInnis-Dittrich, 2016). Further, women over 55 are prescribed more mood-altering drugs than younger women and more than men of any age (Blow & Barry, 2002; Simoni-Wastila & Yang, 2006). Studies have also found that pharmaceutical advertising targets older women resulting in not only physician overprescribing but also older women requesting mood-altering substances from their doctors (Stevens, Andrade, & Ruiz, 2009). Relatedly, women are more likely to exhibit drug dependence later in life (Shibusawa & Sarabia, 2015).

Conceptual Framework: Ageism, Life Course, and Intersectionality

Ageism

Coined by Robert Butler (1969), ageism, defined as negative ageist beliefs, has been linked to negative outcomes for older adults not only because ageism influences how people view and interact with older adults in their personal lives but also because of how it guides professional decision-making in choosing an area of focus. Ageism is linked to high rates of isolation, loneliness, and depression, increased occurrences of injury and illness, and shortened life expectancy among older adults whose personal relationships often suffer with advancing age. Moreover, ageism is linked to a reluctance to join fields of gerontology and geriatrics among helping professionals (Reardon, 2012). This contributes to service gaps created by workforce shortages and skills gaps stemming from lack of cultural competence that reflects a failure to take the impact of age into account. Ageism can also contribute to insufficient funding to address issues of substance misuse among older adults. Moreover, ageism adds to fears about the future self and one's own aging process and is associated with poor intergenerational relations (Nelson, 2005). As a result, older adults are often increasingly underserved and isolated at the same time as their needs grow with advancing age, opening the door for significant risks, such as substance misuse.

Life Course Perspective

Because it explores how advantages and disadvantages accumulate across the life span, life course theory is well positioned to shed light on late-life experiences of diverse older adults. Life course theory suggests that diversity of experience throughout life contributes to diversity among older adults. Moreover, it argues that differences are worthy of close attention by social workers who need to understand a wide range of human experiences in order to effectively provide services and make policies in support of vulnerable populations (Vincent & Velkoff, 2010). Life course theory supports identification of transitions and trajectories in the lives of individuals, including transitions into later adulthood, by examining processes of aging, social contexts, cultural meanings, and the influences of historic period and cohort (Bengtson, Putney, & Johnson, 2005). Moreover, life course theory takes into account race, class, and gender as influential and intersecting factors across the life span (Stoller & Gibson, 2000).

Intersectionality

Furthering key concepts of life course theory, intersectionality theory posits that biological, social, and cultural factors, such as race, class, gender, religion, sexual orientation, and gender identification, interact in specific ways that not only sustain processes of oppression and power but also result in the concurrent experience of multiple levels of discrimination (Mattson, 2014; McCall, 2005; Murphy, Hunt, Zajicek, Norris, & Hamilton, 2009). Building on Black-feminist critical race theory, scholar and activist Kimberle Crenshaw (1991) developed intersectionality as a lens to view social issues with appreciation for the complex contribution of multiple identities. Crenshaw (1991) argued that it is not enough to view each identity in isolation, nor is it enough to simply add identities together, but rather all identities impact one another in numerous ways.

When biases against gender, sexual orientation, socioeconomic class, ethnicity, culture, and religion collide, persons can be marginalized on many levels at once (Hulko, 2009; McCall, 2005; Twigg & Martin, 2015). When age is added as an additional variable, cumulative disadvantages become significant, including health and quality of life disparities in late life, such as higher incidences of chronic illnesses, increased rates of depression, shorter life expectancy, and less utilization of available resources and services. This last point is significant because service utilization has been associated with improved outcomes in terms of physical and mental health, social support, and perceived well-being (Kolb, 2014). Combined, ageism, life course theory, and the intersectionality perspective provide a deeper understanding of the causes and consequences of substance misuse among older adults. Moreover, the theoretical framework suggests ways to better meet these clients' needs.

Providing Care: Assessment and Treatment

Assessment

Signs of substance misuse-related trouble include memory trouble after having a drink or taking medication; loss of coordination, walking unsteadily and frequent falls; unexplained bruises; and having trouble concentrating. Changes in behaviors such as sleeping or eating more or less, mood swings, failing to bathe, increased irritability, sadness, and depression can also be signs. In addition, wanting to spend more time alone and at home; retreat from family, friends, and social occasions; and loss of interest in activities previously thought enjoyable can also be indications of trouble (McInnis-Dittrich, 2016).

Despite these signs, detection of substance misuse can be elusive due to the isolation with which many older adults live (Shibusawa & Sarabia, 2015). Moreover, the signs can also suggest other health and social issues, thus leaving substance misuse undiagnosed. These assessment challenges indicate the need for focused screening to make an accurate assessment. One way to improve assessment is to incorporate screening for risky substance use as a part of regular primary medical care. Researchers have found success in reducing problematic substance use among older adults by incorporating screening tools and brief interventions into primary care (Schonfeld et al., 2015). Integrating a screening tool within a primary care visit not only embraces current best practices by adopting a more holistic approach to care but also reduces stigma associated with substance abuse treatment, which continues to be viewed as a moral failure rather than a mental health or social predicament (McInnis-Dittrich, 2016).

Commonly used screening tools deemed appropriate for older adults include the Alcohol Use Disorders Identification Test (AUDIT), the CAGE, and the Short Michigan Alcohol Screening Test – Geriatric Version (SMAST-G). Screening for problematic substance use during primary care visits suggests a shift toward a public health approach to the problem of substance misuse among older adults. One model supported by over 300 empirical studies as well as organizations such as SAMHSA and the World Health Organization (WHO) is the Screening, Brief Intervention, and Referral to Treatment (SBIRT). SBIRT aims to identify substance use that is harmful or risky to one's health and address any concerns with a brief intervention utilizing skills common to motivational interviewing. Social workers, or other trained health professionals, approach discussing substance use in a nonjudgmental, empathic, and client-centered way only concerned with reducing the risks associated with substance use. Using a brief intervention of approximately 20 min, social workers can identify any risks and have a focused nonjudgmental discussion with an older adult on a plan to reduce those risks, which may or may not include abstinence. Most often, clients can reduce their use in frequency or quantity to significantly diminish their health risks. Conversely, those requiring a higher level of care can be given a referral to appropriate treatment (Schonfeld et al., 2015).

Once an older adult is screened and evidence suggests that further assessment is warranted, a more thorough and comprehensive evaluation process begins, which can lead to diagnosing a substance use disorder. The commonly used *Diagnostic and Statistical Manual of Mental Disorders*, 5th Edition (DSM-5), outlines diagnostic criteria for substance use disorders but should be used cautiously with older adults (Farkas, 2014). For example, tolerance and withdrawal issues may have to be adjusted due to the impact of the aging body on the process. Loss of muscle mass and slowing digestion can significantly impact both tolerance and withdrawal in older adults (Blow & Barry, 2012).

Treatment: Brief, Private, and Personal

Research is only now beginning to take the experiences of older adults into account, where substance abuse is concerned. What little there is suggests that primary care settings, which are the preferred sites for older adults seeking health care, are the best points of entry for substance misuse care. These settings are perceived as more private and confidential, and as better shielding clients from stigma, than clinics (Schonfeld et al., 2015). In addition, brief interventions, such as SBIRT, promote positive outcomes among older adults (Schonfeld et al., 2015). The combination of private, short, and personalized sessions may be the best fit for this cohort, especially older women who associate more stigma to substance abuse problems than men of all ages and younger women (Shibusawa & Sarabia, 2015). In addition, women, in particular, benefit from individualized treatment approaches. Women report that specific information about how a particular substance is negatively affecting one's body has a larger impact than a general warning about the negative health effects of all substances (Shibusawa & Sarabia, 2015). Further, maintaining a therapeutic stance that is empathic and supportive increases the likelihood that an older client will engage with treatment and follow through with recommendations (National Institute on Alcohol Abuse and Alcoholism [NIAAA], 2005).

In addition, service providers need to take life stage into account. Identifying and addressing stressors that are related to the aging process, such as loss and bereavement and making referrals to age-appropriate services such as Alcoholics Anonymous for seniors and Services and Advocacy for GLBT Elders (SAGE), can promote better treatment outcomes. Further, maintaining a flexible treatment program that meets the changing physical, psychological, and social needs of the clients is essential. Particularly relevant to diverse neighborhoods such as Inwood-Washington heights, providing treatments that are culturally and linguistically appropriate for diverse older adults is crucial, and having a culturally competent, prepared workforce is crucial as well.

Case Study: Washington Heights and Inwood

With 71% of Washington Heights and Inwood residents identified as Latino, it is vital to become familiar with the perceptions and experiences of older Latino adults in regard to substance use. Research suggests that cultural values common to the Latino community can function as a protective factor both in avoiding substance use and in recovering from a substance use disorder (Flores et al., 2014). For example, the cultural value of familismo stresses putting the family before individual needs, creating a strong support system, and providing a protective factor against developing a substance use disorder. However, studies reveal that as Latinos acculturate, familismo decreases along with its protective properties (Prado, Szapocznick, Maldonado-Molina, Schwartz, & Pantin, 2008). Building on the cultural value of familismo is personalismo, which is defined as warmth and connection to others. This supportive connection can also function as a protective factor, promoting the development of a support system that can function during times of stress (Smith, Sudore, & Perez-Stable, 2009). Conversely, if Latinos are more acculturated with disorganized or disconnected family relationships, the absence of these connections can contribute to greater vulnerability where both developing a substance use disorder and failing to recover from substance misuse are concerned (Cloud & Granfield, 2008). Knowledge of this context when addressing the problem of substance misuse among older Latinos can inform a more nuanced approach to assessment and treatment.

Located in upper Manhattan, the adjacent neighborhoods of Washington Heights and Inwood share similar demographics, social service needs, and more. Among a population reaching over 195,000, 71% of Washington Heights and Inwood residents are Latino and 48% are foreign born, hailing primarily from Latin America, Eastern Europe, and Russia. About 13% of the neighborhood residents, or about 28,000 people, are over 65, and almost one in four households counts one or more senior citizens among them. Average life expectancy is 83 (diNapoli & Bleiwas, 2015).

Notably, there are no statistics recording substance use among persons older than 65 living in Washington Heights and Inwood. However, statistics capturing the effects of health issues that can be related to substance misuse paint a community portrait with significant concerns stemming from substance use. In 2015, 1055 alcohol-related hospitalizations were recorded, and 779 drug-related hospitalizations were reported. Further, conditions often associated with drug and alcohol abuse, such as HIV, stroke, mental health diagnoses, diabetes, and premature death, underscore the prevalence of the issue (diNapoli & Bleiwas, 2015).

Service providers in the helping professions, including social workers, nurses, and senior center staff, report that substance misuse among older adults residing in the area is on the rise (McGovern, 2016). They attribute this to several causes. These include residents' trauma histories, immigration histories, domestic violence, and poverty. In addition, practitioners identify gentrification and intergenerational conflict as significant issues affecting quality of life among the neighborhoods' older residents. Growing rates of isolation, displacement, and lack of social support contribute to substance misuse (McGovern, 2016). While they report noticing increased occurrences of substance misuse among their older clients, practitioners are at a loss for assessing and treating clients they suspect of substance misuse.

Discussion

There are several reasons why substance misuse among older adults continues to flummox practitioners. Substance abuse is often discovered at work or in social circumstances, but older adults are often more isolated, having retired from work, engaging with smaller social circles, and often experiencing shrunken worlds. These can shield them from the eyes of potential care providers, contributing to unhealthy habits and poor outcomes (McInnis-Dittrich, 2016). Moreover, masking conditions often confound diagnosis. Symptoms of substance misuse often present as age-related conditions such as insomnia, gastrointestinal problems, sexual dysfunction, forgetfulness, dementia, and depression.

Age-based biases among formal and informal care partners also play a part in services and knowledge gaps continuing to affect vulnerable older clients (Rosen, Heberlein, & Engel, 2013). Service providers report hesitating to confront the older adult or refer him/her for treatment because of beliefs about late life. Beliefs such as older adults should not be forced to give up a life-long habit that is one of the few pleasures left for them to enjoy and forcing abstinence would be cruel at this stage of life and can interfere with decision-making among helping professionals (McGovern, 2016). In addition, the mistaken assumption that alcohol and substance abuse treatment is not effective for older adults despite evidence that older adults have better outcomes from treatment than younger adults continues to plague service provision (SAMHSA, 2016).

Viewing substance misuse among older adults from a life course and intersectionality perspective argues for adding age to the roster of identity factors that can negatively affect late-life outcomes. Moreover, it highlights the impact on health of a lifetime of multiple interacting identities, each with its own disadvantages, privileges, power, and social status (Rosenthal, 2016). Combining life course and intersectionality perspectives highlights how feelings of discrimination based on identity factors including age, as well as experiences of institutionalized forms of discrimination, accrue with advancing age and contribute to substance use disorders (Keyes, Hatzenbuehler, & Hasin, 2011). Significantly, belonging to multiple minority identities can result in intersectional invisibility, perpetuated among helping professionals who do not recognize, accept, or understand issues among older diverse clients (Purdie-Vaughns & Eibach, 2008). Viewed through the lens of ageism, life course theory, and the intersectionality perspective, it becomes apparent that service and knowledge gaps persist when meeting the needs of substance-misusing older adults.

Implications and Next Steps

There are implications for social work, mental health, and substance abuse professionals. Expanding social work educational goals, addressing recruitment into fields of gerontology and geriatrics, and implementing policies that support health equity across age groups are three areas that can contribute to better outcomes for substance-misusing older adults.

Where education is concerned, an initial recommendation is to extend the definition of cultural competence to include age. Embedding gerontology in core courses across the curricula of helping professions such as social work, nursing, health sciences, and more, integrating AGHE competencies into practice curricula, and implementing them in practice settings can increase age competency among practitioners and future practitioners. Further, courses that cover substance abuse could adopt a focus on its impact across the life span. Practitioners trained in age competency can contribute to developing and implementing a greater range of age-appropriate services to better meet older client needs. These might include Alcoholics Anonymous for seniors and flexible treatment programs that take the changing physical, psychological, and social needs of older clients into account.

Further, efforts extending beyond current policies may need to be implemented to meet rising service gaps. Specifically, recruiting from among mid-life students and mid-career practitioners may be more effective in filling service gaps than trying to reach traditional (younger) college students and early career practitioners. The potential benefits are twofold. Continuing education and training tailored to increasing scope of practice among seasoned social workers can renew workers' interest in their profession and reduce attrition, while also better meeting client needs (Poulin & Walter, 1993; Woodhead, Northrop, & Edelstein, 2014).

Worker burnout is a long-term issue among social workers and other health professionals practicing with older adults. Often the most experienced practitioners end up leaving the field (Poulin & Walter, 1993; Woodhead et al., 2014). Significantly, both job and client satisfaction ratings improve when the age gap between worker and client shrinks among clients 65+. Training professionals for a wide range of settings, including senior centers, medical practices, housing complexes, and more, can make a positive difference in both practitioners' and clients' lives.

In addition to service gaps, knowledge gaps about a wide range of experiences affecting diverse older adults persist. For example, little is known about the cumulative impact of war experiences, domestic violence, sexual abuse, and other trauma on substance use among older adults. Future lines of inquiry need to explore these content areas and to make use of methods tailored to their capacities and life stage. Increasing inclusivity in research to promote knowledge-building about the experiences of older adults in general could contribute to improved outcomes for this population. Ultimately, the combination of competence building among social workers and policy development that promotes health equity across the life span can address service and knowledge gaps that contribute to significant health and social justice disparities affecting some of the most vulnerable clients, older substance users.

References

Administration on Aging. (2014). *A profile of older Americans: 2014.* Washington, DC: Administration on Aging, Administration for Community Living, U.S. Department of Health and Human Services.

Bengtson, V. L., Putney, N. M., & Johnson, M. L. (2005). The problem of theory in gerontology today. In M. L. Johnson (Ed.), *The Cambridge handbook of age and ageing* (pp. 3–20). Cambridge, UK: Cambridge University Press.

Benshoff, J. J., Harrawood, L. K., & Koch, D. S. (2003). Substance abuse and the elderly: Unique issues and concerns. *Journal of Rehabilitation, 69*(2), 43–48.

Blow, F. C., & Barry, K. L. (2002). Use and misuse of alcohol among older women. *Alcohol Research & Health, 26*, 308–315.

Blow, F. C., & Barry, K. L. (2012). Alcohol and substance misuse in older adults. *Current Psychiatry Reports, 14*, 310–319.

Bogunovic, O. (2012). Substance abuse in aging and elderly adults. *Psychiatric Times.* Retrieved from http://www.psychiatrictimes.com/geriatric-psychiatry/substance-abuse-aging-and-elderly-adults/page/0/3.

Butler, R. (1969). Age-ism: Another form of bigotry. *The Gerontologist, 9*(4), 243–246.

Center for Substance Abuse Treatment. (1998). Chapter 2 – Alcohol. In *Substance abuse among older adults.* Rockville, MD: Substance Abuse and Mental Health Services Administration (US). (Treatment improvement protocol (TIP) series, No. 26.). Available from: https://www.ncbi.nlm.nih.gov/books/NBK64412/.

Cloud, W., & Granfield, R. (2008). Conceptualizing recovery capital: Expansion of a theoretical construct. *Substance Use & Misuse, 43*(12/13), 1971–1986.

Crenshaw, K. (1991). Mapping the margins: Intersectionality, identity politics, and violence against women of color. *Stanford Law Review, 43*, 1241–1299.

diNapoli, T., & Bleiwas, K. (2015). *An economic snapshot of Washington Heights and Inwood.* New York, NY: Office of the State Comptroller.

Farkas, K. J. (2014). Assessment and treatment of older adults with substance use disorders. In S. L. S. Straussner (Ed.), *Clinical practice with substance abusing clients* (3rd ed., pp. 421–441). New York, NY: Guilford Press.

Flores, D. V., Torres, L. R., Torres-Vigil, I., Bordnick, P. S., Ren, Y., Torres, M. I., et al. (2014). From "kickeando las malias" (kicking the withdrawals) to "staying clean": The impact of cultural values on cessation of injection drug use in aging Mexican-American men. *Substance Use & Misuse, 49*, 941–954.

Hulko, W. (2009). The time and context-contingent nature of intersectionality and interlocking oppressions. *Affilia, 24*(1), 44–55.

Kalapatapu, R. K., & Sullivan, M. A. (2010). Prescription use disorders in older adults. *American Journal of Addiction, 19*(6), 515–522.

Kerr-Correa, F., Igami, T. Z., Hiroce, V., & Tucci, A. M. (2007). Patterns of alcohol use between genders: A cross-cultural evaluation. *Journal of Affective Disorders, 102*, 265–275.

Keyes, K. M., Hatzenbuehler, M. L., & Hasin, D. S. (2011). Stressful life experiences, alcohol consumption, and alcohol use disorders: The epidemiologic evidence for four main types of stressors. *Psychopharmacology, 218*(1), 1–17.

Kolb, P. (2014). *Understanding aging and diversity: Theories and concepts.* New York, NY: Routledge.

Mattson, T. (2014). Intersectionality as a useful toll in anti-oppressive social work and critical reflection. *Affilia, 29*(1), 8–17.

McCall, L. (2005). The complexity of intersectionality. *Journal of Women in Culture and Society, 30*(3), 1771–1800.

McGovern, J. (2016). *Keynote address: Older adults and substance abuse: Prevalence, assessment and approaches to care.* Washington Heights and Inwood Council on Aging annual conference.

McInnis-Dittrich, K. (2014). *Social work with elders: A biopsychosocial approach to assessment and intervention*. Boston, MA: Pearson Education.

McInnis-Dittrich, K. (2016). *Social work with elders: A biopsychosocial approach to assessment and intervention* (4th ed.). Boston, MA: Pearson Education.

Murphy, Y., Hunt, V., Zajicek, A., Norris, A., & Hamilton, L. (2009). *Incorporating intersectionality in social work practice, research, policy and education*. Washington, DC: NASW Press.

National Institute on Alcohol Abuse and Alcoholism (NIAAA). (2005). *Social work education for the prevention and treatment of alcohol use disorders: Older adults and alcohol problems*. Retrieved from http://pubs.niaaa.nih.gov/publications/Social/Module10COlderAdults/Module10C.html.

National Institute on Alcohol Abuse and Alcoholism (NIAAA). (2016). *Social work education for the prevention and treatment of alcohol use disorders: Older adults and alcohol problems*. Retrieved from http://pubs.niaaa.nih.gov/publications/Social/Module10COlderAdults/Module10C .html

Nelson, T. (2005). Ageism: Prejudice against our feared future self. *Journal of Social Issues, 61*(2), 207–221.

Nunes, E. V., & Levin, F. R. (2004). Treatment of depression in patients with alcohol or other drug dependence: A meta-analysis. *JAMA, 291*, 1887–1896.

Office of Alcohol and Substance Abuse Services. (2016). *Alcohol's affects on the body*. https://www.oasas.ny.gov/admed/fyi/fyiindepth-elderly.cfm.

Pape, P. A., & Sarabia, S. E. (2014). Assessment and treatment of women with substance use disorders. In S. L. S. Straussner (Ed.), *Clinical practice with substance abusing clients* (3rd ed., pp. 442–465). New York, NY: Guilford Press.

Poulin, J., & Walter, C. (1993). Burnout in gerontological social work. *Social Work, 38*(3), 305–310.

Prado, G., Szapocznick, J., Maldonado-Molina, M. M., Schwartz, S. J., & Pantin, H. (2008). Drug use/abuse prevalence, etiology, prevention, and treatment in Hispanic adolescents: A cultural perspective. *Journal of Drug Issues, 38*(1), 5–36.

Purdie-Vaughns, V., & Eibach, R. P. (2008). Intersectional invisibility: The distinctive advantages and disadvantages of multiple subordinate-group identities. *Sex Roles, 59*(5), 377–391.

Reardon, C. (2012). The changing face of older substance abuse. *Social Work Today, 12*, 8–11.

Rosen, D., Heberlein, E., & Engel, R. J. (2013). Older adults and substance-related disorders: Trends and associated costs. *ISRN Addiction, 2013*, 4. http://www.hindawi.com/journals/isrn/2013/905368/.

Rosenthal, L. (2016). Incorporating intersectionality into psychology: An opportunity to promote social justice and equity. *American Psychologist, 71*(6), 474–485.

Satre, D. D., Sterling, S. A., Mackin, R. S., & Weisner, C. (2011). Patterns of alcohol and drug use among depressed older adults seeking outpatient psychiatric services. *American Journal of Geriatric Psychiatry, 19*(8), 695–703.

Schonfeld, L., Hazlett, R. W., Hedgecock, D. K., Duchene, D. M., Burns, L. V., & Gum, A. M. (2015). Screening, brief intervention, and referral to treatment for older adults with substance misuse. *American Journal of Public Health, 105*(1), 205–211.

Shibusawa, T., & Sarabia, S. E. (2015). Social work practice with older adults with substance/alcohol abuse problems. In D. B. Kaplan & B. Berkman (Eds.), *The handbook of social work in health and aging* (2nd ed., pp. 397–406). New York, NY: Oxford University Press.

Simoni-Wastila, L., & Yang, H. K. (2006). Psychoactive drug abuse in older adults. *The American Journal of Geriatric Pharmacotherapy, 4*(4), 380–394.

Smith, A. K., Sudore, R. L., & Perez-Stable, E. J. (2009). Palliative care for Latino patients and their families: Whenever we prayed, she wept. *JAMA: The Journal of the American Medical Association, 301*(10), 1047–1057.

Stevens, S. J., Andrade, R. A., & Ruiz, B. S. (2009). Women and substance abuse: Gender, age, and cultural considerations. *Journal of Ethnicity in Substance Abuse, 8*, 341–358.

Stoller, E., & Gibson, R. C. (Eds.). (2000). *World of difference: Inequality in the aging experience* (3rd ed.). Thousand Oaks, CS: Pine Forge Press.

Substance Abuse and Mental Health Services Administration. (2016). *Aging, medicines and alcohol.* http://store.samhsa.gov/shin/content//SMA12-3619/SMA12-3619.pdf.

Substance Abuse and Mental Health Services Administration. (2016b). *Age- and gender-based populations.* Retrieved from https://www.samhsa.gov/specific-populations/age-gender-based.

Twigg, J., & Martin, W. (2015). The challenge of cultural gerontology. *The Gerontologist, 55*(3), 353–359.

Vincent, G., & Velkoff, V. (2010). *The next four decades: The older population in the United States: 2010 to 2050.* Washington, DC: US Census Bureau.

Woodhead, E., Northrop, L., & Edelstein, B. (2014). Stress, social support, and burnout among long-term care nursing staff. *Journal of Applied Gerontology, 35*(1), 1–22.

World Health Organization. (2016). http://www.who.int/ageing/en/.

Wu, L. T., & Blazer, D. G. (2011). Illicit and nonmedical drug use among older adults: A review. *Journal of Aging and Health, 23*(3), 481–504.

Chapter 9
Addiction and Stigmas: Overcoming Labels, Empowering People

Jenny Mincin

Introduction

"The stigma of drug misuse keeps people from seeking treatment. Words like 'junkie,' 'addict' and 'druggie' can hurt, damaging self-image and standing in the way of recovery. Addiction is not a choice. It's a chronic disease similar to diabetes, heart disease and arthritis"
State Without Stigmas

Stigmas associated with substance misuse and labels such as "drug addict" or "alcoholic" can serve as barriers to care, cost people their lives, destroy communities and families, and create levels of shame and despair. Lloyd (2012) defines stigma as "a long-lasting mark of social disgrace that has a profound effect on interactions between the stigmatized and the unstigmatized. Factors governing the extent of stigmatization attached to an individual include the perceived danger posed by that person and the extent to which she/he is seen as being to blame for the stigma" (Lloyd, 2012, p. 85). Stigmas run deep when it comes to addiction, from current addicts to those in treatment to those in recovery. For example, those in recovery may constantly be asked why they don't drink creating a sense of marginalization. Or, there may be an individual who uses opioids, but is too ashamed to seek help because he or she may be seen as a "drug addict."

As a result of labeling and stigmas, people may often wait years before admitting they have a problem. Recovery should be a source of pride and serve as an example to others seeking help for addiction. However, the opposite has happened. Misinformation, misunderstanding, and a complex mix of stereotypes play a role in creating stigmas in the addiction population. In this chapter, we will explore how stigmas have had a negative impact on the lives of people with substance use disorder and examples of programs that focus on destigmatization.

J. Mincin (✉)
SUNY Empire State College, Human Services, Saratoga Springs, NY, USA
e-mail: jenny.mincin@esc.edu

© Springer International Publishing AG 2018   125
T. MacMillan, A. Sisselman-Borgia (eds.), *New Directions in Treatment, Education, and Outreach for Mental Health and Addiction*, Advances in Mental Health and Addiction, https://doi.org/10.1007/978-3-319-72778-3_9

Stigma and the Social Problem of Addiction

Drug use, particularly in the United States, has a long history of acceptance and vilification (Shiner & Winstock, 2015). The concept of deviance and "deviant behavior" is a social problem that is rooted in the colonial history of the United States dating back to the Puritans in Massachusetts (Erikson, 1966). In the United States, historically social problems have been seen through the medical lens and perceived as "deviant" behaviors that were pathologized as well as seen as individuals departing from what the dominant culture deems as acceptable social norms and behaviours (Brown, 2015; Feagin & Feagin, 1997; Stanley Eitzen & Baca-Zinn, 2003). The idea that an individual engages in "deviant behavior" and must therefore be punished is engrained in our society. Society decides what is deviant through its moral codes, religious ethics, and legal frameworks and policies (Palamar, 2013; Piven & Cloward, 1993; Shiner & Winstock, 2015; Yeomans, 2014). According to Tierney, Petak and Hahn (1988), "a condition such as mental illness, or physical disability, does not exist objectively as a trait of an individual so much as it is produced through a combination of factors: the way others in society react to and treat the individual is relegated; and the options that society makes available to the individual" (p. 17).

Regulation vis-a-vis laws and policies also contributes to who is labeled deviant and what is acceptable. Alcohol and tobacco are legal in the United States, and now marijuana is increasingly becoming legal. The process of legalization (or adversely making a behavior or substance illegal) legitimizes (or delegitimizes) the behavior (or substance) (Shiner & Winstock, 2015). For example, we see patterns with medically prescribed substances (opioids, amphetamines, etc.) then being used for non-medical purposes leading to the substance becoming illegal. Once a substance is illegal, the behavior of using it becomes illegal and creates stigmas and marginalization. These categories and labels are powerful. Stigmas influence an individual's ability to access help as well as how policy makers will approach an issue. As recent studies show, people who use drugs and alcohol are seen as engaging in deviant behavior, and it is seen as a moral failing that may lead to becoming addicted to alcohol or other substances (Bowden & Goodman, 2015; Dean & Rud, 1984; Kennedy-Hendricks et al., 2017; Lloyd, 2012; Mattoo et al., 2015; Robin, 2009).

When society labels a person as deviant or having moral "failings," it is perceived as a character flaw rather than a disorder that a person can recover. For example, people tend to view someone recovering from a broken leg or cancer differently than someone recovering from opioid misuse or alcoholism. This perspective influences how we treat and perceive the individual. The person recovering from cancer will likely receive broad support from the medical community, family, neighbors, and friends. Rarely do people with substance misuse garner the same level of support and empathy. Desmon and Marrow (2014) found that substance misuse is viewed more negatively than mental illness. The study revealed that substance misuse is seen as a "moral failing" as opposed to a treatable illness (Desmon & Marrow, 2014).

Labels Once a person is labeled, or placed in a category, society offers parameters in which that person functions. Within the symbolic interaction theory is the labeling theory. The labeling theory, according to Patton, states "that what people are called has major consequences for social interaction" (Patton, 2002, p. 113). Negative labels, such as "drug addicted" or "low functioning," can have negative emotional ramifications on people being labeled as such; there is power in words and how we define people (Patton, 2002; Tucker & Simpson, 2011). Further, the critique of the medical model is that the approach is often limiting, even pejorative, and excuses society from becoming an open, inclusive one (Tierney, Petak, & Hahn, 1988).

Contrary to the stereotypes often portrayed, people with substance use disorder (SUD) are a vital, significant, and contributory part of the population with each person having a range of abilities and accomplishments just as those without SUDs. Further, people with SUDs are not homogeneous, but rather a diverse group of people from various backgrounds offering many different skills and contributions to society when supported and able to access services. The moral judgements placed on people with substance use disorder and the incorrect assumption that people with substance issues cannot recover further impede the individual's motivation and self-esteem (Desmon & Marrow, 2014). Dangerously, social policy and resource decisions are made on this assumption. How society constructs "addiction" has real, direct consequences for treatment and potential recovery.

Efforts to Destigmatize Addiction

In recent years, and specifically in the face of the current opioid epidemic, communities and governments are coming together to fight stigma, inform the public, and advocate for more resources, treatments, and access to services. This section outlines some key initiatives throughout the United States that focus on anti-stigma campaigns, educational outreach programs, and advocacy. Media and public service announcements can play an important role in advocating for the needs of people with substance issues and destigmatizing mental illness and SUDs. Below are two examples of successful stigmatization campaigns.

Anti-Stigma Toolkit

In 2012, the Danya Institute, funded in part by SAMHSA, developed the *Anti-Stigma Toolkit: A Guide to Reducing Addiction-Related Stigma (The Danya Institute,* 2012). It is an effective guide that helps people engage in stigma-breaking activities. The toolkit addresses stigmas within the person who is using, stigmas within the health community, and stigmas within society, all barriers to treatment and recovery. The focus is on "breaking the silence" about SUDs. According to the toolkit, "Speaking out is central to the prevention and reduction of stigma. On the most basic level, stigma prevention involves people in recovery, treatment providers and advocates, and people concerned about stigma speaking out. There is power in people telling their stories" (The Danya Institute, 2012, p. 9).

Mental Health First Aid

The National Council on Behavioral Health (NCBH) is a national behavioral health association that brings together 2800 mental health and addiction organizations across the country to promote education, training, and advocacy. Its mission is to work toward "all Americans having access to comprehensive, high-quality care that affords every opportunity for recovery" (NCBH, 2018). The NCBH brought a psychoeducational program, Mental Health First Aid (MHFA), to the United States. MHFA was started in Australia and is now in 20 countries. MHFA is an eight-hour training program that teaches participants, "how to identify, understand and respond to signs of mental illnesses and substance use disorders" (MHFA, 2018). Over 1 million people in the United States have been trained, and there are currently over 11,000 instructors (MHFA, 2018).

Mental Health First Aid Educational Model MHFA is an evidence-based educational model. Just as CPR training assists people in identifying and knowing when to act if someone is injured or is having a heart attack, MHFA teaches participants to identify and know how to assist someone who is in emotional distress, having a crisis, or in recovery. The training includes modules on depression, anxiety, psychosis, and substance use and substance use disorder. Substance use is a topic that is integrated through the 8-hour training, as often there are coexisting conditions, such as anxiety disorder and alcoholism or depression. The curriculum emphasizes understanding mental illness and SUD and breaking down stigmas based on the premise that stigma is a significant reason people with mental illness and SUD do not seek help (MHFA, 2018).

Impact Since MHFA is an evidence-based educational intervention, the organization engages in program evaluation to collect data to measure the impact of the training. Peer-review studies show that MHFA participants grow their knowledge of mental illness and SUD, identify a number of professional and self-help resources for individuals with mental illness and SUD, and show an increase in mental wellness themselves (MHFA, Mental Health First Aid Research, 2018). Significantly, the research shows, "that the program reduces the social distance created by negative attitudes and perceptions of individuals with mental illnesses" (MHFA, 2018).

MHFA is an education program specifically designed to educate people about mental illness and addiction and what they can do to help someone they know. Anyone can take the course and will receive a certification. MHFA's curriculum is designed to be accessible to practitioners and lay people alike. It teaches proven techniques at how to approach people with mental illness and SUD, includes hands-on scenarios, and equips participants with the knowledge and confidence to recognize mental illness and substance misuse in others and themselves. It makes it okay to know someone or be someone with a mental health or SUD. Because the curriculum is evidence-based and accessible, it has a high success rate. It is an empowerment model that emphasizes what people can do to help themselves and each other. The motto is "There is always hope for recovery." When contrasting this with recent studies which showed those surveyed believed that people with SUD had a small chance of recovery, MHFA is changing the narrative (Desmon & Marrow, 2014).

State Without Stigmas

The State of Massachusetts is addressing the growing opioid epidemic, and other substance misuse with targeted campaign and SUD services outreach initiative. The public media campaign, State Without Stigmas, is an anti-stigma initiative that provides information on what SUD is, advocacy for people who misuse drugs or have a substance use disorder, and provides information to policy makers through the Governor's Opioid Working Group (State Without Stigmas, 2018).

Thrive NYC

The New York City Department of Health and Mental Hygiene has initiated a comprehensive mental health program called Thrive NYC. Among the 54 initiatives is the media outreach component, "Today I Thrive." The aim of the public media campaign is to, "publicly reshape the conversation around mental health by sharing positive messages about resiliency and recovery and the City's new resources to connect New Yorkers to services" (Thrive NYC, Thrive NYC Year One Update, 2017). Today I Thrive is a comprehensive approach that includes paid media, public media campaigns on public transportation, and public city spaces. In addition, there is a dedicated outreach team and partners with the faith-based community throughout New York City. A year into the public campaign, it is estimated that over four million people have been reached (Thrive NYC, Thrive NYC Year One Update, 2017).

Links to Anti-Stigma Efforts

- Anti-Stigma Toolkit: http://www.attcnetwork.org/regcenters/productDocs/2/Anti-Stigma%20Toolkit.pdf
- Mental Health First Aid: https://www.mentalhealthfirstaid.org/cs/
- State Without Stigma: http://www.mass.gov/eohhs/gov/departments/dph/stop-addiction/state-without-stigma/
- Thrive NYC: https://thrivenyc.cityofnewyork.us/

Conclusion

From the existing literature, we see that stigmas continue to run deep and have an impact on treatment and recovery. More research needs to be conducted to consider not only where and why stigmas exist but how can we overcome stigmas making direct links to social policy and additional resources to bolster outreach, services, treatment models, and supportive ongoing recovery. In addition, evaluating educational model to test the efficacy of how they change stigmas and stereotypes as well as increase empathy and understanding should be considered.

Debunking myths about SUDs and educating individuals, families, and communities are practical ways to reduce stigma and increase understanding and support. National programs that promote understanding, build resilience, and break down barriers, such as Mental Health First Aid, can go a long way at reducing stigma and increasing people with SUD's chances of accessing needed services (Lloyd, 2012).

> "Many people know someone who struggles with addiction, or who is in treatment or recovery.
>
> - We can all be part of the solution.
> - We can take a stand against stigma.
> - We can support treatment opportunities.
> - We can encourage people in recovery.
> - Most importantly, we can talk about addiction amongst our friends and family members to hopefully address the misperceptions about addiction, treatment options and long-term recovery.
> - Each of us can commit to not using hurtful or damaging words about those who face addiction." – State Without Stigma

Additional Resources to Anti-Stigma Campaigns

- Developing a Stigma Reduction initiative, SAMHSA: http://store.samhsa.gov/shin/content/SMA06-4176/SMA06-4176.pdf
- Say it Forward Anti-Stigma Campaign, Movement for Global Mental Health: http://www.globalmentalhealth.org/say-it-forward-anti-stigma-campaign-uses-truth-break-chains-stigma
- Stigma-Free, National Alliance for Mental Health: https://www.nami.org/stigmafree
- Time to Change, Global Anti-Stigma Campaigns: https://www.time-to-change.org.uk/about-us/what-we-do/global-anti-stigma-alliance/global-campaigns

References

Bowden, K., & Goodman, D. (2015). Barriers to employment for drug dependent postpartum women. *Work, 50*(3), 425–432.

Brown, S. (2015). Stigma towards marijuana users and heroin users. *Journal of Psychoactive Drugs, 47*(3), 213–220.

Dean, J. C., & Rud, F. (1984). The drug addict and the stigma of addiction. *International Journal of Addictions, 19*(8), 859–869.

Desmon, S., & Marrow, S. (2014, October 1). *Drug addiction viewed more negatively than mental illness, Johns Hopkins study shows. While both are treatable health conditions, stigma of addiction much more pronounced, seen as 'moral failing,' researchers say.* Hub. Retrieved from: https://hub.jhu.edu/2014/10/01/drug-addiction-stigma/

Erikson, K. T. (2004 [1966]). *Wayward puritans: A study in the sociology of deviance, Revised Edition.* Boston: Allyn and Bacon.

Feagin, J. R., & Feagin, C. B. (1997). *Racial and ethnic Relations.* New York: Pearson.

Kennedy-Hendricks, A., Barry, C. L., Gollust, S. E., Ensminger, M. E., Chisolm, M. S., & McGinty, E. E. (2017). Social stigma toward persons with prescription opioid use disorder: Associations with public support for punitive and public health–oriented policies. *Psychiatry Online, 68*(5), 462–469.

Lloyd, C. (2012). The stigmatization of problem drug uses: A narrative literature review. *Drugs: Education, Prevention, and Policy, 20*(2), 85–95.

Mattoo, S., Sarkar, S., Gupta, S., Nebhinani, N., Parakh, P., & Basu, D. (2015). 5. Stigma towards substance use: Comparing treatment seeking alcohol and opioid dependent men. *International Journal of Mental Health & Addiction, 13*(1), 73–81.

MHFA, Mental Health First Aid Research. (2018). Retrieved from: https://instructors.mental-healthfirstaid.org/mental-health-first-aid-research

National Center on Behavioral Health. (2018). *Mission statement and leadership.* Retrieved from: https://www.thenationalcouncil.org/about/national mental-health-association/

Palamar, J. J. (2013). An examination of beliefs and opinions about drug use in relation to personal stigmatization towards drug users. *Journal of Psychoactive Drugs, 5*(5), 367–373.

Patton, M. Q. (2002). *Qualitative research and evaluation methods.* New York, NY: Sage.

Piven, F. F., & Cloward, R. (1993). *Regulating the poor: The functions of public welfare.* New York: Vintage.

Robin, R. (2009). Stigma, social inequality, and alcohol and drug use. *Drug and Alcohol Review, 24*(2), 143–155.

Shiner, M., & Winstock, A. (2015). Drug use and social control. The negotiation of moral ambivalence. *Social Science Medicine, 138*, 248–256.

Stanley Eitzen, D., & Baca-Zinn, M. (2003). *Social problems.* New York, NY: Allyn and Bacon.

State Without Stigmas. (2018). Retrieved from: http://www.mass.gov/eohhs/gov/departments/dph/stop-addiction/state-without-stigma/what-isstigma.html

The Danya Institute. (2012). *Anti-stigma toolkit: A guide to reducing addition-related stigma.* Retrieved from: http://www.attcnetwork.org/regcenters/productDocs/2/Anti-Stigma%20 Toolkit.pdf

Thrive NYC. (2017). *Thrive NYC year one update.* Retrieved from: https://thrivenyc.cityofnewyork.us/wp-content/uploads/2017/02/Thrive_Year_End_Updated-1.pdf

Tierney, K. J., Petak, W. J., & Hahn, H. (1988). *Disabled persons and earthquake hazards.* Denver, Colorado: Institute of Behavioral Science.

Tucker, J. A., & Simpson, C. A. (2011). The recovery spectrum: From self-change to seeking treatment. *Alcohol Research & Health, 33*(4), 371–379.

Yeomans, H. (2014). *Alcohol and moral regulation: Public attitudes, spirited measures, and Victorian hangovers.* Bristol, UK: Policy Press.

Part II
Practice

Chapter 10
Addiction in the Community: The Role of Emergency Services

Thalia MacMillan

Your ambulance is called to the scene of an unresponsive male in his 30s. His parents found him in the bathroom on the floor around 7 a.m. and reported that he wouldn't wake up. His father reports that the patient voluntarily checked himself out of a rehab center and called them at 3 a.m., then showing up to their house around 5 a.m. Upon walking into the bathroom, EMS saw several needles on the floor, including one sticking out of the patient's arm; the patient's father tried to hide all of these from you. The parents were hesitant to say much about the patient's medical history, medication use, or drug past.

It has been estimated that every 19 min, an individual will die of an opioid overdose in their community (CDC, 2012). From 2002 to 2015, there was a 2.2-fold increase in the number of deaths related to substance use (National Institute on Drug Abuse [NIDA] 2017b, c). As stated in other chapters, the percentage of individuals within our community who partake in substance use is on the rise. Close to 10% of the population aged 12 or older has used an illicit drug in the past month; this includes marijuana, cocaine, heroin, hallucinogens, inhalants, or prescription-type psychotropic medications that are misused (i.e., pain relievers, tranquilizers, stimulants, and/or sedatives) (Substance Abuse and Mental Health Services Administration [SAMHSA], 2013). Further, substance use among all age-groups, racial groups, socioeconomic status, and genders is increasing (NIDA, 2017b); substance use is not limited to one particular demographic or area of the country.

As the above scenario and sobering statistics illustrate, substance use is happening within communities across the United States. It is key to get emergency services to individuals in need as soon as possible, as it is not always possible for clients to get to the emergency room under their own auspices. With the advent of the Emergency Medical System (EMS), or emergency care/services provided through ambulance services, emergency room care has been extended into the community (Limmer & O'Keefe, 2015). Emergency services within the community frequently

T. MacMillan (✉)
SUNY Empire State College, Community & Human Services, New York, NY, USA
e-mail: thalia.macmillan@esc.edu

© Springer International Publishing AG 2018
T. MacMillan, A. Sisselman-Borgia (eds.), *New Directions in Treatment, Education, and Outreach for Mental Health and Addiction*, Advances in Mental Health and Addiction, https://doi.org/10.1007/978-3-319-72778-3_10

represent the first-line response to provide care. Close to two-thirds of the care provided within the community is provided by volunteer ambulance corps, particularly within suburban and rural areas (National Association of Emergency Medical Technicians [NAEMT], 2017). Unfortunately, many individuals do not call for help when needed or seek help when problems present early, which potentially increases health-care costs and the outcomes of such care when it is provided (NIDA, 2017a, b). In the case of substance use, as many of the scenarios in the chapter will illustrate, emergency services are typically not requested until a severe health event occurs, such as an overdose or a severe reaction. Keep in mind, emergency services in the community represent a mediator between the person being at home and getting them to the emergency room.

This chapter will explore the role of emergency services within the community from the perspective of the emergency service provider; these perspectives may include the emergency medical responder (EMR), emergency medical technician (EMT-B), or paramedic. An understanding of the symptoms associated with drug use and its classification within emergency services will be explored. Further, the responsibilities of the provider, ethical issues associated with providing care, types of care provided, the interaction of agencies, and factors that may affect care will be explored. Scenarios are provided throughout the chapter to illustrate situations that may be faced by emergency services, the issues that may arise, and the type of assumptions that may be present.

Classification of Drug Use Within Emergency Services

Emergency providers are required to have a complete understanding of anatomy and physiology: anatomy as it relates to the body structure itself and physiology as it relates to the functions of the body. By having an understanding of both anatomy and physiology, the provider is able to determine what is affecting normal levels of functioning in the patient. In the emergency service field, alcohol and substance use are classified as poisons to the body. A poison is classified as any substance that has the potential to harm the body by altering its normal functions (Limmer & O'Keefe, 2015). Alcohol and substances may cause harm to the body by interfering with the normal biochemical processes that occur, which in turn impacts an individual's ability to function (Limmer & O'Keefe, 2015). As a provider, it may not be clear the extent of the impact that is occurring; however, what is evident is that the individual is in need of assistance and that multiple physiological systems can be involved.

A thorough assessment of the individual is needed as it will reveal the extent of damage from substance use. By ingesting, inhaling, or injecting some type of substance or poison, the bodily systems may or may not be able to react in a way to protect functioning. For example, individuals who chronically abuse alcohol often present to emergency providers as someone who may have blood sugar issues, gastrointestinal issues, or poor nutrition (Limmer & O'Keefe, 2015). Only by conducting a thorough assessment of the individual, which includes amount of the substance ingested, length of time, food and nutrition history, medical issues present, etc., will an emergency provider be aware of all of the issues that may be present.

While we could make globalizations about what changes we could expect, the fact of the matter is that everyone is different and should be assessed in that same spirit. It is necessary to understand that any assessment can be impacted by numerous factors, such as advanced age and/or hormonal changes (e.g., pregnancy) (Kessler et al., 2005). Children and adolescents have different levels of functioning than adults and, as a result, may respond very differently to substances (Elkins, McGue, & Iacono, 2007). Further, lifestyle and environmental factors also play a role and need to be taken into account in an assessment (Hughes & Eliason, 2002; Kessler et al., 2005).

Symptoms Associated with Substance Use

You are called by the police to a scene in the middle of town. The man is acting paranoid and is extremely restless. He oscillates between being sad to very excited to depressed. He is having difficulty remembering what happened that day and if he took any substances. He was running in and out of traffic; however, the police was able to sit him down temporarily on the side of the road.

In order to understand the symptoms associated with substance use, there is a need to understand the different types of substances and/or classes. The one common threat among all of these substances is that they have the potential to alter a person's thinking and judgment (NIDA, 2017a). While the emergency provider does not always need to know the specific drug, knowing the class of drug can be extremely beneficial to knowing how to treat the patient. Emergency providers often use drug classifications and categories to organize their knowledge. Knowing the effects of each class of drugs helps the provider know what to look for in the assessment. As you can see in the chart, each type of drug has the potential to cause a multitude of effects.

Class	Specific drugs	Possible effects
Alcohol	Alcohol	Depressant effect Altered perceptions Volatile behavior Sleep disturbances Muscle relaxation
Uppers	Amphetamines Cocaine Desoxyn (black beauties) Dextroamphetamine Methamphetamine (speed, crank, meth, crystal, diet pills) Ritalin Preludin	Excitement in the user Use to relieve fatigue Create feelings of well-being Increased pulse and breathing rates Rapid speech Dry mouth Dilated pupils Sweating Going without sleep Restless, hyperactive, uncooperative

(continued)

Class	Specific drugs	Possible effects
Downers	Barbiturates (rainbows) Amobarbital (blue devils, bars) Pentobarbital (yellow jackets) Secobarbital (red devils) Methaqualone (Quaalude) Sedatives (tranquilizers, sleeping pills, valium)	Relaxing Sense of euphoria Hallucinations Causes respiratory depression Sluggish/sleep, lack coordination of body and speech Low pulse and breathing rates
Narcotics	Codeine (often in cough syrup) Demerol Dilaudid Fentanyl Heroin Methadone Morphine Opium Paregoric Acetaminophen with codeine	Produces stupor or sleep Relieves pain Changes many of the normal activities of the body Intense state of relaxation or feeling of well-being Pinpoint pupils Causes respiratory depression Depressed level of consciousness Reduced pulse Lower skin temperature
Mind-altering drugs	LSD (acid, sunshine) Mescaline (peyote) Morning glory seeds PCP (angel dust) Psilocybin (magic mushrooms) Hash/marijuana THC	Mind-affecting drugs Intense state of excitement or distortion of perception Has stimulant properties Fast pulse rate Dilated pupils Flushed face Hallucinations Not aware of time or the environment Aggressive or timid behavior
Volatile chemicals	Amyl nitrate (snappers) Butyl nitrate Cleaning fluid Furniture polish Gasoline Glue Nail polish remover Typewriting correction fluid (white-out)	Initial rush and then act as a depressant Dazed or temporary loss of contact with reality Swollen membranes in nose and mouth "Funny feeling" or "tingling" in the head Changes in heart rhythm

Source: NIDA (2017a)

It should be kept in mind that any list of substances is limited by the information that is current at that time. Unfortunately, new types of substances are "popping up" every year and will not be listed on this table. The effects of any new drug, and the resulting treatment for it, will need to be researched; further, treatments for the substances that are known need to be continually examined for their effectiveness. An additional factor to keep in mind about the intake of substances is that the effects seen in the field can be affected by the dosage utilized, the strength of the substance, body physiology, and total time of use (e.g., alcohol ingested over a 4-hour period of time versus a 1-h period of time) (Limmer & O'Keefe, 2015; NIDA, 2017a).

Polydrug use, or using different substances at the same time, is a frequent problem and has a high risk of consequences (Mccabe, Cranford, Morales, & Young, 2006). One of the most common combinations is using alcohol and another drug/illegal substance at the same time (Mccabe et al., 2006). When substances are combined, the effects felt may be devastating on an individual's health. For example, an individual who drinks and takes painkillers may experience a double depressant type of effect, such that the individual could experience severe sleep disturbances, very low pulse rate, low respirations, and lack of coordination.

Responsibilities of the Emergency Provider and Interaction with Other Agencies

Emergency services and providers within the community are faced with on-the-spot critical decision-making. Information should be taken from those who are present on the scene and through an assessment of the patient. This information is then synthesized to make an appropriate decision as to what type of care should be provided to the patient. Typically, the following sets of steps are conducted:

- Upon arriving on the scene, the emergency provider immediately does an assessment of the scene. Is it safe for the provider, the patient, and the crew? Are there other individuals around? Are needles or bottles present?
- Examine the patient and conduct an initial assessment:

  - Establish responsiveness and mental status – Is the patient alert and oriented? Are they confused? Are they responsive to only voice, pain, or not at all?
  - Airway – Does the patient have a patent airway? Meaning do they have anything blocking the airway?
  - Breathing – Is the patient breathing? Is something depressing their breathing?
  - Circulation (pulse and bleeding) – Does the patient have a pulse?

- Begin emergency care if needed:

  - Does the airway need to be cleared?
  - Does the patient need oxygen? (to help with breathing)
  - Can anyone vouch for the patient's mental status? Is this their normal mental status or is it different somehow?
  - Is CPR needed (if there is no pulse)?

- Provide medications/interventions if appropriate:

  - Oxygen
  - Naloxone (i.e., Narcan)

- Take a set of vitals.
- Conduct a primary assessment of the body.

- Protect the patient from self-injury if possible.
- Transport the patient as soon as possible to the emergency room.
- Perform reassessment and vital signs.
- Transfer care to the emergency room.
- Advocate for your patient at the emergency room.

As noted by Limmer and O'Keefe (2015), there is no specific order to these steps. One of the best skills that the provider can have is to utilize their senses when providing care and to specifically notice what they see, smell, hear, and observe about the situation (Richmond, 2017). For example, even though a provider may not see any drug paraphernalia directly in view, they may smell something suspicious in the patient's room.

Depending on the safety of the scene and the patient's status, one of the above steps may come before another. In all cases, however, scene safety of the crew takes precedence. In order to ensure this, the police will typically work hand in hand with emergency medical care. The police can help to ensure the crew and patient are safe. In some cases, before taking vitals or conducting an assessment, the emergency provider may need to protect the patient from themselves; in cases such as these, soft restraints may be needed or the presence of the police. As noted above, different types of substances affect individuals very differently. As such, not everyone should be assessed the same way.

Ethical Issues

You are part of your town's volunteer ambulance squad. Your town is classified as small in nature; truly the saying "everyone knows your name and your business" holds true. Your ambulance is dispatched to a home of a woman in her 20s who has a known criminal history and has dealt drugs in the past. You have been called to the house before, as the woman has overdosed once before. Many people on the squad are hesitant to go to the house or to help the woman.

The emergency provider has a scope of practice by which their role is defined. This encompasses the regulations, ethical considerations, protocols, certifications, and educational requirements needed to treat patients (National Highway Traffic Safety Administration [NHSTA], 2007). As with any other profession, emergency service providers follow a code of ethics, and their role in providing emergency care should not be over- or underestimated (National Association of Emergency Medical Technicians [NAEMT], 2013; Winston & Moskop, 2014). The code of ethics and conduct has been updated over the years in an effort to stay current in the field. Regardless of the reason for why care is being provided, such as the use of drugs versus a stomach issue, the patient deserves to be treated with dignity and respect (Winston & Moskop, 2014).

One of the key tenets of the code of ethics for emergency providers is to do no harm and provide quality care to all individuals who are in need, regardless of the reason (NAEMT, 2013). Ensuring that the patient will not be harmed further through the provision of emergency care is essential. In order to achieve this, the provider must complete an assessment of the situation and individual in order to determine what type of care is needed. This also speaks to the standard of care that is expected; when on the scene with multiple providers, one provider can assume that the other providers will provide the same level of care and has the same requisite knowledge.

A second ethical tenet is that of consent. Permission is needed from the patient in order to treat them; this is also known as expressed consent. In circumstances where the patient in unresponsive or is in an altered mental state, care can be provided through implied consent (Ripley et al., 2012). In cases where the patient has taken a mind-altering substance, like a hallucinogen, and is not aware or rational, the emergency provider can provide care until the point that the patient is able to make rational decisions.

A third ethical tenet is confidentiality. As with any other type of medical profession, all information gathered should not be shared with anyone except the emergency room (American College of Emergency Physicians, 2011). No information should be shared with family, friends, or on social media. In cases of substance abuse, for some it may be tempting to "gossip" and discuss a recent emergency call, but this violates the patient's right to privacy.

A fourth ethical tenet is that of continuing education. As information, policies, protocols, procedures, and diagnoses evolve over time, it is important to keep up to date (NAEMT, 2013). In the field of substance use, what we know about substances, their effects on the body, and how we treat them continues to change rapidly. As such, it is important to keep updated as a provider. Many emergency services require monthly and yearly trainings.

One thing to keep in mind is that all emergency providers have a duty to act. This means that they have an obligation to provide care to a patient once they arrive at a scene (Wolfberg, 2013). To begin care and then stop it would represent abandonment. Ultimately once care is initiated, the patient needs to be transferred to another health-care provider who has equal or greater medical training. Typically, this means that the emergency provider would transfer care to the nurses and doctors at the emergency room.

Type of Care Provided

Your ambulance is treating a 35-year-old male at his home. He was found unconscious on his bed by a friend who came to check on him. There are about 20 bottles of various types of alcohol in the patient's living room and several in his bedroom. On the floor, you see many different types of pills but no containers. You approach the patient and he tries to punch members of the ambulance crew. When anyone tries to administer treatment, the patient spits at them or tries to hit them. Members of the crew notice that the patient does seem to be experiencing medical issues though, as he is very confused and is diaphoretic or sweating profusely.

When providing emergency care and treatment to a patient, one should never underestimate simple types of care. Individuals under the influence of substances can be extremely confused and not fully aware of what is going on. If this is the case, the emergency provider can do simple things that may make the most difference. For example, if the patient is conscious, the best thing the provider can do is to stay alert in cases of unpredictable behavior, treat the patient in a calm manner, maintain eye contact with the patient, treat the individual with respect, and speak directly to the patient (Limmer & O'Keefe, 2015).

Additional types of care can be specific to the needs of the patient. The assessment and steps detailed above can reveal the medical needs of the patient. In some cases, oxygen needs to be administered. In other cases, where an individual has overdosed on some type of opioid, has decreased respiratory depression (less than 8 breaths per minute), and is responding to voice or pain, naloxone (i.e., Narcan) may need to be administered to the patient (Barton et al., 2009).

As noted above, there is a need to find out as much information about the patient as possible. Typically, substance use is not done in a vacuum, and the individual may have other health conditions or be taking some type of regular medication. In order to provide the best care possible, this type of information is needed. For example, if the patient is abusing alcohol and is diabetic, it is important to ascertain the patient's blood sugar level as part of the assessment. Additionally, if a patient has some type of cardiac history and is taking methamphetamine, it is important to assess if the patient is experiencing any symptoms such as increased pulse or difficulty breathing.

Factors Affecting Care

The ambulance is called to a home where a family resides. You are asked to treat a 68-year-old woman. She only speaks Russian; unfortunately, no one on your crew speaks Russian. The patient's daughter speaks it and offers to translate. She reports that her mother took two Ambien for sleep and seems to be more groggy than normal. You notice on the bedside there is a bottle of melatonin and a bottle of Tylenol PM. You ask the patient if she has taken any of these; the daughter translates the question to her mother. The mother reported that she took one Ambien, but also several melatonin and two Tylenol PM.

Age, culture, lifestyle, and environmental factors can potentially impact the dynamic between the patient and the emergency provider (Flores, Rabke-Verani, Pine, & Sabhawal, 2002). Failure to take cultural context and language into account may lead to inaccurate assessment of symptoms or issues; miscommunication between the provider, patient, and family; and an inaccurate provider understanding of substance abuse symptoms, dosage taken, type of substance taken, or other factors or cause anxiety in the patient if they do not know what is being conducted and why (Flores et al., 2002).

One thing that should not be overlooked at all times is the patient's right to be treated with respect and dignity. This might be especially true in small towns where there is often an assumption that "everyone knows each other's business." Many patients have concerns that people will know find out they are receiving help. Many are anxious as to how others will react when they are viewed in an ambulance. In these instances, we should reassure patients of their privacy and that no information will be shared.

Conclusion

Emergency care is rising to meet the needs of the community with respect to substance use. Knowing what types of drugs, the possible effects of such substances, and how emergency services can assist is crucial in helping the community. Emergency providers are bound by a code of ethics and conduct to help those in their community. Cultural, linguistic, lifestyle, medical, and environmental factors must be taken into account for an accurate assessment and provision of care to a patient. Emergency care providers must strive to continue to learn about the different types of substances that individuals abuse, the symptoms that they present with, and the best type of care that can be provided as a result.

References

American College of Emergency Physicians. (2011, April). *Code of ethics for emergency physicians.* Retrieved online at www.acep.org/Content.aspx?id=29144.

Barton, E. D., Ramos, J., Colwell, C., Benson, J., Baily, J., & Dunn, W. (2009). Intranasal administration of naloxone by paramedics. *Journal of Prehospital Emergency Care, 6*(1), 54–58.

Center for Disease Control (CDC). (2012). CDC grand rounds: Prescription drug overdoses — a U.S. Epidemic. *Weekly, 61*(1), 10–13.

Elkins, I. J., McGue, M., & Iacono, W. G. (2007). Prospective effects of attention-deficit/hyperactivity disorder, conduct disorder, and sex on adolescent substance use and abuse. *Archives of General Psychiatry, 64*(10), 1145–1152.

Flores, G., Rabke-Verani, J., Pine, W., & Sabhawal, A. (2002). The importance of cultural and linguistic issues in the emergency care of children. *Pediatric Emergency Care, 18*(4), 271–284.

Hughes, T. L., & Eliason, M. (2002). Substance use and abuse in lesbian, gay, bisexual and transgender populations. *Journal of Primary Prevention, 22*(3), 263–298.

Kessler, R. C., Berglund, P., Demler, O., Jin, R., Merikangas, K. R., & Walters, E. (2005). Lifetime prevalence and age-of-onset distributions of DSM-IV disorders in the National Comorbidity Survey Replication. *Archives of General Psychiatry, 62*(6), 593–602.

Limmer, D., & O'Keefe, M. F. (2015). *Emergency care* (13th ed.) Upper Saddle River, NJ: Pearson.

Mccabe, S. E., Cranford, J. A., Morales, M., & Young, A. (2006). Simultaneous and concurrent polydrug use of alcohol and prescription drugs: Prevalence, correlates, and consequences. *Journal of Studies on Alcohol, 67*(4), 529–537.

National Association of Emergency Medical Technicians. (2013, June) *National Association of Emergency Medical Technicians EMT oath and code of ethics*. Retrieved online from www. naemt.org/about_us/emtoath.aspx.

National Association of Emergency Medical Technicians; NAEMT. (2017). *EMS statistics*. Retrieved online at: http://www.naemt.org/About_EMS/statistics.aspx.

National Highway Traffic Safety Administration. (2007). *National EMS scope of practice model*. Washington, DC: NHTSA.

National Institute on Drug Abuse. (2017a). *Commonly abuse drugs charts*. Retrieved on the World Wide Web: https://www.drugabuse.gov/drugs-abuse/commonly-abused-drugs-charts.

National Institute on Drug Abuse. (2017b). *Trends and statistics*. Retrieved on the World Wide Web: https://www.drugabuse.gov/related-topics/trends-statistics.

National Institute on Drug Abuse. (2017c). *Overdose death rates*. Retrieved on the World Wide Web: https://www.drugabuse.gov/related-topics/trends-statistics/overdose-death-rates.

Richmond, N. (2017). Listening to our patients. *Journal of the Emergency Medical Services, 42*(8) [online].

Ripley, E., Ramsey, C., Prorock-Ernest, A., Foco, R., Luckett, S., & Ornato, J. P. (2012). EMS providers and exception from informed consent research: Benefits, ethics, and community consultation. *Journal of Prehospital Emergency Care, 16*(4), 425–433.

Substance Abuse and Mental Health Services Administration; SAMHSA. (2013). *Results from the 2013 national survey on drug use and health: Summary of national findings*. Retrieved online at: https://www.samhsa.gov/data/sites/default/files/NSDUHresultsPDFWHTML2013/Web/NSDUHresults2013.pdf.

Winston, B., & Moskop, J. C. (2014). A review of the updated NAEMT code of ethics. *Journal of Emergency Medical Services, 39*(6), [online].

Wolfberg, D. (2013). Pro Bono: Are you always on call? *Journal of Emergency Medical Services, 38*(3), [online].

Chapter 11
Substance Use During and After Major Crisis and Disaster: A Practitioner's Guide

Jenny Mincin

While many people may need additional support during and after a disaster, people with substance use disorders often have specific needs including access to support networks and medical and mental health services. However, these needs are often unknowingly overlooked or misunderstood. There are many facets to understanding how substance use issues may manifest as well as how to be responsive to people with substance use issues both during and after a disaster. For practitioners, understanding the most recent research on substance use disorders (SUD) and the context of disasters and crisis is critical to providing effective and supportive services to those in need.

This chapter will focus on the two primary areas: (1) needs of people in recovery from SUD during and after disasters and (2) people who are substance users and not in recovery. Ways of working with and supporting people with SUD will also be explored. This chapter will also seek to illustrate what disasters are, the systems by which disaster mental health professionals are expected to function in, and the context for which practitioners will be working. Disaster and crisis, by its very nature, is chaotic and destabilizing. Often, practitioners will be working in less than optimal environments. Maintaining flexibility and a team environment enables practitioners to effectively implement disaster mental health services including for people with SUD.

J. Mincin (✉)
SUNY Empire State College, Human Services, Saratoga Springs, NY, USA
e-mail: jenny.mincin@esc.edu

© Springer International Publishing AG 2018   145
T. MacMillan, A. Sisselman-Borgia (eds.), *New Directions in Treatment,
Education, and Outreach for Mental Health and Addiction*, Advances in Mental
Health and Addiction, https://doi.org/10.1007/978-3-319-72778-3_11

Definitions

Defining Disabilities and Substance Use Disorder

People with SUD who are in recovery are considered a part of the disability community. People with disabilities are an important and significant part of the general population. According to the 2012 census, there are close to 50 million people with disabilities, which is approximately 19% of the total population in the United States (U.S. Census, 2012). It is estimated that of the 50 million who have identified themselves as having a disability, 28% of them are 65 years and over. It is common for people to have coexisting (comorbidity) disabilities including physical, mental health, and substance use disorder. For the purposes of this chapter, substance use will be defined both in terms of people who use alcohol and/or drugs and those with an addiction problem with alcohol and/or drugs.

Though accurate numbers can be challenging to collect because of underreporting, according to the National Institute on Alcohol Abuse and Alcoholism (NIAAA), roughly 24.7% of people over the age of 18 reported engaging in "binge drinking" in the past 6 months and 6.7% reported engaging in "heavy drinking" over the past 6 months (National Institute on Alcohol Abuse and Alcoholism [NIAAA], 2016). The NIAAA estimates that over 16 million adults over the age of 18 have an alcohol use disorder (AUD); though this number is likely to be low because of underreporting. Estimates of self-report are also likely to be low as the substances being used are often illegal. Estimates from the Substance Abuse and Mental Health Services Administration (SAMHSA) indicate that 9.4% of respondents aged 12 and over had reported drug use in the past month (National Institute on Drug Abuse, 2016 (NIDA, 2015; SAMHSA, 2014)).

Opioid use and addiction have significantly increased in recent years with an estimated 33,000 people who were killed in 2015 in the United States (Bosman, 2017). The number of deaths from opioid use have quadrupled between the years 1999 and 2014; the United States is in the midst of an opioid epidemic (U.S. Health and Human Services [HHS], 2014a, 2014b). West Virginia, New Hampshire, Kentucky, Ohio, and Rhode Island lead the country in deaths due to opioid overdose (Centers for Disease Control [CDC], 2016a, 2016b). In some communities, opioid use is so prevalent that it has become the number one killer (Bosman, 2017; CDC, 2016a, 2016b; HHS, 2016).

Defining Disasters

A disaster is defined as a catastrophic event of severe magnitude that impacts public safety and human resources and overwhelms affected communities (James & Gilliland, 2017; Quarentelli, 2006; Stebnicki, 2017). In 2016, there were nearly 50 major, nationally declared disasters declared in the United States (Federal Emergency Management Agency [FEMA], 2014). The American Red

Cross responds to nearly 65,000 local disasters annually (American Red Cross). According to the US Federal Emergency Management Agency (FEMA), there are three general categories of disasters: natural (i.e., weather events such as hurricanes), technical (i.e., system failures such as blackouts), and civil (i.e., such as riots, terrorist attacks, and transportation strikes) (FEMA, 2014; James & Gilliland, 2017; Quarentelli, 2006). Disasters can occur in two different ways: forecasted (such as coastal storms) and spontaneous (such as explosions, school shootings, and plane crashes) (FEMA, 2014; James & Gilliland, 2017).

Traditionally, disaster response was a "lights and sirens" event in which first responders (fire and police) handled most aspects of the crisis. Emergency management has evolved over the years and is now an integrated model that includes first responders, logistics, human services, and the integration of special and vulnerable needs populations. The expectation is that emergency planning, response, and recovery will have an inclusive approach and be in compliance with the Americans with Disabilities Act (ADA) of 1990 as well as implement a strength-based approach to working with victims (FEMA, 2014). This is important for both emergency managers and human service practitioners to understand when working with people with SUD. Specifically, emergency managers and crisis counselors must be in compliance with the ADA, and mental health practitioners should be trained in disaster mental health interventions, such as psychological first aid. FEMA currently implements ADA-compliant disaster guidelines, and the guidelines are integrated throughout the federal response system (FEMA, 2014). While the strength-based approach and resiliency model are not legally mandated, there is an expectation that disaster workers and crisis counselors alike will use the strength-based framework when developing and implementing disaster related programs (FEMA, 2014)

The FEMA Strategic Plan 2014–2018 specifically places disaster service delivery as a top priority (FEMA, 2014). Disaster service delivery includes the provision of human services and attending to people with special needs and disabilities. SUD is a diagnosable illness that is also protected under the Americans with Disabilities Act of 1990. SUD is considered a "cognitive" disability, and, as a result, people with SUD are legally protected against discrimination (Davis et al., 2013). Therefore, the specific needs of people with SUD, along with the needs of people with disabilities at large, should be incorporated into the disaster human service delivery system. FEMA provides frameworks, guidelines, and experiential knowledge about disasters (Manela & Moxely, 2002, p. 13). Legally, the ADA ensures that people with disabilities, including those who are in recovery (not actively using), are protected under the law and therefore must have access to appropriate services during and after a disaster. Disaster services may include shelter and housing, disaster mental health and psychological first aid, employment, and transportation.

Disaster Human Services and Emergency Management

Federally, FEMA is the agency that establishes guidelines and grants for state and local emergency management. The state often administers guidelines and grants to local jurisdictions, and local jurisdictions are expected to carry out the guidelines.

FEMA has a system known as the Federal Response Plan (FRP) of which there are 15 Emergency Support Functions (ESFs), which provide guidelines, agency roles, and responsibilities, and creates structure and common language for emergency management and first response. Disaster Human Services falls under ESF Public Health and Medical Services. If you are a disaster mental health practitioner who is called out on a response, you will report under the public health ESF structure.

Disaster Human Services is an umbrella term for the types of services victims of disaster may need before, during, and after a crisis. Service areas include housing, mental health (termed "disaster mental health" or "psychological first aid"), special needs and disability, volunteer and donation coordination, voluntary agency coordination, health and wellness, immigrant and minority affairs, and outreach and education (HHS, 2014a, 2014b). Disaster Human Services may include the following (HHS, 2014a, 2014b):

1. Ensuring the needs of disaster victims are included and incorporated into the disaster planning process
2. Coordination and implementation of services during a disaster response.
3. Implementation and oversite of recovery efforts
4. Engagement in the mitigation process as it pertains to human services including disaster mental health and disaster case management

According to the US Department of Health and Human Services:

> Human services (also known as social services) support the social and economic well-being of individuals and families and their ability to maintain activities of daily living in a safe, healthy manner. Disaster human services are an extension of non-disaster human services programs and systems but with attention to two fundamental priorities in response and recovery: ensuring continued service delivery when emergency events disrupt services and addressing unmet human services needs created or exacerbated by the disaster. (2014)

Formal Networks of Disaster Mental Health Practitioners Nationally, there are several agencies that deploy disaster mental health practitioners during disasters and are a part of the National Crisis Response Team. These agencies include the American Red Cross, National Organization for Victims Assistance, Federal Emergency Management Agency, Medical Reserve Corps, and State and Local emergency management agencies (James & Gilliland, 2017). Generally, these organizations will have disaster plans in place that includes disaster mental health deployment teams and training. It is critical to be trained in standard, evidence-based disaster mental health models including critical ISM, crisis counseling, and psychological first aid. In addition to these certification trainings, understanding the needs of specific populations that will need additional accommodations is paramount. This includes people with SUD and mental health issues. Similar to crisis intervention models, these interventions are aimed at lessening stress and anxiety in victims of disaster as well as enabling practitioners to assess victims to see if further assistance is needed.

Realities of Working in a Disaster As a disaster mental health practitioner, it is important to recognize that many systems will be compromised during a major crisis (Cole, 2017). When disaster or major crisis strikes, many of the services that are normally offered can be disrupted. For example, older people who receive Meals on Wheels may go days or even weeks without being able to receive food services.

For people with SUD, they may not be able to access support groups, get to therapy, or access medications, which is especially critical if they also have a diagnosed mental illness. Awareness of treatment plans, outreach in shelters and recovery centers, and knowing what services will be available during and after disasters and crises can help save lives.

Inclusion of Mental Health and Addiction

The National Council on Disability (NCD; 2006) released a report in 2006 outlining how the government failed to assist people with psychiatric disabilities during Hurricanes Katrina and Rita identifying major violations of the law on several accounts including discrimination during evacuations. Psychiatric disabilities include (but are not limited to) people with autism, dementia, schizophrenia, depression, anxiety, and SUD. People with psychiatric disabilities may live in adult homes or live independently and go to specific facilities to receive services. These services were wiped out as a result of the storm. Specifically, some individuals with psychiatric disabilities "had difficulty comprehending the evacuation messages and other essential communications and some were treated roughly because they could not follow the instructions." There was also loss of life because of paratransit failures (NCD, 2006).

The NCD report findings also indicate that the mismanagement of evacuating people with psychiatric disabilities resulted in losing residents, mistreatment, and inappropriate institutionalization. In addition, the report found that people with psychiatric disabilities were turned away from general population shelters *because* they had a mental illness, a clear violence of section 504 of the ADA and blatant discrimination (NCD, 2006). According to the report:

> Disaster response plans often did not include protocols to evacuate people with psychiatric disabilities. During evacuations, emergency officials physically lost residents of group homes and psychiatric facilities many of who are still missing. Others have not or cannot return home because essential supports have not been restored or because the cost of living has increased too much. When people with psychiatric disabilities arrived at evacuation locations – ranging from state parks to churches – those locations often were not prepared to meet the medical and mental health needs of the evacuees with psychiatric disabilities. Many people with psychiatric disabilities never made it to evacuation shelters because they were inappropriately and involuntarily institutionalized. Some of these people still have not been discharged, despite evaluations that indicate they should be. (NCD, 2006)

Psychological Responses to Disaster: Normal Reactions to an Abnormal Situation

People who have gone through a disaster or major crisis may experience several different physical, emotional, and mental signs and symptoms, most of which tend to be within in the normal response range. Chart 11.A outlines different feelings and symptoms victims and disaster response and recovery workers may experience during and immediately following a disaster.

Chart 11.A Examples of post-disaster symptoms

Psychological	Physical	Mental
Irritability	Feeling tired or drained	Hard time concentrating
Feeling anxious and unsafe	Hypervigilance	Memory loss
Feeling depressed and sad	Loss or gain of appetite	Mind is racing
Blaming self or others	Headaches	Confusion
Grief	Stomach issues including nausea	Easily distracted

During a disaster, resources are severely limited. For people with SUD, they may experience similar loss as other victims including loss of home, loved ones, and community (Halpern & Tramontin, 2007; Miller, 2012). In addition to this loss, people with SUD may not have access to the types of services and support systems that help them maintain their recovery including not having access to mental health and healthcare professionals, 12-step support groups, community and/or religious centers, and friends and family. Immediately following a disaster, service delivery is halted or severely reduced. Victims of disaster often find themselves either in a shelter, hotel, or with friends or family who have temporarily taken them in. In addition to shelters and other temporary housing, victims will need to access disaster assistance services in recovery centers or disaster assistance centers. These are the settings in which disaster mental health professionals will be administering support services and referrals.

Over time, the effects of the disaster start to diminish, but gaps may emerge as systems begin to go back to normal. For example, community and mental health clinics may not be functioning or have been destroyed all together and need to be rebuilt. In addition, while some victims of disaster will start to feel more settled over time, others may continue to struggle with the effects of the disaster and emerging trauma.

Risk Factors

Disasters and crisis affect everyone in different ways. However, there are certain risk factors that can increase during disasters. For people who are in recovery, the possibility of a relapse can go up. People with preexisting substance use and addiction are at a higher risk for either relapse or increased usage during and after a disaster. Not everyone who has been through the devastation of a disaster will develop a substance use disorder. Likewise, not everyone who is in recovery from substance use disorder will go back to using. As much as disasters can increase the chances of a person in recovery to use again, it can also have the effect of reinforcing the person's recovery. It is important to encourage the person to attend support groups, speak with friends and family, and stay connected to the aspects of his/her life that help the person stay in recovery.

Since disasters have the potential to cause mental health issues, it is important for practitioners to look for and accurately assess when a person is increasing substance use after a disaster and as a means of coping with illnesses such as posttraumatic stress disorder. Just because someone did not have a substance use disorder prior to the disaster does not mean she/he will not develop one. PTSD, depression, and anxiety can increase the risk for developing a substance use disorder more broadly. PTSD, anxiety, and depression that develop in a person post-disaster increase the risk for increased substance use (as a coping mechanism) and even lead to a SUD.

Resiliency Model

It is generally accepted that in crisis and disaster, one primary intervention model used is the resiliency model. In fact, and as discussed earlier in this chapter, FEMA has incorporated a victim-centered, resiliency model in its national framework (FEMA, 2014; Hermann, 1997; Mller, 2012; Stebnicki, 2017). Resiliency is rooted in the strength-based approach and focuses on how victims survived the traumatic event; it utilizes the strengths of the survivor to overcome trauma and live a meaningful life. The strength-based approach, or strengths perspective, was developed by Saleeby (1996) as a different approach from the more diagnostic model (Mattaini & Lowery, 2007). According to Saleeby (1996), the strength-based approach developed as a technique in working with people with severe mental health conditions and has grown to work with other vulnerable populations such as the elderly, youth at risk, and even communities. It also is closely aligned with resilience, wellness, integration, and psychosocial approaches and is a primary model used in disaster mental health. The strength-based approach was developed, in part, as a response to the individual, pathology, and deficit approach that seems prevalent in the medical models (Saleeby, 1996).

Mattaini and Lowery (2007) stated: "The strengths-based approach, although not denying problems or oppression, begins with and works with the client's strengths, which have often been largely or entirely ignored in traditional practice" (p. 45). Specifically, the strength-based approach focuses on how people survived traumatic experience and builds upon that as well as the notion that people can be resilient, which is similar to more integrated models. Saleeby (1996) stated:

> Practicing from a strengths-based perspective does not require social workers to ignore the real troubles that dog individuals and groups. Schizophrenia is real. Child sexual abuse is real. Pancreatic cancer is real. But in the lexicon of strengths, it is as wrong to deny the possible as it is to deny the problem. The strengths-based perspective does not deny the grip and thrall of addictions and how they can morally and physically sink the spirit and possibility of any individual. But it does deny the overwhelming reign of psychopathology as civic, moral and medical categorical imperative. (p. 297)

During a disaster, it is critical that the human service practitioner assesses an individual's mental health especially if substance use is suspected. Early intervention is key to lowering the risk for relapse or increased usage and in fact may prevent the development of a substance use disorder in individuals who had no prior history of one.

Crisis Intervention, Psychological First Aid, and Long-Term Treatment

During a disaster, disaster mental health and psychological first aid (PFA) are the primary mental health response models (Jacobs et al., 2016; McCabe et al., 2014; Salon, 2016; Stebnicki, 2017). It is not appropriate to implement an assessment and treatment model as it is problematic on several levels. In a disaster environment, you are often not in a clinical setting with the types of resources you can normally access, such as social service agencies, hospitals, detox units, and clinics (Halpern & Tramontin, 2007; Miller, 2012). In fact, many resources are stretched as a result of the disaster and often businesses are closed. This includes access to mobile crisis, medical facilities, clinicians, and medications. In addition, during a disaster there may be several hundred or thousands of victims, like with large-scale disasters such as Hurricane Katrina. Identifying individuals in the most distress becomes a key objective. Distress may include substance use. Often, the practitioners will not have the resources or time to use a treatment model. In this case, a treatment model can over-pathologize individuals (Halpern & Tramontin, 2007; Miller ,2012). Diagnosis is to be done by a licensed clinician when the immediate effects and dangers of the disaster have begun to abate. Not everyone who experiences a disaster will develop a substance use disorder. Diagnosing during the disaster can be dangerous, can yield inaccurate results, and is not a proven effective method of providing mental health support. The exception to this is if an individual approaches disaster personnel and self-discloses that they have a substance use disorder or other mental illness. That person may need assistance managing the stress of the situation (which is a normal reaction) or need medication. Otherwise, PFA is the appropriate, evidence-based intervention in a disaster environment.

As a disaster mental health practitioner, you will want to conduct quick, evidence-based assessments, such as the psychological first aid assessment (Brymer et al., 2006; Halpern & Tramontin, 2007; Miller, 2012) and the triage assessment system (James & Gilliland, 2017). The assessment will need to be implemented within the setting you are in, which may be a crammed shelter or a victim's damaged home. In a major crisis or disaster, assessments focus on immediate needs, not long-term treatment and therapy (Brymer et al., 2006; James & Gilliland, 2017). The assessments are specifically designed to be implemented in nontraditional therapeutic settings such as shelters, homes, coffee shops, and disaster assistance centers. Quick assessments require the practitioner to focus on the physical, mental, and emotional states of individuals in an effort to understand the level of distress the person may or may not be in as result of a crisis. Using clear, direct language in a calm and comforting manner is at the core of rapid assessment in major crises and disaster (Brymer, et al., 2006).

Below is a chart that includes key concepts from psychological first aid (Miller, 2012; Stebnicki, 2017) but takes into consideration specific needs of people with SUD and what disaster mental health workers should look for and how to approach (Brymer et al., 2006; James & Gilliland, 2017). In the reference section of this chapter, you can find a link to the psychological first aid assessment worksheet and the triage assessment form.

Quick Assessment Suggestions for SUD in Major Crisis and Disaster

Goal	Observe	Approach	Engage
Assess if someone is in distress or crisis	Is the person crying or showing other signs of distress?	Calm demeanor and comforting tone	How are you doing? Do mind if I sit here with you? Is there something I can do?
Assess if someone needs additional help such as medical attention	Is the person shaking or showing other physical signs of distress?	Even-toned, but alert; appear confident	Do you need assistance? Is everything ok? How can I help?
Ensure the person knows they are not alone and support is there if needed	Does the person seem irritated? Is the person alone or with other people? Are they agitated or do they look worried?	Gentle eye contact, calm tone	I am noticing….You are sitting alone….You seem anxious… let me find out if there are any recovery support groups here….Can I help facilitate a phone call….I am available to stay with you and listen….
Diffuse a potential hostile situation or eruption	Is the person angry? Appear hostile? Lashing out at people?	Clear and straightforward language, calm demeanor	I'm noticing you seem upset, is there something I can help you with? How about we sit down and talk about what might be bothering you? This is a stressful time, I understand how upsetting this might be so let's think of ways to deal with how you are feeling
Help the person achieve a level of stability or equilibrium despite the major crisis or disaster. If the person is in recovery, focus on supporting staying clean and sober. If the person is in a harm reduction program	Does the person need to talk to someone?	Stay in the moment; do not ask about or bring up trauma; this is not an assessment for mental illness	Is there something you can do now that might help you? Are you hungry or thirsty? Can we take a walk to the other side of the shelter? Would you like to help us out here at the shelter? Do you feel like using or drinking? Do you feel like you need something to get you through this?

In a crisis, it is important to help individuals define their immediate needs and personal immediate goals. If the person with SUD has awareness of their needs, let them guide the process. Engaging questions such as "what do you need right now" can help them think of their own resiliency, enable them to have a sense of control in a situation that feels out of control, and allow them to have ownership of their recovery (Brymer et al., 2006; Halpern & Tramontin, 2007; James & Gilliland, 2017; Miller, 2012) (Fig. 11.1).

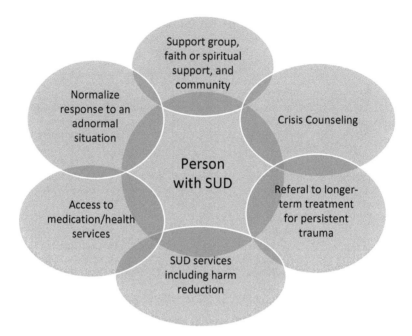

Fig. 11.1 Factors that can contribute to healing after a disaster

Assessing Substance Use Disorders in Disasters

Utilizing the strength-based, resiliency model, the practitioner will want to gather prior information and experiences from an individual's past including the coping mechanisms that the individual uses in times of crisis (Mincin, 2012; Ryan et al., 2008). This probing can help establish if there are any immediate substance use issues. Keep in mind that as a practitioner working in a disaster environment, you may be conducting rapid assessments and basic intake in nonclinical environments including shelters, homes, or disaster assistance centers. Intake questions may include what he or she has been exposed to in the past and survived, known, or understood; chronic ailments; family dimensions and dynamics; and the political and social structure that all come into relevance (Halpern & Tramontin, 2007; Miller, 2012; Mincin, 2012; Ryan et al., 2008). Questions are focused on how people have managed the stress and trauma such as "How did you manage and cope with the events in your life thus far?" The medical- or trauma-focused model looks at the effects of the trauma itself rather than the whole person and how he or she may have survived that trauma (Correa, Velez, & Gifford, 2010; Mincin, 2012). Saleeby (1996) stated that: "Having assessed the damage, social workers need to ensure that the diagnosis does not become the cornerstone of the person" (p. 303).

While social workers should incorporate practice grounded in evidence-based practice, there is also a balance with fully understanding the perspectives, experiences, and strengths that each individual brings to the healing process.

Engaging in disaster mental health practice includes both integration of evidence-based debriefing, SBA and PFA models, as well as flexibility and a commitment to assisting victims through the initial crisis period. Remaining open to the needs of people with SUD while consistently assessing for harm to self or others is a critical aspect to supporting people with substance use issues and disorders.

People in Recovery

For people who are in recovery or in a harm reduction program, encouraging them to continue to stay with their program is important. The following are critical supports:

1. Keep in mind that while a disaster or crisis may increase the risk for people in recovery to relapse, it does not mean that they will relapse. In fact, with solid support and access to support services, the person may stay in their recovery program and heal from the trauma because they already have support systems in place. This is important to remind the client. The person in recovery knows how to reach out for help and can use the tools from their recovery program to help keep them in recovery and cope with the aftereffects of the disaster or crisis. Pointing out the positive aspects to their recovery and reminding them of tools they may already have can give strength, hope, and resiliency.
2. Ask if they feel like drinking or using. Screen for suicide risk if appropriate.
3. In a shelter environment, it could be possible to find a safe space so that people in recovery or in harm reduction can hold meetings and support each other.
4. Asking individuals what they need to maintain their recovery is also important.
5. Incorporate them into the game plan and solutions.
6. Educate people on the common signs and symptoms of disasters.
7. Look for signs of potential relapse.
8. Assist with access to mental health professionals and healthcare providers if the individual is on withdrawal medications and/or drug treatment for mental illness. Keep in mind that it is not uncommon for a person with SUD to also have a diagnosis of mental illness.
9. If a person does relapse, do not shame them or judge them. Accept it and encourage them to go back to their recovery program (Fig. 11.2).

Substance Users Not in Recovery

For people who are heavy users or grappling with the addiction and not in a recovery program, vigilance is critical. First, workers must ensure the safety of others in disaster assistance centers and shelters. If the person is intoxicated, reach out to other disaster personnel and security. While you do not want to escalate a situation, it is important that the person who is intoxicated does not harm herself or others.

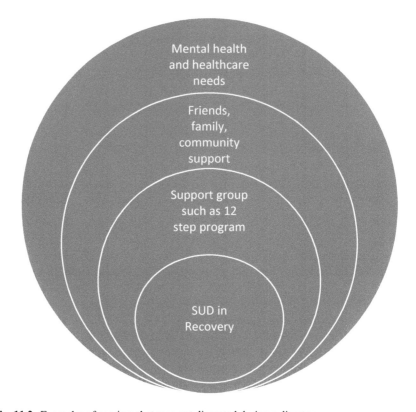

Fig. 11.2 Examples of services that may get disrupted during a disaster

When a person is under the influence, often coping mechanisms and judgement are severely impaired. The person should be monitored, and practitioners should not handle the situation alone. Guidance includes:

1. If the person is under the influence, consider removing him or her from the larger group of victims. Ensure you use a buddy system whereby a team of disaster workers take turns monitoring the person, and notify security so that if the person does become erratic or even violent, security will be prepared and respond quickly.
2. Screen for suicide risk. Active using is a risk factor for suicide.
3. If you discover someone is an active user during an intake, you can probe them regarding their substance use. NIDA suggests asking straightforward questions: do you use drugs and/or alcohol? If so, how many times a week? How many drinks do you have in 1 day? How many times do you use in a day?
4. Be sure to have local mental health and addiction clinic referrals as well as 12-step program information on hand. This is an opportunity to provide education to the client about alcohol and substance abuse.
5. Impress upon the client that disasters can sometimes increase alcohol and substance use. As trauma, stress, and anxiety do not start to diminish, it is not uncommon to turn to substances to help with coping (Halpern & Tramontin, 2007;

Herman, 1997; Miller, 2012). Explain that over the short term, using drugs and/ or alcohol may appear to help, but over the long term, this can cause additional problems including health issues and exacerbate mental health illness.

6. If you suspect someone in a shelter or recovery center is overdosing, seek medical assistance immediately. They may be able to administer Naloxone (i.e., Narcan) as well as other lifesaving interventions. Otherwise, you may need to call for an ambulance, which may or may not be able to respond depending on how overwhelmed the medical system is as a result of the crisis or disaster.

7. Do not threaten or try to force the person to get help or quit using alcohol or drugs. This will only make the person defensive, feel judged, and could drive them further into their SUD. Rather, encourage them to learn more about possible solutions, ask them about how they feel about their alcohol and substance use, and give them hope that they can reduce their use or stop altogether. The power and choice is with the individual, not the disaster mental health practitioner.

Naloxone (Narcan) and Buprenorphine (Bupe) In the event of an overdose, naloxone can be administered if it is available at the shelter or location where you are providing disaster mental health services. Naloxone can reverse the effects of opioid overdose and save a person's life (HHS, 2016; NYC DOH, 2016). Buprenorphine (bupe) can help with withdrawal symptoms and is considered a part of the harm reduction intervention model. In an emergency, people who are utilizing bupe as a part of their treatment plan may need help accessing this medication.

Substance Use Disorder and Increase in Substance Use After a Disaster

After a disaster, it is common to have heightened feelings and have physical reactions to the events. Some people may find they are drinking more than usual a few weeks or months following a disaster. They may be able to recognize this and return to their normal levels of drinking. Others may find they continue to struggle with the aftereffects of a disaster and use drinking and drugs as a way to cope with the tragic event. This could develop into a substance use disorder even if the client did not have a SUD prior to the disaster. During the recovery phase, disaster mental health practitioners have an opportunity to look for signs of alcohol and substance use in clients, conduct outreach, and refer and educate the client. Guidance includes:

1. If you suspect a client may be using alcohol and/or drugs that is new after the disaster or crisis, utilize an alcohol and drug use screening tool to assist will assessing severity.

2. Screen for suicide risk.

3. Have appropriate referrals for the client. He or she may be dealing with trauma from the event, past trauma, and/or mental illness, and increased substance use may partially relate to the trauma of the event. It is critical to refer the client to someone who understands trauma and PTSD.

Cultural Diversity and Inclusion

Access to services and resources vary from community to community, neighborhood to neighborhood. For example, communities that have higher rates of poverty often have less resources for and access to health and mental health services. The same is true during disasters. In fact, it has been consistently shown that vulnerable communities are impacted in different ways and with increased dire outcomes (Halpern & Tramontin, 2007; Miller, 2012). People with disabilities, who have higher rates of poverty than people without disabilities, die at higher rates (Davis et al., 2013; Quarentelli, 2006). Further, vulnerable communities often take longer to recover (because of lack of resources) and tend to have less access to recovery and rebuilding programs and services (Cutter, 2006; Fordham et al., 2010; Halpern & Tramontin, 2007; Miller, 2012).

People who are in a vulnerable group include people of color, people with disabilities (which can include people with substance use disorder), immigrants, non-English speakers, and aging and older people (Fordham et al., 2013; Thomas et al., 2013). In addition, factors such as socioeconomic class and gender (particularly women and girls and gay, bisexual, lesbian, transgender) can be a vulnerability. Vulnerabilities can be comorbid in that they can coexist. For example, a Latino woman who has a substance use disorder and lives in poverty. In this scenario, providing services in culturally and linguistically appropriate ways can make the difference between assisting a survivor or leaving a survivor feeling isolated and misunderstood. For a person who is living in poverty and dealing with a substance use disorder, losing a home or job due to a disaster can have multiple effects on the survivor. If the person cannot access services and resources to assist with mental health and substance use challenges, or help find a new home or job, they risk relapse and perhaps even homelessness. Disaster mental health practitioners need to acknowledge and understand the full person: what her life was like prior to the disaster and how that will impact her during and post-disaster. All of these factors should be considered in the immediate crisis plan as well as referrals and the longer-term crisis assessment and action planning (Fordham et al., 2013; Stebnicki, 2017).

In addition to the aspects of a person's life that might make recovery from a disaster more challenging, it is critical to incorporate the person's strengths. This is where the SBA and resiliency models are particularly effective. Taking the Latino woman as an example, the disaster mental health practitioner can incorporate her culture, beliefs, community, family, and her substance abuse recovery into the crisis counseling process. It is important to find out where she gathers her strength. Does she belong to a religious organization? If so, encourage her to use her faith as a foundation for healing and coping. Perhaps she may even want to volunteer at the shelter if she is bilingual and assist with the response process. Perhaps she will want to hold a 12-step group in the shelter to support other people with SUD. In each of us lies strengths and challenges or areas for growth (Stebnicki, 2017). Our diversity can, at time, make us more socially vulnerable. But, our diversity is also a powerful source of strength, hope, and healing especially during times of tragedy, significant loss, and trauma (Stebnicki, 2017).

Conclusion

This chapter briefly outlines some of the needs of people with comorbid substance use disorders and mental health diagnoses during times of major crisis and disaster. As practitioners, understanding the needs of people with SUD and how to best support them during a major crisis or disaster is a specific skill. Administering disaster mental health is an especially challenging career but a vital one. Learning more about disaster mental health, crisis interventions, and the fundamentals of SUD can help you support someone in a time of need.

Further Information for Practitioners

This section offers additional online resources for mental health practitioners.

Training

1. You can access free emergency management training at the Federal Emergency Management Agency's (FEMA) Emergency Management Institute (EMI) website. Practitioners can learn about the foundations of emergency management as well as become trained on how nongovernmental agencies integrate into emergency response. FEMA EMI: https://www.fema.gov/pdf/about/odic/fnss_guidance.pdf.
2. The National Child Traumatic Stress Network (NCTSN) offers a free, online training in psychological first aid. You can also access other crisis training platforms on the website. PFA Training: https://learn.nctsn.org/enrol/index.php?id=38.

Assessment Tools and Forms

1. The Substance Abuse and Mental Health Services Agency (SAMHSA) provides an alcohol use screening tool called AUDIT. You can access the tool here: http://www.integration.samhsa.gov/AUDIT_screener_for_alcohol.pdf.
2. Psychological first aid assessment worksheet: http://www.nctsn.org/sites/default/files/pfa/english/7-appendix_d_provider_worksheets.pdf.
3. Triage assessment form: http://www.wctcca.com/uploads/1/1/2/3/11232275/triage_asssessment_form_crisis_intevention.pdf.

Local Disaster Scenario:
What are Your Next Steps?

You are working in a shelter after a massive fire destroyed three apartment buildings leaving over 200 people without a home or possessions. The apartment building complex included one building that is a "NORC" (Naturally Occurring Retirement Center) while the other two buildings are mixed family and individuals. Roughly 90% of residents in the NORC are 65 and older, but because it is a NORC and not an assisted living center, there are no official services other than a community room where residents gather for social engagement. Many residents of the NORC go elsewhere in the community or services, including medical care and support groups.

You notice an older woman sitting by herself and not with other residents from the NORC. You decide to approach her. As you near her, you notice she has tremors and looks like she is in distress. She is 64 years old. You introduce yourself and she quietly says hello and her name is Beth. You initially engage in small talk and ease into asking her about the tremors and if she is ok. She says that she thinks he is ok, but that she used to be in recovery from drinking and recently had relapsed. Beth has been wanted to go back to recovery, but then the fire happened and now she is not feeling well and not sure what to do.

What are your next steps?

1. What are your initial in-take questions? What key information do you need to gather?

2. Are you considering her cultural, religious, and ethnic background? How would you go about doing that while being respectful?

3. How would you frame your questions using the strengths-based model?

4. What indicators would you look for to determine if Beth is in a crisis state or in need of additional support services?

References

American Red Cross. http://www.redcross.org/about-us/our-work/disaster-relief

Bosman, J. (2017, January 6). *Inside a killer drug epidemic: A look at America's Opioid Crisis.* Retrieved from: https://www.nytimes.com/2017/01/06/us/opioid-crisis-epidemic.html?rref=co llection%2Ftimestopic%2FPrescription%20Drug%20Abuse&action=clickcontentCollection= timestopics&region=stream&module=stream_unit&version=latest&contentPlacement=3&pgt ype=collection&_r=1

Centers for Disease Control. (2016a, December 16). *Death overdose death data.* Retrieved from: https://www.cdc.gov/drugoverdose/data/statedeaths.html

Centers for Disease Control. (2016b, December 30). Increases in drug and opioid-involved over-dose deaths — United States, 2010–2015. *Morbidity and Mortality Weekly Report 65*(50–51), 1445–1452. Retrieved from: https://www.cdc.gov/mmwr/volumes/65/wr/mm655051e1. htm?s_cid=mm655051e1_w

Cutter, S. (2006). *The geography of social vulnerability: Race, class, and catastrophe.* Retrieved from: http://understandingkatrina.ssrc.org/Cutter/

Federal Emergency Management Agency. (2015). *Crisis counseling assistance and training program.* Retrieved from: https://www.fema.gov/recovery-directorate/crisis-counseling-assistance-training-program

Federal Emergency Management Agency. (2016). *Disaster declarations for 2016*. Retrieved from: https://www.fema.gov/disasters/grid/year/2016

Halpern, J., & Tramontin, M. (2007). *Disaster mental health theory and practice*. Belmont CA: Brooks/Cole Publishing.

Herman, J. (1997). *Trauma and recovery: The aftermath of violence – From domestic abuse to political terror*. New York: Basic Books.

Jacobs, G. A., Gray, B. L., Erickson, S. E., Gonzalez, E. D., & Quevillon, R. P. (2016). Disaster mental health and community-based psychological first aid: Concepts and education/training. *Journal of Clinical Psychology*. ISSN: 1097-4679, *72*(12), 1307–1317.

James, R. K., & Gilliland, B. (2017). *Crisis intervention strategies* (8th ed.). Cengage Learning: Boston, MA.

Manela, R., & Moxley, D. (2002). Best practices as agency-based knowledge in social welfare. *Administration in Social Work, 26*(4), 1–24.

Mattaini, M. A., & Lowery, C. T. (2007). Foundations of social work. In M. Mattani, C. Lowery, & C. Meyer (Eds.), *The foundations of social work practice: A graduate text* (4th ed.). Washington, D. C: NASW Press.

McCabe, O. L., Everly, G. S., Jr., Brown, L. M., Wendelboe, A. M., Hamid, N. H., Tallchief, V. L., & Links, J. M. (2014). Psychological first aid: A consensus-derived, empirically supported, competency-based training model. *American Journal of Public Health, 104*(4), 621–628.

Miller, J. L. (2012). *Psychosocial capacity building in response to disasters*. New York: Columbia University Press.

Mincin, J. (2012). Unpublished paper. *Strengths and weakness of the U.S.-based refugee resettlement program: A survey of International Rescue Committee employee perceptions*. New York: NYGraduate Center, City University of New York.

National Institutes on Alcohol Abuse and Alcoholism. (n.d.). *Alcohol use disorder*. Accessed on 1/13/18 from https://www.niaaa.nih.gov/alcoholhealth/overview-alcohol-consumption/alcohol-use-disorders

National Institute on Alcohol Abuse and Alcoholism. (2016, January). *Alcohol facts and statistics*. Retrieved from: https://www.niaaa.nih.gov/alcohol-health/overview-alcohol-consumption/alcohol-facts-and-statistics

National Institute on Drug Abuse. (2015). *Drug Facts*. Accessed on 1/13/18 from https://www.drugabuse.gov/publications/drugfacts/nationwide-trends

Quarentelli, J. L. (2006). *Catastrophes are different from disasters: Some implications for crisis planning and managing drawn from Katrina*. Retrieved from: http://understandingkatrina.ssrc.org/Quarantelli/

Ryan, D., Dooley, B., & Benson, C. (2008). Theoretical perspectives on post-migration adaptation and psychological well-being among refugees: Towards a resource-based model. *Journal of Refugee Studies, 21*(1), 1–18. Oxford, England: Oxford University Press.

Saleeby, D. (1996). The strength perspective in social work practice: Extensions and cautions. *Social Work, 41*(3), 296–305.

Stebnicki, M. A. (2017). *Disaster mental health counseling: Responding to trauma in a multicultural context*. New York: Springer Publishing.

Substance Abuse and Mental Health Services Administration. (2014). *Substance Use and Mental Health Estimates from the 2013 National Survey on Drug Use and Health: Overview of Findings*. Accessed on 1/13/18 from https://www.samhsa.gov/data/sites/default/files/NSDUH-SR200-RecoveryMonth-2014/NSDUHSR200-RecoveryMonth-2014.htm.

U.S. Census. (2012). https://www.census.gov/newsroom/releases/archives/miscellaneous/cb12-134.html

U.S. Health and Human Services. (2014a). *HHS disaster human services CONOPS*. Retrieved from: https://www.acf.hhs.gov/ohsepr/resource/hhs-disaster-human-services-conops-0

U.S. Health and Human Services. (2014b, March 27). *Health and human services concept of operations*. Retrieved from: https://www.phe.gov/Preparedness/planning/abc/Documents/disaster-humanservices-conops-2014.pdf

U.S. Health and Human Services. (2016, June). *The opioid epidemic by the numbers*. Retrieved from: https://www.hhs.gov/sites/default/files/Factsheet-opioids-061516.pdf

U.S. Health and Human Services. (2017, January). *Continuing progress on the opioid epidemic: The role of the affordable care act.* Retrieved from: https://aspe.hhs.gov/pdf-report/continuing-progress-opioid-epidemic-role-affordable-care-act

Walsh, J., Gibsons, A., & Brown, L. M. (2016). Peace of mind's price tag: The psychological costs of financial stressors on older adults postdisaster. *Translational Issues in Psychological Science, 2*(4), 408–417.

Chapter 12
Addiction, Spirituality, and Resilience

Jennifer Spitz

> The most beautiful people we have known are those who have
> known defeat, known suffering, known struggle, known loss,
> and have found their way out of the depths. These persons have
> an appreciation, a sensitivity, and an understanding of life that
> fills them with compassion, gentleness, and a deep loving
> concern. Beautiful people do not just happen.
> —Elizabeth Kubler-Ross

Introduction

Substance abuse is a disease that is difficult to understand. It is often simply thought of as a bad choice. Its consequences are severe and unintended, and the road to recovery can be long and winding. Most chronic relapsing diseases are not judged and critiqued as is substance abuse. Love, compassion, and support are readily offered by family and friends. These connections provide a sense of future and hope while building the sufferer's confidence in their ability to conquer the challenge. This is rarely true with addiction. Connections are supplanted by alienation, hope is lost, and an already fragile sense of self is further ravaged by shame and guilt. The work of recovery requires reconstructing a sense of self and a meaning and purpose to one's life. This chapter will explore the centrality of this process to sustained recovery. Themes of attachment, spirituality, and resilience will be discussed as context for recovery.

In the *Diagnostic and Statistical Manual of Mental Disorders* (5th ed.; DSM-5; American Psychiatric Association, 2013), a diagnostic distinction between substance abuse and dependence has been eliminated. Diagnostic criteria now exist across a continuum. This is a significant and important change. Previous diagnostic

J. Spitz (✉)
SUNY Empire State College, Community & Human Services, Hartsdale, NY, USA
e-mail: Jennifer.Spitz@esc.edu

© Springer International Publishing AG 2018
T. MacMillan, A. Sisselman-Borgia (eds.), *New Directions in Treatment,
Education, and Outreach for Mental Health and Addiction*, Advances in Mental
Health and Addiction, https://doi.org/10.1007/978-3-319-72778-3_12

requirements prohibited a more nuanced assessment which could account for the complexity with which addictive disease often presents. While the disease progresses rapidly for some, resulting in behaviors and consequences that constitute dependence, clinicians are often faced with muddier situations in which they must parse out problematic substance use.

> The client may drink in an episodic or binge pattern or use cocaine, episodically, in large social situations.
>
> Or, the marijuana smoker only partakes when friends make it available.
>
> There's the college student who is using Adderall to improve focus and energy when studying for long hours or the athlete whose Vicodin, prescribed for a sports injury, has become the only source of relaxation and escape.
>
> And the 40-year-old parent of three young children who has one or two (an occasional third) glasses of wine while trudging through the evening routine.
>
> And finally, the young business professional who needs to "let loose" on the weekends and typically ramps up with a few drinks and manages insomnia with a few "roofies."

Are these individuals addicted? Do we base this response on how much, how often, with whom, and when? These inquiries will be made when assessing an individual to determine the nature and extent of their substance use. There is a great deal of interpretation as to the causes of the maladaptive behavior (Magidson, Bornovalova, & Daughters, 2010). For example, is the high school junior missing class and withdrawing from friends because he/she is drinking excessively or is the excessive drinking causing the former? In addiction treatment, such dilemmas often occur early on with clients who view their use as recreational or attribute problematic use to issues other than the possibility of addictive illness. This is when clients are typically labeled as "in denial" or "resistant". However, one could argue that denial is an over applied concept. Ambivalence might be a more appropriate term. What will sobriety mean? What will life look like? "Exercising ambivalence reduces resistance to treatment and change by validating a wide array of possible outcomes through detailed exploration of how a behavior pattern works for a client" (Shaffer & Simoneau, 2001, p. 102). Resistance reduction creates space for a client's ambivalence without an expectation of change. Shaffer (1992) posits that painful ambivalence stimulates denial which emerges from the split between the positive and negative aspects of an addictive behavior pattern. "The addict literally embodies this ambivalence, wanting to change and stay the same simultaneously" (Kemp & Butler, 2013, p. 259). Consider behaviors that can become rituals or habits such as a morning cup of coffee or a favorite reality TV show. Now consider the void left by their extinction. Will there be a replacement and will it be as satisfying? This is difficult to answer! Hence, the dilemma for the individual with a substance use disorder. One can see how fear and uncertainty can cause ambivalence about change.

To maximize the potential for change, we must carefully assess the motivation for it. Motivational interviewing (MI) is a counseling approach that puts this goal at its center, starting where the client is. Motivational interviewing has been defined as "a directive, client centered counseling style for eliciting behavior change by helping clients to explore and resolve ambivalence" (Rollnick & Allison, 2004, p. 105). In this model, the change process is segmented into specific tasks to be accomplished and goals to be achieved (DiClemente, Schlundt, & Gemmell, 2004, p. 104). DiClemente et al. (2004) suggest that there are five stages of change: precontemplation, contemplation, preparation, action, and maintenance. In the precontemplation stage, there is no desire for or intent to change. Many substance abusers enter treatment in this stage, sometimes by legal mandate. In the contemplation stage, one may be aware of a problem but not yet ready to commit to doing something about it. Next is the preparation stage in which some immediate action is taken that leads to small change. In the action stage, the individual is engaged in the process of change and behavior modification. Finally, in the maintenance stage, the goal is integration of change to solidify gains (DiClemente et al., 2004). By identifying where the client lands on this continuum, the counselor can craft targeted interventions that have an increased chance of success (DiClemente et al., 2004).

MI was initially considered an effective model for substance abuse due to its direct and change-oriented approach. It has since become a more widely applied model for dealing with depression, anxiety, and compulsive behaviors (Rollnick & Allison, 2004). Much of its effectiveness lies in the collaborative working relationship between client and counselor in which the client is fully the driver of change. With this in mind, let's expand our lens. What if we thought about the habitual and harmful use of substances as purposeful behavior? After all, why would someone repeatedly engage in dangerous and destructive behavior with diminishing returns? Let's consider an idea, one that research supports; there is a strong connection between substance misuse and attachment (Fletcher, Nutton, & Brend, 2015; Flores, 2006; Höfler & Kooyman, 1996; Khantzian, 2012), and this may be where the clinical journey should begin.

Attachment and Substance Misuse: A Theoretical Perspective

Attachment theory was initially developed by John Bowlby (1958), who became interested in the subject while working with children. Attachment behavior, according to Bowlby (1951, 1958), is an instinctive penchant to seek safety in proximity with a specific individual, the attachment figure (typically mother or primary caregiver), who is perceived to be protective. Bowlby (1951) posits that interactions of genetic, neurobiological, and developmental factors contribute to the regulation of stress resilience, anxiety sensitivity, and personality development. In addition, the primary caregiver's ability to tune into (attunement) and reflect (mirroring) the emotional states of the infant are essential to the development of emotional capacity and competence (Bretherton, 1992). It is through these processes that the infant comes to understand the self as a separate entity with distinct feeling states and ultimately develops understanding of and empathy for the feelings of others. This is the groundwork for emotional self-regulation and identity. Incongruent mirroring leads to mistrust of one's own emotional responses and the need to search the social environment for cues about how to think, feel, and act (Padykula & Conklin, 2010).

Substance use disorders can evolve from the attempt to regulate one's attachment system in an effort to adapt (Padykula & Conklin, 2010). Individuals with substance use disorders suffer because they cannot or do not regulate their emotions, self-esteem, relationships, and behavior (Khantzian, 2012,). Self-regulation difficulties increase vulnerability to substance misuse. These individuals have great difficulty recognizing and tolerating feelings. This is due, in part, to fragile self-esteem and the absence of self-efficacy and competence (Graber, Turner, & Madill, 2016). Therefore, relationships with oneself and others are undeveloped or impaired by the lack of insight and skill necessary to sustain them. Substances become a means of avoidance and distraction. Or, they might provide a false sense of confidence often portrayed as bravado that further undermines relationships. Taking Khantzian's thinking forward, it can be suggested that the substance of abuse becomes the substitute for relationship to oneself and others (Khantzian, 2012). Höfler and Kooyman (1996) argued that an individual might choose a substance as an attachment alternative to relationships. They linked this use of substances-as-relationships to attachment ruptures in childhood, manifesting during the life-transition stage in adolescence. "Because these individuals have an inability to recognize and regulate their own feelings and sense of self, they act as though they do not need close interpersonal relationships" (Khantzian, 2012, p. 112).

Flores (2006) suggests that individuals who struggle with developing intimacy and closeness with others may seek a method in which to self-soothe in times of distress. The relationship with substances can arguably become an attachment, which acts as both an obstacle to and a substitute for interpersonal relationships (Fletcher et al., 2015). A drug can create the feeling of having a secure base, and, within this framework, "addictive behaviors can be understood as misguided attempts at self-repair" (Flores, 2006, p. 112). Substance abuse then becomes the solution, and the consequence of an individual's impaired ability to develop and maintain healthy attachments, effectively "protecting" the individual from relational vulnerability (Fletcher et al., 2015). When the fundamental ability to connect with others is damaged, it is not surprising that some seek external emotional support and regulation from a substance. As the use of substances increases, the individual's ability to interact with others is further impaired, and the cycle of addiction is set in motion (Fletcher et al., 2015, p. 117).

Wedekind et al. (2013) conducted a study of 59 inpatient alcohol-addicted males and females to investigate attachment styles. "The prevalence of the secure attachment style in the sample was 33% and 67% for the insecure attachment style. Differences in the distribution between sexes were not significant. Secure attachment was found in 35% of males and 31% of females. Insecure attachment styles were accordingly found in 65% of males and 69% of females and could be distinguished into 24% dismissive (males 21%, females 31%), 24% ambivalent (males 23%, females 25%), and 19% avoidant (males 21%, females 13%)" (Wedekind et al., 2013). The study validated that subjects with insecure attachment styles have a reduced capability of experiencing reliability, trust, and safety through relationships. Although the sample size is small, the study clearly reinforces research findings on the significant role of attachment in human development and behavior.

Disruption in this process often leads to maladaptive attempts at repair. Addiction can be a manifestation of this. "The difficulty with self-definition implies that addicts have little intimate understanding of themselves in terms of morals, values, beliefs, individuality, interpersonal relationships, and social roles" (Wedekind et al., 2013, p.4).

An important goal of recovery is to "develop a sense of self" (Mustain & Helminiak, 2015, p. 366). This can be a challenging task as demonstrated by a 2009 study that examined the "lived experience" (p. 153) of alcohol addiction utilizing interpretive phenomenological analysis (IPA; Shinebourne & Smith, 2009). IPA is a qualitative method that gives voice to the lived experience of participants (Shinebourne & Smith, 2009). While there is subjectivity in this method, it provides an opportunity "to develop a rich picture of the felt experience, embedded in the world of the participant" (Shinebourne & Smith, 2009, p. 154). This study indicated that alcoholics experience a fractured or split sense of self that is in constant flux with no center or consistency (Shinebourne & Smith, 2009). "The untruth of addiction makes lying to self, then to others, increasingly more comfortable and likely" (Kemp & Butler, 2013). In addition, many losses have left feelings of disconnection and isolation. Recovery of self-identity will require a backward focus to allow "old wounds to recede into an authentic past" (Kemp & Butler, 2014, p. 263). Treatment must then focus on finding a road forward. This is where our discussion of spirituality begins.

Attachment Through Spirituality

"Spirituality is a word, a term, a concept, a process, an outcome, a practice, a search for the sacred, a norm, a value, a status, a state, an experience, a path, an opportunity, a meaning, a buzzword…something different to different people, or, to the same person at different times in his or her life, development and (trans)formation" (Allamani, Einstein, & Godlaski, 2013, p. 1082). Spirituality encompasses the individual's sense of self and sense of mission and purpose in life. "In contrast to religion, spirituality connotes a direct and personal experience of that which each individual considers sacred; this connotation is unmediated by a particular belief system prescribed by dogma or by hierarchical structure…."(Grodzicki & Galanter, 2005, p. 2). Having lost a sense of oneself and their place in the world, as well as many important relationships, the spiritual path is one of self-examination, discovery, and connection. "…recognizing the search for values, meaning, purpose, and a sense of transcendence offers an opportunity for the realization of personal accountability, social integration, positive thinking and emotional balance" (Grodzicki & Galanter, 2005, p. 2). Spirituality can be a protective barrier to the misuse of alcohol and other substances. Research indicates that spirituality is posited to be protective from alcohol and other drug misuse and is a unique component of recovery from substance abuse disorders (Sussman et al., 2013, p. 1204).

Significant events such as divorce, job loss, illness, and addiction raise difficult questions about our place and purpose in the world. "Inherent in traumatic events can be losses of both a concrete nature (e.g., people, possessions, places, safety) and an abstract nature (e.g., self-esteem, self-respect, self-worth)" (Furr, Johnson, & Goodall, 2015, p. 44). They highlight our vulnerabilities and limitations as human beings. "These are matters of 'ultimate anxiety': the anxiety and fate of death, the anxiety of emptiness and meaninglessness and the anxiety of guilt and condemnation" (Pargament, 2007, p. 11). With limited coping resources to tolerate the strong emotions evoked by such events, self-medication becomes an escape. "We use the whole process of addiction to escape unresolved painful feelings such as abandonment, worthlessness and emptiness, but at the same time as we try to escape them; these negative feelings fuel our attempts at addictive self-repair. It's paradoxical and it's a vicious circle, but that's what we do" (Nixon, 2013, p. 14).

Room (2013) questioned whether a connection exists between intoxication and spirituality. She posited that there is a meaningful transaction between addiction, intoxication, and spirituality and a spiritual element to addictive behavior that is relative to the search for connection. In early religious practices, intoxication was a means of connecting with the religious world. Contact with spirits would only come in an intoxicated state (Room, 2013). Today, in some religions and cultures, alcohol is a powerful signifier. Intoxication is only enjoyed with others, and it is through this sense of community that a spiritual connection is made. For others, intoxication can destroy spirituality when it causes disconnection as one withdraws into an isolated subjective experience (Room, 2013).

This idea can parlay into recovery, as well. Alcoholics Anonymous functions as a collective community of support centered around sobriety and spirituality. One attends these meetings for individual recovery as well as commitment to the well-being of the community. "Participation in 12-Step programs may alter members' social networks by increasing the number of acquaintances who support quitting or inoculate members from negative influences" (Gamble & O'Lawrence, 2016, p. 935). Lastly, abstinence can be seen as a spiritual practice or "badge of membership," again highlighting the value of connection through the shared goal of sobriety (Room, 2013). Room's framework offers an interesting lens through which addiction can be understood as a metaphor for one's search for meaning, connection, and purpose.

Resilience Through Spirituality

Resilient people do not let adversity define them. They find resilience by moving towards a goal beyond themselves, transcending pain and grief by perceiving bad times as a temporary state of affairs.... It's possible to strengthen your inner self and your belief in yourself, to define yourself as capable and competent. It's possible to fortify your psyche. It's possible to develop a sense of mastery. —Hara Estroff Marano, Editor-at-Large for Psychology Today

Resilience is the process of adapting well in the face of adversity, trauma, tragedy, threats, or significant sources of stress (Resilience, 2017). It enables us to bounce back from these difficult experiences. Resilience varies among individuals and is influenced by many factors such as personality, ethnicity, culture, and socioeconomic conditions (Seligman, 2011). Resilience is conceptualized not as a quality visible in every situation but as one defined and measured by the context, population, risk, promotive (or protective) factors, and outcome (Schultze-Lutter, Schimmelmann, & Schmidt, 2016). A history of physical, emotional, and/or social trauma will also influence one's degree of resilience. Promoting resilience, particularly among vulnerable populations, is important in reducing the risk of negative mental health outcomes and risky externalizing behaviors such as substance abuse and violence (Graber et al., 2016). Mechanisms that facilitate resilience include effective coping, self-efficacy, self-esteem, strong interpersonal skills, and a supportive friendship network (Graber et al., 2016). Resilient behavior is unique to everyone. Some will succumb to immobilizing emotional difficulty, while others have the ability to utilize physical and psychological measures to return to baseline functioning (Seligman, 2011). Still others demonstrate post-traumatic growth in which they emerge from a trauma physically and emotionally stronger. The ability to restabilize and/or grow from challenging experience demonstrates resilience (Seligman, 2011). Spirituality can be a powerful source of resilience. For those in recovery, spiritual practices instill positive emotions through activities that replace substance use. Individuals who rate themselves higher on spirituality also tend to have better health, less illness, better treatment response, and lower mortality rates (Womble, Labbe, & Cochran, 2013).

Practice Skills/Models

Most recovery models fail to connect the addict self with the recovery self (Nixon, 2013) increasing narcissistic and defensive behaviors. Pathology typically rests upon cognitive distortions, negative thoughts, dysfunctional attitudes, and maladaptive schema (Szabo, Toth, & Pakai, 2014). Grief and loss are also emotional stressors. Integration can be experienced only when individuals feel the vulnerability of the dark emotions that fuel their addiction and come in touch with the authentic self. Doing so without judgment or rejection allows the disparate pieces of the whole to come together (Nixon, 2013). From this emerges a new or renewed purpose. Atonement and reconciliation are important elements of this process. It is through these actions that the burden of shame is lightened (Lyons, Deane, Caputi, & Kelly, 2011). Treatment must focus on grieving, resolving and integrating losses, and developing resilience with which to face future losses (Furr et al., 2015). Life views and beliefs must be newly explicated.

Narrative therapy helps clients examine their lives and presumes many strengths, beliefs, and values that, in a revised narration, can become an empowering personal construct that enables a view of one's problems as separate from themselves.

Empirical studies have shown that narrative therapy has been a measurably effective tool against depressive symptoms and interpersonal problems (Vromans & Schweitzer, 2011, p. 5). One of narrative therapy's techniques is to externalize the problem, using language which defines it as influencing the person rather than existing within him. Recovery creates a space for a more adaptive narrative, drawing new conclusions about self and the world. A revised story builds resilience in that it engenders gratitude, hope, and healing. Events of the past can be interpreted as sources of strength and insight that are resources for challenges yet unknown. There is a parallel existence of distress and resilience (Vromans & Schweitzer, 2011).

In an interesting and unique study, oral narrative strategies were demonstrated to enhance psychological well-being. Participants utilized the narrative structure of fairy tales to elicit metaphorical meaning that would help to solve problems and increase well-being. The focus was on the psychoeducational content of traditional fairy tales, their problem-solving approach, and the process of maturation experienced by their characters (Ruini, Masoni, Ottolini, & Ferrar, 2014). Participants discussed the meaning they extracted and shared their own interpretation and value of the message. Themes addressed included resilience capacities, wisdom, and character strengths. This concept was applied to help clients write their own story. The intent of the exercise was the shift in thinking to make new connections to causal relationships, problem-solving, and new meaning in the story. "…their emotions were projected in a fictional, impossible setting, and this provided them with the right distance from problems, connected with a more effective cognitive engagement in problem solving" (Ruini et al., 2014, p. 7). The intent and value of narrative approaches is the empowerment it offers to the author who can reconstruct meaning and purpose in difficult times. The discovery of dormant strengths and untapped resilience is critical. A more adaptive self-image and improved relationships become real possibilities. Understanding the causes of maladaptive behavior allows for better decision-making and redefinition of beliefs and values. Discovering strength in one's struggle is perhaps one of the gifts of recovery.

Culture as Context

Client narratives provide a lens through which to view the influence of culture. This is a critical context in understanding how substance use may be culturally situated. However, a focus solely on race and/or ethnicity often ignores disparities that exist in regard to other aspects of identity (e.g., gender, socioeconomic status, disability, and sexual orientation) (Fisher-Borne, Cain, & Martin, 2015) and these must be considered. Culture also shifts over time in keeping with the sociopolitical landscape and, therefore, requires ongoing attunement. Cultural humility is a newer construct that emphasizes accountability over mastery. This means "a commitment to self-reflection that is active and responsible" (Fisher-Borne et al., 2015). Cultural humility acknowledges power inequities in practitioner-client relationships and suggests awareness on the part of providers about the influence of cultural values and structural forces (Fisher-Borne et al., 2015) that shape client experiences and opportunities. It is essential for practitioners to be aware of the impact of their own beliefs and practices, as well as privilege and power on interactions with clients. Substance misuse or substance use disorders add another layer, as they, too, create an identity.

Substance use disorder most often exists in a context of pain. Its roots are deep in experiences of abandonment, rejection, loss, betrayal, humiliation, abuse aggression, and punishment. Feelings of worthlessness, inadequacy, and emptiness are compounded by shame, guilt, fear, and anger caused by the self-destructive vortex that is addiction. Pain resolution is a primary purpose of substance use (Kim-Lok Oh, Megat Ahmad, Bahari, & Voo, 2016). Instantaneous relief is achieved but quickly becomes elusive. The end is no longer justified by the means. Early steps into recovery serve the very same purpose. Honesty, accountability, and empowerment bring trust, faith, and relationship, and the pain gradually ebbs.

Conclusion

We have examined the relationship of addictive illness to attachment impairments and disruptions and explored spirituality as a source of both connection and resilience. These are important elements in treatment plans. Further mixed methods research which provides both quantitative and qualitative data would be beneficial in developing targeted interventions that address the biopsychospiritual needs.

References

Allamani, A., Einstein, S., & Godlaski, T. (2013). A review of the many meanings of an unseizable concept. *Substance Use and Misuse, 48*, 1081–1084.

American Psychiatric Association. (2013). *Diagnostic and statistical manual of mental disorders* (5th ed.). Washington, DC: Author.

Bowlby, J. (1951). Maternal care and mental health. World Health Organization Monograph (Serial No. 2).

Bowlby, J. (1958). The nature of the child's tie to his mother. *The International Journal of Psychoanalysis, 25*, 19–52.

Bretherton, I. (1992). The origins of attachment theory: John Bowlby and Mary Ainsworth. *Developmental Psychology, 28*, 759–775.

DiClemente, C. C., Schlundt, D., & Gemmell, L. (2004). Readiness and stages of change in addiction treatment. *The American Journal on Addictions, 13*(2), 103–119.

Fisher-Borne, M., Montana Cain, J., & Martin, S. L. (2015). From mastery to accountability: Cultural humility as an alternative to cultural competence. *Social Work Education, 34*(2), 165–181.

Fletcher, K., Nutton, J., & Brend, D. (2015). Attachment, a matter of substance: The potential of attachment theory in the treatment of addictions. *Clinical Social Work Journal, 43*, 109–117.

Flores, P. J. (2006). Conflict and repair in addiction treatment: An attachment disorder perspective. *Journal of Groups in Addiction & Recovery, 1*(1), 5–26.

Furr, S. R., Johnson, D., & Goodall, C. S. (2015). The prevalence of grief and loss in substance abuse treatment. *Journal of Addictions and Offender Counseling, 36*(1), 43–56.

Gamble, J., & O'Lawrence, H. (2016). An overview of the efficacy of the 12-step group therapy for substance abuse treatment. *Journal of Health and Human Services Administration, 39*(1), 142–160.

Graber, R., Turner, R., & Madill, A. (2016). Best friends and better coping: Facilitating psychological resilience through boys' and girls' closest friendships. *British Journal of Psychology (London, England: 1953), 107*(2), 338–358.

Grodzicki, J., & Galanter, M. (2005). Spirituality and addiction. *Substance Abuse, 26*(2), 1–4.

Höfler, D. Z., & Kooyman, M. (1996). Attachment transition, addiction and therapeutic bonding— An integrative approach. *Journal of Substance Abuse Treatment, 13*(6), 511–519.

Kemp, R., & Butler, A. (2013). Love, hate and the emergence of self in addiction recovery. *Existential Analysis, 25*(2), 257–268.

Kemp, R., & Butler, A. (2014). Love, hate and the emergence of self in addiction recovery. *Existential Analysis, 25*(2), 257.

Khantzian, E. J. (2012). Reflections on treating addictive disorders: A psychodynamic perspective. *American Journal on Addictions, 21*(3), 274–279.

Kim-Lok Oh, A., Megat Ahmad, P. H., Bahari, F. B., & Voo, P. (2016). Pain resolving in addiction and recovery: A grounded theory study. *Grounded Theory Review, 15*(2), 8–24.

Lyons, G. C., Deane, F. P., Caputi, P., & Kelly, P. J. (2011). Spirituality and the treatment of substance use disorders: An exploration of forgiveness, resentment and purpose in life. *Addiction Research & Theory, 19*(5), 459–469.

Magidson, J. F., Bornovalova, M. A., & Daughters, S. B. (2010). Drug abuse. In D. L. Segal & M. Hersen (Eds.), *Diagnostic interviewing* (pp. 251–281). New York: Springer.

Mustain, J. R., & Helminiak, D. A. (2015). Understanding spirituality in recovery from addiction: Reintegrating the psyche to release the human spirit. *Addiction Research & Theory, 23*(5), 364–371.

Nixon, S. J. (2013). Executive functioning among young people in relation to alcohol use. *Current Opinion in Psychiatry, 26*(4), 305–309.

Padykula, N. L., & Conklin, P. (2010). The self-regulation model of attachment trauma and addiction. *Clinical Social Work Journal, 38*(4), 351–360.

Pargament, K. (2007). *Spiritually integrated psychotherapy: Understanding and addressing the sacred.* New York: The Guilford Press.

Resilience. (2017). *American Psychological Association.* Retrieved from http://www.apa.org/help-center/road-resilience.aspx

Rollnick, S., & Allison, J. (2004). Motivational interviewing. In N. Heather & T. Stockwell (Eds.), *The essential handbook of treatment and prevention of alcohol problems* (pp. 105–115). West Sussex, UK: Wiley.

Room, R. (2013). Spirituality, intoxication and addiction: Six forms of relationship. *Substance Use & Misuse, 48*(12), 1109–1113.

Ruini, C., Masoni, L., Ottolini, F., & Ferrari, S. (2014). Positive Narrative Group Psychotherapy: The use of traditional fairy tales to enhance psychological well-being and growth. *Psychological Well Being, 4*(1), 1–13.

Sara Jo Nixon, Executive functioning among young people in relation to alcohol use. Current Opinion in Psychiatry 26 (4):305-309(2013) should be included.

Schultze-Lutter, F., Schimmelmann, B., & Schmidt, S. (2016). Resilience, risk, mental health and well-being: Associations and conceptual differences. *European Child & Adolescent Psychiatry, 25*(5), 459–466.

Seligman, M. E. (2011). Building resilience: What business can learn from a pioneering army program for fostering post-traumatic growth. *Harvard Business Review, 89*(4), 100.

Shaffer, H. J. (1992). The psychology of stage change: The transition from addiction to recovery. In J. H. Lowinson, P. Ruiz, R. B. Millman, & J. Langrod (Eds.), *Substance abuse: A comprehensive textbook* (2nd ed., pp. 100–105). Baltimore: Williams and Wilkins.

Shaffer, H. J., & Simoneau, G. (2001). Reducing resistance and denial by exercising ambivalence during the treatment of addiction. *Journal of Substance Abuse Treatment, 20*, 99–105.

Shinebourne, P., & Smith, J. (2009). Alcohol and the self: An interpretative phenomenological analysis of the experience of addiction and its impact on the sense of self and identity. *Addiction Research and Theory, 17*, 152–167.

Sussman, S., Milam, J., Arpawong, T. E., Tsai, J., Black, D. S., & Wills, T. A. (2013). Spirituality in addictions treatment: Wisdom to know...what it is. *Substance Use & Misuse, 48*(12), 1203–1217.

Szabo, J., Toth, S., & Pakai, A. (2014). Narrative group therapy for alcohol dependent patients. *International Journal of Mental Health and Addiction, 12*(4), 470–476.

Vromans, L., & Schweitzer, R. (2011). Narrative therapy for adults with major depressive disorder: Improved symptom and interpersonal outcomes. *Psychotherapy Research, 21*, 4–15.

Wedekind, D., Bandelow, B., Heitmann, S., Havemann-Reinecke, U., Engel, K. R., & Huether, G. (2013). Attachment style, anxiety coping, and personality-styles in withdrawn alcohol addicted inpatients. *Substance Abuse Treatment, Prevention and Policy, 10*(8), 1–7.

Womble, M. N., Labbe, E. E., & Cochran, C. R. (2013). Spirituality and personality: Understanding their relationship to health resilience. *Psychological Reports, 112*(3), 706–716.

Chapter 13
A Framework for Addressing Spirituality in the Treatment of Substance Use Disorders: The Three-Legged Stool

E. Gail Horton and Naelys Luna

Since the 1930s, spirituality has been recognized as an important factor in recovery from substance use disorders (SUD) as evidenced by the important place it has held in 12-step support groups such as Alcoholics Anonymous. These groups are based on the assumption that SUD is both a spiritual and a physical disease, and they emphasize spiritual principles and practices to increase meaning in their members' lives (Chen, 2006; Jarusiewics, 2000). A body of research concerning relationships between spirituality and recovery from SUD has been growing over the past decade in response to social work and mental health professionals' increasing interest in how it can help them to treat their clients more successfully (Cook, 2004). Research has found spirituality to be associated with maintenance of abstinence (Kelly, Stout, Magill, Tonigan, & Pagano, 2011; Piderman, Schneekloth, Pankratz, Stevens, & Altschuler, 2008) and reduced relapse into heavy drinking (Robinson, Cranford, Webb, & Brower, 2007). In addition, recent studies have found negative relationships between spirituality and symptoms of comorbid depressive symptomatology (Diaz et al., 2011; Diaz, Horton, McIlveen, Weiner, & Williams, 2011; Diaz, Horton, & Malloy, 2014).

Furthermore, clients themselves are apparently interested in incorporating spirituality into their recovery processes. For example, Arnold, Avants, Margolin, and Marcotte (2002) found that among a sample of HIV-positive inner-city drug users, a large majority expressed interest in treatment with a focus on spirituality. Another study similarly found that respondents indicated that they wanted more of an emphasis on spirituality in treatment (Galanter et al., 2007). In addition, these respondents indicated that their spiritually-based 12-step self-help groups were more helpful to their recovery process than was outpatient substance abuse therapy and that their spiritual lives were even more important to them than having a job.

E. Gail Horton • N. Luna (✉)
Florida Atlantic University, School of Social Work, Boca Raton, FL, USA
e-mail: Ndiaz10@fau.edu

© Springer International Publishing AG 2018
T. MacMillan, A. Sisselman-Borgia (eds.), *New Directions in Treatment, Education, and Outreach for Mental Health and Addiction*, Advances in Mental Health and Addiction, https://doi.org/10.1007/978-3-319-72778-3_13

Fig. 13.1 The three-
legged stool framework

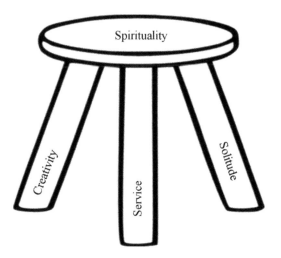

Some individuals, particularly those with dual diagnoses, may need help in developing a spiritual life, either from peers in their 12-step support groups or from their therapists (Polcin & Zemore, 2004). Research, however, has not yet provided much concrete guidance concerning what form this help should take. One reason for this gap in the knowledge base may be that the term *spirituality* has not been defined clearly, and thus efforts to operationalize spirituality in treatment have been seriously hampered (Cook, 2004). In this chapter, we will present a theoretical model based on the multidimensional nature of spirituality that will support clinical practitioners in their efforts to provide interventions to their clients in substance abuse treatment and other mental health settings. We call it the three-legged stool, spirituality being the "seat" of the stool and the three "legs" supporting the seat being *creativity*, *service*, and *solitude* (Fig. 13.1).

The three-legged stool framework has emerged slowly over our years of teaching and research, and it finally coalesced as we began to present our research results at national and international conferences. While teaching courses in chemical dependence, it became obvious to one of us (EGH) that most substance abuse textbooks offer very little information on the importance of spirituality to human development. Nor do they provide suggestions concerning which spiritual interventions might provide a focus to assist individuals with substance use problems to gain or maintain sobriety. Recognizing this dearth of information concerning the importance of spirituality in the treatment of SUD, we began to formulate a model that could offer some direction to practitioners interested in incorporating it into their treatment. It is, however, important to note that the framework we are suggesting is just in the initial stages of development and has not yet been tested empirically.

We will begin our presentation of the three-legged stool framework with a review of the literature concerning spiritual interventions in the treatment of substance abuse. We will then discuss definitions of spirituality found in the literature that inform our model. Next, we discuss the three-legged stool model in detail, justifying the inclusion of creativity, service, and solitude by presenting the conceptual and empirical literature associated with each leg. Lastly, we will acknowledge limitations of the framework and suggest possible future research to improve and/or validate it.

Spirituality and Substance Use Disorder Treatment Outcomes

White and Whiters (2005) have noted the historical roots of faith-based recovery spread well back into the eighteenth century in the USA. By the 1930s, Alcoholics Anonymous (AA), a self-help program strongly influenced by evangelical Christian ideology (Dermatis & Galanter, 2015), was established and growing. Despite the long history of attempts to use spirituality to address SUD, spirituality as an intervention in the treatment of alcohol and drug problems has not been well studied (Miller & Bogenschutz, 2008), and the results of the studies that have been conducted are not uniformly positive. For example, researchers have found direct positive relationships between spirituality and abstinence measures (Piderman et al., 2008; Robinson et al., 2007; Robinson, Krentzman, Webb, & Brower, 2011; Sterling et al., 2007) as well as the positive mediating effects of spirituality between drinking outcomes and AA attendance (Kelly et al., 2011; Zemore, 2007a). Other researchers, on the other hand, have found no such mediating effects (Magura et al., 2003; Tonigan, in Owen et al., 2003; Tonigan, in Longabaugh et al., 2005).

Very little research has explored relationships between spirituality and co-occurring substance use and mental health disorders even though it has been known for many years that co-occurring disorders can complicate the treatment of SUD (Claus & Kindleberger, 2002; McLellan, Luborsky, Woody, O'Brien, & Druley, 1983; Weisner, Matzger, & Kaskutas, 2003). One early study found that spirituality was equally important to patients and their service providers and that those service providers frequently underestimated how important spirituality was to their patients (McDowell, Galanter, Goldfarb, & Lifschutz, 1996). These researchers did not, however, explore treatment outcomes in their sample. Polcin and Zemore (2004) examined psychiatric severity and spirituality among a sample of individuals attending 12-step self-help groups and found that while severity of co-occurring psychiatric symptoms was not related to length of sobriety, it was significantly negatively related to measures of spirituality. They explained this unexpected finding by pointing out that their sample consisted of individuals attending a self-help group and may not have been receiving treatment for their psychiatric issues.

The reasons for these mixed results concerning associations between spirituality and positive treatment outcomes are not yet fully understood. However, it is possible that a persistent lack of agreement on how to define and operationalize the term spirituality may be at least partially to blame. In the next section, we discuss various definitions as found in the literature and explain how spirituality is operationalized in the three-legged stool framework.

Defining Spirituality

Cook (2004) has provided an excellent example of the depth and breadth of the problem of defining spirituality as it relates to the treatment of SUD. He undertook a review of all books and articles published between 1922 and 2001 that focused on spirituality and SUD. Among the 265 publications that he identified, he found a total of 13 conceptual components of spiritualty: relatedness, transcendence, humanity, core/force/soul, meaning/purpose, authenticity/truth, values, non-materiality, (non)religiousness, wholeness, self-knowledge, creativity, and consciousness. Given this, it can easily be seen why it has been so difficult for researchers to measure the concept.

Researchers have over time used a broad variety of instruments to measure different aspects of spirituality. One early study measured spirituality by asking respondents about their perceptions of God as being more or less controlling vs. loving (Benson & Spilka, 1973). Continuing this linking of spirituality and religious thought, in the 1990s one study explored the quality of participants' relationship with God (Hall & Edwards, 1996). About that same time, Piedmont (1999) noted that all religions recognize "the capacity of individuals to stand outside of their immediate sense of time and place to view life from a larger, more objective perspective" (p. 988), calling this capacity spiritual transcendence. His research determined three dimensions of transcendence – prayer fulfillment (joy and contentment resulting from prayer), universality (unity and purpose in life), and connectedness (personal responsibility to others).

In the early 2000s, researchers began to move away from the traditional view of spirituality as being necessarily religious in nature. One group constructed a scale, the Spirituality Index of Well-being, that specifically excluded measures of religious practices, beliefs, and support (Daaleman & Frey, 2004; Frey, Daaleman, & Peyton, 2005). They noted along with other researchers (e.g., Piderman et al., 2008; Seidlitz et al., 2002) that spirituality appears to be multidimensional in nature, with religion being just one of the dimensions. They decided to focus on factors associated with the "nonreligious spiritual propensity" (p. 559) to ask and find answers to major existential questions having to do with purpose and meaning in life.

Several groups of researchers have noted a close relationship between religion and spirituality but have also identified distinct differences between the concepts. For example, Seidlitz et al. (2002) argued that the term spirituality tends to include personal experiences of the Transcendent, while religiousness tends to include institutional beliefs and practices. These researchers devised an instrument (the Spiritual Transcendence Index) to measure "experiences of transcending one's ordinary psychological experiences and life circumstances" (p. 441). They argued that this transcendence results in a cognitive component (purpose and meaning in life) and an affective component (feelings of spiritual communion). Their scale was similar to one devised earlier by Paloutzian and Ellison (1982) (the Spiritual Well-being Scale) that included aspects of existential well-being (purpose and meaning in life) and religious well-being (connectedness to God).

Other authors have also noted the distinctions between spirituality and religion. From his review of writings concerning spirituality and SUD, Cook (2004) constructed a definition of spirituality as being "a distinctive, potentially creative and universal dimension of human experience" (p. 548) that involves a relationship with oneself, with others, or with something transcending self that provides fundamental purpose and meaning to life. Hodge and McGrew (2005) found that college students tended to define spirituality as a belief in and connection with God or a Higher Power, while the term religion tended to mean the practice of that spirituality (rituals, worship). Canda and Furman (2010) defined spirituality as being "a universal quality of human beings and their cultures related to the quest for meaning, purpose, morality, transcendence, well-being and profound relationships with ourselves, others and ultimate reality" (p. 5). In contrast, they defined religion as being "an institutionalized . . . pattern of values, beliefs, symbols, behaviors and experiences" (p. 76) manifested in particular cultures and communities.

The legs of the three-legged stool framework (creativity, service, and solitude) emerged directly out of the definitions discussed above. Creativity is seen as being a quality present in all human beings that both allows the expression of the core/force/soul and provides a connection with the Transcendent. Service is seen as a way to build existential purpose and meaning by moving beyond the tendency to focus only on self and connecting positively with others in the broader community. Solitude is also seen as a way to develop purpose and meaning through a deepening of their relationship with self and something beyond self through solitary prayer and meditation. We also believe that this development of solitude practices will close the circle by promoting individuals' expression of their innate creativity.

Below, we will discuss the theoretical and empirical literature pertaining to the three legs of our suggested framework as they relate to the treatment of SUD.

Creativity

Although we consider this first leg of the stool, creativity, to be an important route to self-knowledge and existential purpose and meaning in life for individuals with substance use disorders, there is very little in the SUD literature to date that addresses its value in treatment. Cropley (2006) suggested that Maslow, May, and Rogers, some of our earliest and most influential mental health practitioners and theoreticians, saw creativity as being "a form of self-expression. .. that is intimately connected with personal dignity, expression of one's inner being, self-actualization and the like" (p. 125). Siegel (2012), a well-known and respected author on interpersonal neurobiology, has argued that creativity is "a way of being in which life emerges in new and fresh combinations of inner experiences and outer explorations" (p. 17–18) that supports both mental and physical health. Therefore, in our three-legged stool framework, creativity is understood to be the emergence of clients' fresh, new ideas that may arise either consciously or unconsciously. The creative process allows the inner self (core/force/soul) to be expressed and supports the development of purpose and meaning in life.

Our review of the literature concerning creativity and SUD identified articles that focused on two types of creative therapy – creative arts therapy and play therapy. Unfortunately, researchers in the creative arts and play therapy fields have not yet documented the effectiveness of these modalities in rigorous research. All of the studies we identified were simply descriptions of their work with individual clients, and none were supported by quantitative or qualitative data and analysis. However, we feel comfortable in discussing them because the authors of these small studies were clearly convinced that their clients had benefitted from the creative activities or play that they documented. In the subsections below, we present the conceptual and empirical support that we identified concerning these creative modalities.

Creative arts therapy According to the National Coalition of Creative Arts Therapies Associations (at http://www.nccata.org/#), creative arts (or recreational) therapy utilizes a wide variety of creative activities such as writing (both prose and poetry), dance and movement, music, painting and drawing, and drama. These activities are used in the treatment of individuals ranging in age from children in neonatal nurseries to the elderly in nursing homes.

Although no empirical research to date has explored the value of the creative arts as a spiritual intervention, there is some theoretical support for its inclusion in our three-legged stool framework. Armstrong (1993), Damianakis (2001), and Edwards (2000) have all held that creative activities are closely associated with spirituality in the literature. For example, Damianakis (2001) argued that any writing that is original to the writer (writing not limited to poetry or fiction) is creative writing and, as such, an inherently spiritual act. Furthermore, he linked this kind of writing to Maslow's (1968) concept of self-actualization, arguing that creativity is a source of self-transcendence that leads to "a deeper sense of eternity, connection to others and the cosmos" (p. 26). Oreskovic and Bodor (2010), on the other hand, have noted that the abuse of substances can actually damage the parts of the brain that maintain balance of thoughts and emotions, thus impairing creative solutions to life problems.

There have been only five peer-reviewed studies that have focused on creative arts interventions for individuals with substance use issues (Feen-Calligan, 2007; Johnson, 1990; Julliard, 1995; Matto, 2002; Reiland, 1990). A broad range of creative activities were explored in these articles. However, all of the studies had methodological limitations related to study design and sample size, making it impossible to make statistically significant correlations or causal connections between the interventions used and treatment outcomes. The earliest studies described the use of drawing (Reiland, 1990); poetry, art, dance, and music/drama performance therapies (Johnson, 1990); and multimedia collage and role-plays (Julliard, 1995). Later studies combined art therapy and cognitive behavioral therapy (Matto, 2002) and art and creative journaling (Feen-Calligan, 2007). These creative activities were offered to clients in varied treatment settings: detox (Feen-Calligan, 2007), inpatient (Matto, 2002; Reiland, 1990), partial hospitalization (Johnson, 1990), and intensive outpatient (Julliard, 1995). Despite the methodological shortcomings of these studies, in every case the authors clearly believed that the creative activities were beneficial to their clients by increasing their self-awareness (Matto, 2002; Reiland, 1990), breaking through denial and understanding their powerlessness over their use of substances (Julliard, 1995; Matto, 2002), overcoming recovery-related shame (Johnson, 1990), and increasing problem-solving capabilities and connectedness to the Transcendent (Feen-Calligan, 2007).

In summary, although creative arts interventions have not yet been empirically validated, both theoretical and preliminary research suggest that creative arts therapy may be a useful adjunct to other SUD treatment modalities. We believe that these interventions may result in an increase in spirituality as clients gain knowledge of self and are able to express their core/force/soul, experience relatedness to their Higher Power, and develop purpose and meaning in life.

Play therapy McDargh (1986) has noted that play can be defined as

> the capacity for relaxed, spontaneous, and unguarded experiencing of the self's agency and creativity in acting upon the world. In play, the [individual] tries on roles, tests limits, explores the world, experiments with emotions that outside the space of play would be too daunting or problematic or anxiety provoking. (p. 259)

Play therapy has not generally been thought of as a spiritual intervention. However, McDargh has pointed out that play is inherently spiritual for many people, since for them "it is the inner representation of God that is the effective guarantor of play. ... that evokes the environment within which emotional refueling can take place, and the self restored and recuperated" (p. 259).

There are many activities that fall under the umbrella of play therapy. According to Schaefer (2003) these activities could include role-play, psychodrama, verbal play (humor), playing with dolls, board games, and sand tray. Indeed, Amatruda (2003) found that sand tray helped her clients presenting with grief, depression, and trauma to find their center, to achieve a sense of wholeness, and to forge a connection to the divine.

Unfortunately, as with the literature on creative arts therapy, research on the use of play therapy techniques with individuals in treatment for substance use issues is extremely scant. However, one small qualitative study was conducted using a sample of four male repeat offenders mandated into substance abuse treatment (Monakes, Garza, Wiesner, & Watts, 2011). This study found that in conjunction with cognitive behavioral therapy, the use of Adlerian sand tray therapy was perceived by the clients as having provoked insights that allowed them to delve deeper into their issues than talk therapy alone. In addition, the sand tray exercises helped them to reevaluate their lifestyles and set meaningful goals for change.

Similarly, Avrahami (2003) and Treadwell, Kumar, and Wright (2010) have attempted to use psychodrama in conjunction with cognitive behavioral therapy in the treatment of SUD. They found that psychodrama helped their clients to recognize and correct their faulty thinking patterns. Similarly, Somov (2008) reported that residential clients found psychodrama to be a useful way to practice relapse prevention skills and to make concrete and realistic treatment termination plans.

Ramseur and Wiener (2003) also found psychodrama to be useful in developing relapse prevention skills. In addition they found that it helped to build trust and interdependence among group members.

Although the research mentioned above was unable to determine a causal relationship between the use of play therapy techniques and improvement in client functioning, the studies are strongly suggestive of a relationship between creativity/play and the self/core/soul aspect of spirituality. Therefore, we include play therapy in the three-legged stool framework for its potential to promote connectedness to core self, to others, and to the Transcendent.

Service

The second leg of our three-legged stool framework is service. It has long been assumed that service to others is a fundamental element of a strong spiritual life (Sher & Straughan, 2005). Within the 12-step recovery community, service is seen as being fundamental to long-term abstinence (Humphreys, 2004; Tonigan, 2007). Indeed, in research on helping behaviors in AA, Zemore (2007b) argued that, given the importance of helping activities in virtually all major religions, helping others is "the behavioral expression of a spiritual orientation" (p. 447). Zemore and Pagano (2008) noted that spirituality and service are tightly intertwined in 12-step programs such as AA, as evidenced by their assumption that helping other alcoholics is fundamental to the spiritual growth of the helper. They defined service as being any voluntary action that is intended to provide emotional or instrumental help to another individual or to the broader community with no expectation of external reward. We base our concept of service in the three-legged stool framework on this definition by Zemore and Pagano.

Unlike the gap in the literature concerning creativity and substance abuse, there are several methodologically sound studies in the literature that have found service to be beneficial to relapse prevention (Pagano, Friend, Tonigan, Scott, & Stout, 2004; Pagano, Zemore, Onder, & Stout, 2009; Witbrodt & Kaskutas, 2005; Zemore, Kaskutas, & Ammon, 2004). For example, Witbrodt and Kaskutas (2005) conducted a longitudinal randomized control design study of individuals diagnosed with substance use disorder. They discovered that involvement in 12-step related service was a better predictor of 1-year posttreatment abstinence than any of the other variables in the study. The other variables included eight variables concerning 12-step work (e.g., having a sponsor and attendance at meetings) and ten variables concerning participants' social networks (e.g., number of friends who actively support sobriety and who maintain complete abstinence).

Similarly, Pagano et al. (2004) found a significant inverse relationship between self-reported AA-related helping behaviors and the probability of relapse 1 year after treatment completion among a large sample of individuals diagnosed with alcohol use disorder. However, since the study did not include a control group, a causal relationship could be established. In addition, Zemore et al. (2004) have found significant relationships between in-treatment helping behaviors and both posttreatment 12-step involvement and lower rates of binge drinking.

Zemore and Kaskutas (2004), however, have shown that not all forms of service are equally beneficial. They explored relationships between spirituality and three forms of helping – recovery helping (i.e., helping other alcoholics with their recovery), life helping (helping others with non-recovery-related issues), and community helping (community projects such as fundraising, soup kitchens, mentoring youth, etc.). Longer abstinence was significantly predicted by more time spent in community helping activities, less time spent in recovery helping activities, and higher levels of spirituality (measured as daily experiences of God and connectedness with others and the universe). In addition, they found significant positive relationships among spirituality and all three kinds of helping behaviors. They suggested that their findings were consistent with the view that helping is an expression of spirituality and that helping others may be giving individuals recovering from SUD a sense of purpose and meaning in their lives that could help them avoid relapse.

Research on helping as an adjunct to spiritual development has focused exclusively on 12-step recovery groups, and no research to date has explored its place in a non-twelve-step therapeutic setting. However, Piliavin and Siegl (2007) have found strong evidence for a strong association among individuals in the general population between positive well-being and volunteering. Since it appears to increase both purpose and meaning in life and connectedness to others and thus can potentially be used to increase spirituality, we are comfortable in including service as one of the elements of our framework.

Solitude

In formulating our three-legged stool framework, we chose the term *solitude* very intentionally and thoughtfully. It is important when discussing solitude to understand the difference between it and aloneness. Bernstein (2012) has distinguished between the terms by noting that aloneness carries a connotation of frightening disconnection and abandonment. Solitude, on the other hand, connotes a sense of comfort when not in the company of others.

In our framework, the term solitude refers to activities related specifically to contemplative practices. Contemplation has been defined as: "deep reflective thought; the state of being considered or planned; religious meditation; or a form of Christian meditation or prayer in which a person seeks to pass beyond mental images and concepts to a direct experience of the divine" (https://en.oxforddictionaries.com/definition/contemplation). In the current context, we are specifically interested in contemplative activities that allow opportunities for deep reflection and for a direct experience of the divine (though we do not limit this opportunity to Christian practices). Interest in meditation and prayer as possible prevention and intervention techniques has steadily increased since the mid-1990s when research focused on use of faith, spiritual practices, and religious beliefs in the prevention and treatment of mental health issues (see Larson & Larson, 1994; Larson, Sherill, & Lyons, 1994).

Although we recognize that prayer and meditation may be included in the corporate activities conducted within religious or group spiritual settings, our concept of solitude is meant to access the more personal and internal experience of spirituality specified in the definitions of spirituality constructed by Cook (2004) and Canda and Furman (2010). This focus is not meant to suggest that corporate religious/spiritual rituals and practices should in any way be discouraged among those individuals in recovery who are interested in them and find them useful. However, we are interested in practices that specifically encourage the quieting of the mind that allows individuals to access their core self and their Higher Power through attentive and reflective silence.

Meditation Although all major religions practice some form of meditative practice, the most common type of meditation found in the research literature, mindfulness meditation (Brown, Ryan, & Creswell, 2007), has its roots in Buddhist practices (Marlatt, 2002). Mindfulness has been defined as "paying attention in a particular way – purpose, in the present moment, and without judgment" (Kabat-Zinn, 1994). According to Briere (2015), the object of mindfulness meditation is to "maintain awareness of, and openness to, immediate experience – including internal mental states, thoughts, feelings, memories, impinging elements of the external world – without judgment and with acceptance" (pp. 14–15).

Mindfulness meditation is thought to help substance-dependent clients tolerate their current negative experiences, such as craving (Marlatt & Chawla, 2007). Speaking specifically about individuals in recovery, Marlatt (2002) argued that mindfulness meditation can help clients to develop a distinctly different relationship with their thoughts and feelings through a process called "urge surfing" (p. 47). Instead of trying to avoid or change the thoughts and feelings associated with craving, clients are encouraged to allow the urge to build, crest, and then pass away like a wave. Briere (2015) explains that the utility of this process lies in its ability to help the client learn that it is possible to simply notice thoughts and feelings as "time-limited intrusions of history, internally generated phenomena" (p. 20) that do not have to be acted on.

Results concerning the effectiveness of mindfulness meditation on treatment outcomes have shown mixed results. For example, Bowen et al. (2006) conducted a longitudinal study concerning the use of a 10-day Vipassana meditation course (a form of mindfulness meditation) among incarcerated men with histories of alcohol and/or illicit drug abuse. They looked for differences between course participants and other inmates who received treatment as usual. Results indicated that 3 months after release from prison, men in the meditation group reported significantly less substance use and lower levels of psychiatric symptoms than those in the treatment as usual group. In addition, meditators also reported higher levels of alcohol-related internal locus of control and higher levels of optimism.

In contrast, another longitudinal study found no significant differences in urine toxicology reports between individuals receiving standard substance abuse treatment and individuals receiving standard treatment plus mindfulness meditation (Alterman, Koppenhaver, Mullholand, Ladden, & Baaime, 2004). However, they did find that the meditation group had fewer medical problems posttreatment than the non-meditation group.

Although empirical research on the value of mindfulness meditation in the treatment of substance use disorders remains somewhat sparse, there are a number of empirically tested mindfulness-based therapeutic models being used to treat other mental health issues. For example, mindfulness-based stress reduction (MBSR; Miller, Fletcher, & Kabat-Zinn, 1995) utilizes both formal meditation practices (such as body scans, loving-kindness meditation, walking, yoga, and sitting meditations) and informal practices (such as becoming more aware while eating, talking, listening, and during stress) (Magyari, 2015) to help individuals manage their stress levels.

Clinicians have begun to recognize the value of these mindfulness practices in combination with cognitive behavioral techniques. Mindfulness-based cognitive therapy (MBCT; Teasdale et al., 2000), for example, utilizes MBSR techniques in combination with traditional cognitive behavioral therapy in the treatment of depression and anxiety, disorders that are highly comorbid with substance use disorders. Acceptance and commitment therapy (ACT; Hayes, Strosahl, & Wilson, 1999) was also developed to help clients understand their thought processes, teaching clients to distinguish between three types of thoughts – descriptive, evaluative, and distortion – and encouraging them to observe their thoughts rather than to avoid them. Similarly, dialectical behavior therapy (DBT; Linehan et al., 2002) combines mindfulness with cognitive behavioral techniques to address the dysfunctional thinking common among borderline personality disorder clients.

One drawback in discussing these mindfulness-based therapies in the context of the three-legged stool framework is that none of them have been considered to be spiritual interventions. However, as the developers of mindfulness-based interventions mentioned above have suggested, meditation and contemplation may help individuals detach from the dysfunctional thinking that has been supporting their problematic use of substances. This detachment may help them gain access to both their core selves and the Transcendent.

Prayer According to Juhnke, Watts, Guerra, and Hsieh (2009), prayer is a traditional component of 12-step programs as evidenced by its inclusion in the 11th step: "we have sought through prayer and meditation to improve our conscious contact with God as we understood him, praying only for knowledge of His will for us and the power to carry that out" (Alcoholics Anonymous World Services, 2001, p. 59). In addition, individuals in recovery commonly use the Serenity Prayer (Niebuhr & Brown, 1987) within many of these groups. This long-standing tradition of prayer within the recovery community is an effort to increase an individual's connectedness with the Transcendent.

From a very different perspective based on attachment theory, Jankowski (Jankowski & Sandage, 2011) has argued that God may be conceptualized "as a member of the client's relational system" (p. 241). He suggested that an individual's attachment behavioral system may be activated through a specific prayer form – contemplative prayer. Contemplative prayer is thought to be a very personal spiritual expression through which hope could develop in response to the sense of felt security within the individual's relationship with God. From this security, improvements in other relationships in the individual's life may also be strengthened.

Unlike the literature on meditation discussed in the section above, there is no empirical validation of contemplative prayer as an intervention for substance use issues. However, there are some studies exploring relationships between prayer and improvements in mental health problems that are frequently comorbid with substance use disorder diagnoses. For example, in an early study of the use of contemplative prayer, Finney & Malony (1985) found that when prayer was incorporated into psychotherapy, participants reported a decrease in negative feelings and a slight increase in spirituality. More recently, Maltby, Lewis, and Day (2008) found that meditative prayer predicted lower levels of depression, anxiety, somatic complaints, and social dysfunction. In addition, of particular importance in the context of the three-legged stool framework, it also predicted higher levels of existential well-being (purpose/meaning), one of the components of spirituality as defined here.

From the discussion of contemplative practices presented above, we believe we are justified in including solitude as a leg in our three-legged stool framework. It appears to have the potential to increase spirituality in individuals with substance use issues by improving connectedness to both others and to the Transcendent. In addition, it may also have the potential to increase existential purpose and meaning in life.

Limitations and Future Directions for Research

There is one caution that needs to be mentioned in regard to the three-legged stool framework, having to do with competency. According to the National Association of Social Worker Code of Ethics (2008), practitioners should not work outside of their area of professional competence. We believe that it is important that any practitioner who would like to use the three-legged stool framework in their treatment recognize that this framework as envisioned by us is not a form of spiritual direction. Spiritual direction is generally considered to be a ministry offered by a particular religious organization (see, e.g., http://www.leadershiptransformations.org/selah.htm or http://www.sdiworld.org/resources/formation-and-training-programs) and requires specific training not usually provided in mental health and substance abuse and misuse educational programs. The three-legged stool is meant to increase spirituality as defined earlier in this chapter, not religiosity.

Related to the professional competency issue mentioned above is the issue of cultural competency. Since this framework has not yet been empirically validated, we do not know if it would be more or less beneficial to different cultural groups. Alterman et al. (2004) have suggested that meditation may be more effective in addressing substance use in some groups of individuals rather than in others. Future studies could explore how creativity and service might also vary among culturally diverse groups.

Our explication of the three-legged stool framework above suggested how the legs could be used to address individuals in treatment for SUD but did not mention how the model might be used to help dually diagnosed individuals. Unfortunately, there is currently no literature on which to base any suggestions for using the framework with that population. Cranford, Nolen-Hoeksema, and Zucker (2011) have noted that approximately 1.2 million people are diagnosed with co-occurring alcohol and mental health disorders every year. Future research could explore whether the three-legged stool framework would be useful in treating this especially vulnerable population. Research could also compare individuals at different levels of treatment (e.g., outpatient, partial hospitalization, and residential). Comparisons of individuals in substance abuse treatment versus individuals who are not in treatment regarding the usefulness of creativity, service, and solitude in addressing spirituality needs would also be valuable.

One of the major limitations to our proposed three-legged stool framework is the lack of methodologically sound research supporting the use of creativity, service, and/or solitude in the treatment of SUD. To date, research has not included rigorous quantitative or qualitative methods but instead has been primarily descriptive and has focused on case studies. However, we have recently conducted a pilot study using qualitative methods to examine the perceptions of residential substance abuse clients regarding services they received that focused on creativity (art therapy, music therapy, expressive writing, psychodrama, and recreational therapy), service (peer leadership, reaching out to newcomers, and community service projects), and solitude (meditation/relaxation, acupuncture, tai chi, qi gong, yoga, and cranial sacral massage) (Horton et al., unpublished manuscript). It should be noted that the agency where the research was conducted did not use the three legged stool framework to structure its services. Rather, we simply explored how their current services supported (or did not support) our framework. Our findings, though certainly not definitive, were encouraging; the themes associated with all three of the three-legged stool elements indicated increases in clients' perceptions of their connectedness to self, others, and the Transcendent. However, only a few indicated an increase in the purpose and meaning dimension. It is our hope that the three-legged stool framework presented in this paper will result in further, more methodologically sound research.

We believe that future research should also consider the possibility that there are more than three legs to the stool. That is, it may be valuable to consider other possible constructs that could increase spirituality. For example, forgiveness is a factor that has been shown to be associated with both spirituality and substance abuse treatment outcomes (Lyons, Dean, & Kelly, 2010; Lyons, Deane, Caputi, & Kelly, 2011) and would fit well with the prayer and meditation component. Likewise, self-compassion has shown promise in increasing spirituality and may developed through mindfulness practice (Bernie, Speca, & Carlson, 2010). As researchers and clinicians use the three-legged stool framework over time, other possibilities and combinations may also occur.

In the interest of rigorous research, it would be valuable to explore associations between spirituality and the legs of the stool. For example, do contemplative practices have a direct impact on the levels of spirituality or does it mediate the connection between the individuals and his or her Higher Power? If self-compassion were included as a leg, would it increase spiritual growth or would it be increased through spiritual growth?

Most importantly, future research could also explore the possibility associations between the three-legged stool framework and positive treatment outcomes. Especially valuable would be longitudinal research with several years of follow-up.

Conclusion

The purpose of this paper was to present the three-legged stool to the SUD treatment community for consideration as a framework for increasing spirituality among individuals in treatment for substance use issues. In this framework creativity, service and solitude act as the "legs" that support a "seat" of spirituality. We believe that this framework can be utilized to build spirituality among individuals in treatment for substance use issues. It should be emphasized that in our discussion of the framework, we have not intended to suggest that the three-legged stool is the only model that could address spiritual development; indeed, there is at this time no empirical validation of the framework. Rather, we hope that our presentation of the framework will open up a conversation about how spirituality among individuals in treatment can be increased and that it will encourage others to test this and other possible models that could help these individuals. It is also hoped that our and others' research efforts will spur therapists in the SUD and mental health treatment fields to target the development of spirituality during and after treatment as they work to improve clinical outcomes.

References

Alcoholics Anonymous World Services. (2001). *Alcoholics Anonymous: The story of how many thousands of men and women have recovered from alcoholism* (4th ed.). New York: Author.

Alterman, A. I., Koppenhaver, J. M., Mullholand, E., Ladden, L. J., & Baaime, M. J. (2004). Pilot trial of effectiveness of mindfulness meditation for substance abuse patients. *Journal of Substance Use, 9*(6), 259–268.

Amatruda, K. (2003). Somatic consciousness in adult sand-play therapy. In C. E. Schaefer (Ed.), *Play therapy with adults* (pp. 233–270). Hoboken, NJ: Wiley.

Armstrong, K. (1993). *A history of God: The 4,000-year quest of Judaism, Christianity and Islam.* New York: Ballantine Books.

Arnold, R. M., Avants, S. K., Margolin, A., & Marcotte, D. (2002). Patients' attitudes concerning the inclusion of spirituality into addiction treatment. *Journal of Substance Abuse Treatment, 23*, 319–326.

Avrahami, E. (2003). Cognitive behavioral approach in psychodrama: Discussion and example from addiction treatment. *The Arts in Psychotherapy, 30*(4), 209–216.

Benson, P., & Spilka, B. (1973). God image as a function of self-esteem and locus of control. *Journal for the Scientific Study of Religion, 12*(3), 297–310.

Bernie, K., Speca, M., & Carlson, L. E. (2010). Exploring self-compassion and empathy in the context of mindfulness-based stress reduction (MBSR). *Stress and Health, 26*, 359–371.

Bernstein, J. W. (2012). Commentary on a paper by Danielle Knafo. *Psychoanalytic Dialogues, 22*, 72–75.

Bowen, S., Witkiewitz, K., Dilworth, T., Chawla, N., Simpson, T., Ostafin, B., et al. (2006). Mindfulness meditation and substance use in an incarcerated population. *Psychology of Addictive Behaviors, 20*(3), 343–347.

Briere, J. (2015). Pain and suffering: A synthesis of Buddhist and western approaches to trauma. In V. M. Follette, J. Briere, D. Rozelle, J. W. Hopper, & D. I. Rome (Eds.), *Mindfulness-oriented interventions for trauma: Integrating contemplative practices* (pp. 11–30). New York: Guilford Press.

Brown, K. W., Ryan, R. M., & Creswell, J. D. (2007). Mindfulness: Theoretical foundations and evidence for its salutary effects. *Psychological Inquiry, 18*(4), 211–237.

Canda, E. R., & Furman, L. D. (2010). *Spiritual diversity in social work practice*. New York: Oxford University Press.

Chen, G. (2006). Social support, spiritual program, and addiction recovery. *International Journal of Offender Therapy and Comparative Criminology, 50*, 306–323.

Claus, R. E., & Kindleberger, L. R. (2002). Engaging substance abusers after centralized assessment: Predictors of treatment entry and drop out. *Journal of Psychiatric Drugs, 34*(1), 25–31.

Cook, C. C. H. (2004). Addiction and spirituality. *Addiction, 99*, 539–551.

Cranford, J. A., Nolen-Hoeksema, S., & Zucker, R. A. (2011). Alcohol involvement as a function of co-occurring alcohol use disorders and major depressive episode: Evidence from the National Epidemiologic Survey on alcohol and related disorders. *Drug and Alcohol Dependence, 117*, 145–151.

Cropley, A. (2006). Creativity: A social approach. *Roeper Review, 28*(3), 125–130.

Daaleman, T. P., & Frey, B. B. (2004). The spiritual index of well-being: A new index for quality-of-life research. *Annals of Family Medicine, 2*, 499–503.

Damianakis, T. (2001). Postmodernism, spirituality, and the creative writing process: Implications for social work practice. *Families in Society: The Journal of Contemporary Human Services, 82*(1), 23–34.

Dermatis, H., & Galanter, M. (2015, February). The role of twelve-step-related spirituality in addiction recovery. *Journal of Religion and Health, 21*, (no pagination).

Diaz, N., Horton, E. G., Green, D., McIlveen, J., Weiner, M., & Mullaney, D. (2011). Relationship between spirituality and depressive symptoms among individuals who abuse substances. *Counseling and Values, 56*(1), 43–56.

Diaz, N., Horton, E. G., & Malloy, T. (2014). Attachment style, spirituality, and depressive symptoms among individuals in substance abuse treatment. *Journal of Social Service Research, 40*(3), 313–324.

Diaz, N., Horton, E. G., McIlveen, J., Weiner, M., & Williams, L. B. (2011). Spirituality, religiosity and depressive symptoms among inpatient substance abusers. *Journal of Religion and Spirituality in Social Work: Social Thought, 30*(1), 71–87.

Edwards, C. G. (2000). Creative writing as a spiritual practice: Two paths. In M. E. Miller & S. R. Cook-Greuter (Eds.), *Creativity, spirituality, and transcendence: Paths to integrity and wisdom in the mature self* (pp. 3–23). Stamford, CT: Ablex Publishing Corp.

Feen-Calligan, H. (2007). The use of art therapy in detoxification from chemical addiction. *The Canadian Art Therapy Association Journal, 20*(1), 16–28.

Finney, J. R., & Malony, H. N. (1985). An empirical study of contemplative prayer as an adjunct to psychotherapy. *Journal of Psychology and Theology, 13*(4), 284–291.

Frey, B. B., Daaleman, T. P., & Peyton, V. (2005). Measuring a dimension of spirituality for health research: Validity of the spirituality index of well being. *Research on Aging, 27*(5), 556–577.

Galanter, M., Dermatis, H., Bunt, G., Williams, C., Trujillo, M., & Steinke, P. (2007). Assessment of spirituality and its relevance to addiction treatment. *Journal of Substance Abuse Treatment, 33*, 257–263.

Hall, T. W., & Edwards, K. J. (1996). The initial development and factor analysis of the spiritual assessment inventory. *Journal of Psychology and Theology, 24*(3), 233–246.

Hayes, S. C., Strosahl, K. D., & Wilson, K. G. (1999). *Acceptance and commitment therapy: An experiential approach to behavior change.* New York: Guilford Press.

Hodge, D. R., & McGrew, C. C. (2005). Clarifying the distinctions between spirituality and religion. *Social Work and Christianity, 32*(1), 1–21.

Humphreys, K. (2004). *Circles of recovery: Self-help organizations for addictions.* Cambridge, UK: Cambridge University Press.

Jankowski, B., & Sandage, S. J. (2011). Meditative prayer, hope, adult attachment, and forgiveness: A proposed model. *Psychology of Religion and Spirituality, 3*(2), 115–131.

Jarusiewics, B. (2000). Spirituality and addiction: Relationship to recovery. *Alcoholism Treatment Quarterly, 18*, 99–110.

Johnson, L. (1990). Creative therapies in the treatment of addictions: The art of transforming shame. *Arts in Psychotherapy, 17*, 299–308.

Juhnke, G. A., Watts, R. E., Guerra, N. S., & Hsieh, P. (2009). Using prayer as an intervention with clients who are substance abusing and addicted and who self-identify personal faith in God and prayer as recovery resources. *Journal of Addictions and Offender Counseling, 30*(1), 16–23.

Julliard, K. (1995). Increasing chemically dependent patients' beliefs in step one through expressive therapy. *American Journal of Art Therapy, 33*, 110–119.

Kabat-Zinn, J. (1994). *Wherever you go, there you are: Mindfulness meditation in everyday life.* New York: Hyperion.

Kelly, J. F., Stout, R. L., Magill, M., Tonigan, J. S., & Pagano, M. E. (2011). Spirituality in recovery: A lagged meditational analysis of Alcoholics Anonymous' principal theoretical mechanism of behavioral change. *Alcoholism: Clinical and Experimental Research, 35*, 454–463.

Larson, D. B., & Larson, S. S. (1994). *The forgotten factor in physical and mental health: What does the research show?* Rockville, MD: National Institute for Healthcare Research.

Larson, D. B., Sherill, K. A., & Lyons, J. S. (1994). Neglect and misuse of the "R word": Systematic reviews of religious measures in health, mental health and aging research. In J. S. Levin (Ed.), *Religion and health: Theoretical foundations and methodological frontiers.* Thousand Oaks, CA: Sage Publications.

Linehan, M. M., Schmidt, H., Dimeff, L. A., Craft, J. C., Kanter, J., & Comtois, K. A. (2002). Dialectical behavior therapy for patients with borderline personality disorder and drug dependence. *American Journal on Addiction, 8*(4), 279–292.

Longabaugh, R., Donovan, D. M., Karno, M. P., McCrady, B. S., Morgenstern, J., & Tonigan, J. S. (2005). Active ingredients: How and why evidence-based alcohol behavioral treatment interventions work. *Alcoholism: Clinical and Experimental Research, 29*, 235–247.

Lyons, G., Deane, F., Caputi, P., & Kelly, P. (2011). Spirituality and the treatment of substance abuse disorders: An exploration of forgiveness, resentment and purpose in life. *Addiction Research and Theory, 19*(5), 459–469.

Lyons, G., Deane, F., & Kelly, P. (2010). Forgiveness and purpose in life as spiritual mechanisms of recovery from substance abuse disorders. *Addiction Research and Theory, 18*(5), 528–543.

Magura, S., Knight, E. L., Vogel, H. S., Mahmood, D., Laudet, A. B., & Rosenblum, A. (2003). Mediators of effectiveness in dual focus self-help groups. *American Journal of Drug and Alcohol Abuse, 29*, 301–322.

Magyari, T. (2015). Teaching mindfulness-based stress reduction and mindfulness to women with complex trauma. In V. M. Follette, J. Briere, D. Rozelle, J. W. Hopper, & D. I. Rome (Eds.), *Mindfulness-oriented interventions for trauma: Integrating contemplative practices* (pp. 140–156). New York: Guilford Press.

Maltby, J., Lewis, C. A., & Day, L. (2008). Prayer and subjective well-being: The application of a cognitive-behavioural framework. *Mental Health, Religion, and Culture, 11*, 119–129.

Marlatt, G. A. (2002). Buddhist philosophy and the treatment of addictive behavior. *Cognitive and Behavioral Practice, 9*, 44–50.

Marlatt, G. A., & Chawla, N. (2007). Meditation and alcohol use. *Southern Medical Journal, 100*(4), 451–453.

Maslow, A. (1968). *Towards a psychology of being*. New York: Van Nostrand.

Matto, H. (2002). Integrating art therapy methodology in brief inpatient substance abuse treatment for adults. *Journal of Social Work Practice in the Addictions, 2*(2), 69–83.

McDargh, J. (1986). God, mother, and me: An object relational perspective on religious material. *Pastoral Psychology, 34*(4), 251–263.

McDowell, D., Galanter, M., Goldfarb, L., & Lifschutz, H. (1996). Spirituality and the treatment of the dually diagnosed: An investigation of patient and staff attitudes. *Journal of Addictive Diseases, 15*(2), 55–68.

McLellan, A. T., Luborsky, L., Woody, G. E., O'Brien, C. P., & Druley, K. A. (1983). Predicting response to alcohol and drug abuse treatment: Role of psychiatric severity. *Archives of General Psychiatry, 40*, 620–625.

Miller, J. J., Fletcher, K., & Kabat-Zinn, J. (1995). Three-year follow-up and implications of a mindfulness-meditation stress reduction intervention in the treatment of anxiety disorders. *General Hospital Psychiatry, 17*(3), 192–200.

Miller, W., & Bogenschutz, M. (2008). Spirituality and addiction. *Southern Medical Journal, 100*(4), 433–436.

Monakes, S., Garza, Y., Wiesner, V., & Watts, R. E. (2011). Implementing Adlerian sand tray therapy with adult male substance abuse offenders: A phenomenological inquiry. *Journal of Addictions and Offender Counseling, 31*(2), 94–107.

National Association of Social Workers. (2008). *Code of ethics of the National Association of Social Workers*. Available at https://www.socialworkers.org/pubs/code/default.asp

Niebuhr, R., & Brown, R. M. (1987). *The essential Reinhold Niebuhr: Selected essays and addresses*. New Haven, CT: Yale University Press.

Oreskovic, A., & Bodor, D. (2010). Addiction and art. *Alcoholism, 46*(1), 9–13.

Owen, P. L., Slaymaker, V., Tonigan, J. S., McCrady, B. S., Epstein, E. E., Kaskutas, L. A., et al. (2003). Participation in Alcoholics Anonymous: Intended and unintended change mechanisms. *Alcoholism: Clinical and Experimental Research, 27*, 524–532.

Pagano, M. E., Friend, K. B., Tonigan, A. S., Scott, J., & Stout, R. L. (2004). Helping other alcoholics in Alcoholics Anonymous and drinking outcomes: Findings from Project MATCH. *Journal of Studies on Alcohol, 65*(6), 766–773.

Pagano, M. E., Zemore, S. E., Onder, C. C., & Stout, R. L. (2009). Predictors of initial AA-related helping: Findings from Project MATCH. *Journal of Studies on Alcohol, 70*, 117–125.

Paloutzian, R. F., & Ellison, C. W. (1982). Loneliness, spiritual well-being and quality of life. In L. A. Paplau & D. Perlman (Eds.), *Loneliness: A sourcebook of current theory, research, and therapy* (pp. 224–237). New York: Wiley Interscience.

Piderman, K. M., Schneekloth, T. D., Pankratz, V. S., Stevens, S. R., & Altschuler, S. I. (2008). Spirituality during alcoholism treatment and continuous abstinence for one year. *Journal of Studies on Alcohol, 68*, 282–290.

Piedmont, R. L. (1999). Does spirituality represent the sixth factor of personality? Spiritual transcendence and the five-factor model. *Journal of Personality, 67*(6), 985–1013.

Piliavin, J. A., & Siegl, E. (2007). Health benefits of volunteering in the Wisconsin Longitudinal Study. *Journal of Health and Social Behavior, 48*, 450–464.

Polcin, D. L., & Zemore, S. (2004). Psychiatric severity and spirituality, helping, and participation in Alcoholics Anonymous during recovery. *American Journal of Drug and Alcohol Abuse, 30*, 577–592.

Ramseur, C., & Wiener, D. (2003). Rehearsals for growth applied to substance abuse growth. In D. Wiener & L. Oxford (Eds.), *Action therapy with families and groups: Using creative arts improvisation in clinical practice* (pp. 107–134). Washington, DC: American Psychological Association.

Reiland, J. D. (1990). A preliminary study of dance/movement therapy with field-dependent alcoholic women. *The Arts in Psychotherapy, 17*, 349–353.

Robinson, E. A. R., Cranford, J. A., Webb, J. R., & Brower, K. J. (2007). Six-month changes in spirituality, religiousness, and heavy drinking in a treatment-seeking sample. *Journal of Studies on Alcohol, 68*, 282–290.

Robinson, E. A. R., Krentzman, A. R., Webb, J. R., & Brower, K. J. (2011). Six-month changes in spirituality and religiousness in alcoholics predict drinking outcomes at nine months. *Journal of Studies on Alcohol, 72*, 660–668.

Schaefer, C. E. (2003). *Play therapy with adults*. Hoboken, NJ: Wiley.

Seidlitz, L., Abernathy, A. D., Duberstein, P. R., Evinger, J. S., Chang, T. H., & Lewis, B. (2002). Development of the spiritual transcendence index. *Journal of the Scientific Study of Religion, 41*, 439–453.

Sher, M. E., & Straughan, H. H. (2005). Volunteerism, social work, and the church: A historic overview and look into the future. *Social Work and Christianity, 32*(2), 97–115.

Siegel, D. (2012). *A pocket guide to interpersonal neurobiology: An integrated handbook of the mind*. New York: Norton & Co..

Somov, P. (2008). A psychodrama group for substance use relapse training. *The Arts in Psychotherapy, 35*(2), 151–161.

Sterling, R. C., Weinstein, S., Losardo, D., Raively, K., Hill, P., Petrone, A., et al. (2007). A retrospective case control study of alcohol relapse and spiritual growth. *American Journal of Addictions, 16*, 56–61.

Teasdale, J. D., Segal, Z. V., Williams, J. M. G., Ridgeway, V., Soulsby, J., & Lau, M. (2000). Prevention of relapse/recurrence in major depression by mindfulness-based cognitive therapy. *Journal of Consulting and Clinical Psychology, 68*, 615–623.

Tonigan, J. S. (2007). Spirituality and Alcoholics Anonymous. *Southern Medical Journal, 100*(4), 437–440.

Treadwell, T., Kumar, V. K., & Wright, J. (2010). Integrating cognitive behavioral with psychodramatic theory and techniques. In S. S. Fehr (Ed.), *Interventions in group therapy* (Revised ed., pp. 395–401). New York: Routledge/Taylor Francis.

Weisner, C., Matzger, H., & Kaskutas, L. (2003). How important is treatment? One-year outcomes of treated and untreated alcoholic dependent individuals. *Addiction, 98*(7), 901–911.

White, W. L., & Whiters, D. (2005). Faith-based recovery: Its historical roots. *Counselor Magazine for Addiction Professionals, 6*(5), 58–62.

Witbrodt, J., & Kaskutas, L. A. (2005). Does diagnosis matter? Differential effects of 12-step participation and social networks on abstinence. *American Journal of Drug and Alcohol Abuse, 31*, 685–707.

Zemore, S. E. (2007a). A role for spiritual change in the benefits of 12-step involvement. *Alcoholism: Clinical and Experimental Research, 31*(10 Suppl), 76s–79s.

Zemore, S. E. (2007b). Helping as healing among recovering alcoholics. *Southern Medical Journal, 100*(4), 447–450.

Zemore, S. E., Kaskutas, L. A., & Ammon, L. N. (2004). In 12-step groups, helping helps the helper. *Addiction, 99*(8), 1015–1023.

Zemore, S. E., & Kaskutas, L. A. (2004). Helping, spirituality and Alcoholics Anonymous in recovery. *Journal for Studies on Alcohol, 65*, 383–391.

Zemore, S. E., & Pagano, M. E. (2008). Kickbacks from helping others: Health and recovery. In M. Galanter & L. A. Kaskutas (Eds.), *Research on Alcoholics Anonymous and spirituality in addictions recovery* (Vol. 18, pp. 141–166). New York: Springer Science + Business Media.

Chapter 14
Resiliency and Culturally- Responsive Practice for Adolescents and Young Adults with Substance Abuse and Mental Health Challenges

Brenda Williams-Gray

Introduction

Adolescence through young adulthood is a period of great developmental growth, challenge, and paradox. With the exception of the first year of life, at no other time does one have such a broad scope of physiological change, as puberty becomes the bridge from childhood to adulthood. The capacity for greater abstract thinking comes from the existential quagmire of questioning who you are, what you believe, and what your purpose is in the world. The developmental tasks of seeking independence, taking risks, and pushing away from parental, familial figures arrive at a time when adult support is most needed. Societal expectations are unclear, as the benchmarks for the transition to adulthood are arbitrary and sometimes counterintuitive; one can enlist in the military, marry, vote, and drive before being of age to drink or smoke.

Diverse adolescents and young adults in urban communities with substance abuse disorders and co-occurring mental health issues are increasingly vulnerable to traumatic events, social problems, and the sociopolitical landscape. Traumatic events such as the death of a parent or loved one, abuse and/or maltreatment, health impairments or disease, familial conflict, out-of-home foster care placement, domestic and community violence, and natural disaster can impact one's psychosocial and ego capacity. Precrisis functioning, family, and community involvement can either create risk compromising their mental health or be protective factors that support resiliency potential (Webb, 2007; Williams-Gray, 2016).

Social problems that increase exposure to physical and psychological stress, such as school bullying and cyberbullying, and bias based on gender, race, ethnicity, and/or sexual identity, can compromise a healthy self-identity and tax one's coping

B. Williams-Gray (✉)
Lehman College/CUNY, Bronx, NY, USA
e-mail: Brenda.williams-gray@lehman.cuny.edu

© Springer International Publishing AG 2018
T. MacMillan, A. Sisselman-Borgia (eds.), *New Directions in Treatment, Education, and Outreach for Mental Health and Addiction*, Advances in Mental Health and Addiction, https://doi.org/10.1007/978-3-319-72778-3_14

capacity. Environmental racism such as inadequate education, housing, unsafe water supplies, food deserts, and poverty creates conditions that increase risk for youth and young adults with substance abuse and co-occurring mental health conditions. These aforementioned social problems potentially add layers of vulnerability to this population because school and the neighborhood become community spaces that cannot be relied upon as a safety net or support system.

Finally, the sociopolitical landscape can have a negative impact on diverse youth in urban communities. The national climate surrounding the 2016 presidential election has exacerbated fear and violence toward immigrant populations who are underrepresented and marginalized. Young men of color and their families continue to worry about community policing that has brought about tragic outcomes. Civil liberties specific to women's health that were once viewed as untouchable are subjected to rollbacks; recent gender identity safeguards are now vulnerable. This societal uncertainty can lead to a loss of faith that institutions of power will use their authority appropriately to provide protection and safety, trickling down to mistrust of the helping professional community. Thus, culturally relevant practice is critical to the engagement and assessment process in working with adolescents and young adults that have substance abuse and co-occurring mental health issues.

Given the aforementioned context, this chapter will provide practitioners with the current trends on adolescent substance use and its relationship to mental and behavioral health. A framework for understanding of how to utilize protective factors to promote resiliency during engagement and assessment for working with diverse adolescents who have substance abuse and co-occurring mental health challenges will be provided. Creating a culturally responsive practice for practitioners will be described. A case example will integrate the use of the resiliency and a culturally relevant framework, which is grounded in social work principles and congruent with theories that guide clinical practice.

Literature Review and Current Trends

Substance Use Risks, Co-occurring Mental Health, and Behavioral Health Indicators

Substance use disorder (SUD) in adolescents and young adults is multidimensional; the layers of complexity include risk factors, comorbidity, and mental health challenges and developmental consequences.

From a developmental standpoint, the optimal time to prevent drug use and its negative consequences is with youth aged 12–14 years old (Marsiglia, 2016). According to the 2015 National Survey on Drug Use and Health (NSDUH), 10.1% of persons 12 years and older used illicit drugs and 7.8% in the past year were diagnosed with a SUD (SAMHSA, 2016). Factors that negated drug use were high perception of risk, prevention programs, and youth perception of parental or peer disapproval. In contrast, easy availability of substances and low perception of risk correlate with an increased likelihood of substance use among adolescents and young adults. Additionally, early initiation of alcohol or drug use is associated with developing SUD.

Regarding the availability to obtain drugs, close to half (46%) of 12- to 17-year-olds suggested that marijuana was easy or very easy for them to access. The ease of access drops for this age group to 8.1% and 12.5% for heroin and cocaine, respectively. Seventy-two percent of 18–25-year-olds indicated that it is easy for them to obtain marijuana, while 15.4% reported that they were able to easily obtain heroin. Slightly over one quarter (26.6%) of the 18–25-year-olds surveyed indicated that access to cocaine was easy (SAMHSA, 2016).

The perceived risk of harm for those 12 years and older was greatest for heroin at 94.2%, cocaine at 87.4%, and lowest for marijuana at 36.3%. Less than half (44.2%) perceived great risk from binge drinking weekly, even in the face of public documentation of health issues and injuries associated with excessive drinking. For the initiation of substance use, the NSDUH survey found that approximately 1.2 million 12- to 17-year-olds use marijuana for the first time, compared to one million for 18- to 25-year-olds. The misuse of pain relievers is defined as "use in any way not directed by a doctor, including use without a prescription of one's own, use in greater amounts, more often, or longer than told to take the drug; or use in any other way not directed by a doctor" (SAMHSA, 2016, p. 9). Misuse of pain relievers was second only to marijuana initiation of use with 2.1 million users aged 12 and over, the average age being 25.8 years. One hundred and twelve thousand (approximately 0.1 million) 12- to 17-year-olds and 663,000 young adults 18–25 used cocaine for the first time in 2015. For heroin, the estimates were 11,000 for 12- to 17-year-olds and 68,000 for 18- to 25-year-olds. Approximately 2.4 million adolescents aged 12–17 used alcohol for the first time as did 2.2 million young adults aged 18–25. Those who were the least likely to perceive risk of harm were the most likely to initiate use (SAMHSA, 2016).

Sinclair and Davis Smith (2016) identified studies that highlighted additional risk impacting urban adolescent substance use. Individual factors are family history of addiction; inadequate ego functioning, i.e., poor impulse control; and a sensation seeking leaning coupled with difficulties with risky behaviors (Robbins and Bryan, 2004; Yanovitzky, 2005). A significant familial risk factor identified by Anthony, Alter, and Jenson (2009) is poor parent-child bonding, which may be greater than the individual risk factors. Finally, peer drug use is a strong influence on urban adolescent substance use, while community detachment, economic scarcity, high crime, and population density are identified as community risks (Clark, Belgrave, & Nasim, 2008). Straussner and Fridman (2016) add school as a potential venue for risk as bullying or poor academic functioning can impact self-worth and contribute to substance use. Additionally, the community is a risk factor if it lacks of meaningful activities and work. From a macro perspective, mass media's glamorizing of substance use and living with racism are key risk factors associated with substance use and abuse.

Straussner and Fridman (2016) address demographics about similarities and differences between urban and non-urban environments. The ease and availability of obtaining prescription and illegal drugs continues to be an ongoing epidemic across the socio-geographic spectrum; drug use in cities is not greater than suburban areas. However, urban communities have greater population density, anonymity for drug dealers, and access to transportation that contribute to the availability and access to drugs. Consistent with the 2015 findings from the Monitoring the Future (MTF) annual survey through the National Institute on Drug Abuse (NIDA), unlike the stereotypes, the rates of substance use are greatest for white youth, least for African-American youth, with Hispanic youth in between. Inner-city youth of color have greater exposure and risk to crack than suburban youth (Johnston, O'Malley, Miech, Backman, & Schulenberg, 2016; Straussner & Fridman, 2016). However, societal penalties and involvement with the criminal justice system are inconsistently applied as one looks at race and class. The incarceration rate disproportionately impacts young Black and Hispanic youth with limited social capital and resources for drug-related offenses that are not criminalized in wealthier, White communities (Warde, 2016). Thus, the impact of SUD can create greater vulnerability to low-income urban youth of color whose treatment options can be thawed by the criminal justice system.

Substance abuse does not happen in a vacuum. Key factors for adolescents and young adults with SUD that have co-occurring mental and behavioral health challenges are histories of violence and adverse childhood experiences (Sinclair & Davis Smith, 2016). Youth with SUD often have co-occurring anxiety, depressive, bipolar, eating and conduct disorders (Waldron & Brody, 2010). The impact of traumatic experiences can play a role in SUD when substance use becomes an intervention of coping or an escape from the experience of trauma, particularly when normative coping processes are not adequate and the young person has not received appropriate treatment. Trauma, such as child abuse and maltreatment; sexual abuse; rape and child trafficking; witnessing domestic, community, and migration violence; environmental disasters; and terrorism, raises the potential for post-traumatic stress disorder (PTSD) symptoms (Garbarino, Dubrow, Kostelny, & Pardo, 1992; Herman, 1997). When adolescents express their pain by acting out, attention is paid to the oppositional and disruptive behaviors; when they act in, an awareness of their depression may be apparent; however, in both cases these symptoms may mask trauma. The priority typically becomes changing the undesirable behavior, and attention to the underlying traumatic events is secondary or not explored, leaving the trauma untreated. Young adults returning from active duty can experience loss of bodily functioning and exposure to atrocities. External wounds are seen and treated, but PTSD symptoms, nightmares, flashbacks, numbing, and emotional constriction may be less apparent. In addition to the relationship to trauma and poor mental health outcomes, behavioral issues emerge from SUD. Critical developmental gains around health self-identity, educational and work aspirations, and role formation can be disrupted by SUD. Likewise, conflicts in family relationships can emerge. Adolescents and young adults with SUD can become a risk for sexually transmitted diseases, HIV/AIDS, pregnancy, violence, overdose, and death (Waldron

& Brody, 2010). The risk factors discussed support how one's ego functions, family dynamics, and community challenges compromise a young person's developmental and coping capacities.

Finally, the challenge in treating dually diagnosed clients is whether to address the SUD or the mental and behavioral health issues concurrently or with a sequential overlap. The presenting problem, mission and priorities of the treating agency, and insurance designated discharge timeframes sometimes dictate how to approach intervening. The severity of competing symptoms, client's current coping, and their input are also important considerations. Social workers and other helping professionals are often left to ponder how to support healthy outcomes for both the substance abuse and mental and behavioral health issues. Integrating a resiliency- based framework, with attention to individual protective factors, into the assessment process can be a useful perspective approach.

Theoretical Model: Resiliency and Protective Factors

Resiliency: Definitions and Models

Knowledge development about resiliency, which explores the optimism in the human spirit regardless of adversity, has origins in psychopathology. Studies about children where there was an expectation of pathology revealed cohorts of children with healthy psychosocial functioning. Lam and Grossman (1997) describe resiliency as:

> the dynamic process involving interaction of biological, psychological and social factors that ameliorate the negative effects of stressful life events to promote successful adaptation over an individual's life. Resilience is conceptualized as protective factors interacting with adversity, such that successful adaptation is promoted. (p. 176–177)

The aforementioned definition addresses developmental resilience, resiliency as strength-based and resiliency as recovery. The developmental approach presents resilience as on a continuum, not as a linear construct endowed at birth. Instead it focuses on the interactive nature between the person and environment which changes and evolves over time. Werner (1993) describes resilient young adults developmentally as approaching college or the work force, with "a positive self-concept and internal locus of control" (p. 504). Developmental assets frame the resiliency needs of children through adolescence fostering a life model perspective (Search Institute, 2017). Research on developmental resilience successfully challenges the long-standing belief that the stages of development are stagnant and inevitable. It contradicts the notions that the only outcome of childhood trauma must be adult psychopathology or that extremely toxic environmental stressors guarantee problematic daily functioning in all life spheres (Saleeby, 2013).

While trauma continues to be a key component in the resiliency literature and research, resiliency frameworks are evolving from a deficit perspective to a normative and strength-based perspective. Saleeby (2013) notes resilience is not a trait; it is the continuing expression of capacity through the intersection or interplay of risks and strengths. Of note is the normalcy of resiliency in the literature. Masten (2001) refers to resilience as "ordinary magic," while Bonanno (2004) highlights the commonality of (and underestimates) resilience and absence of post-traumatic stress disorder (PTSD) in individuals exposed to trauma. Consistent with the strength perspective, this framing of resiliency as part of an individual's capacity for adaptation can then be fostered and supported. As such, trauma or risk is related not only to negative outcomes, but to protective capacities that support well-being and recovery. This thinking supports rejecting the notion that segments of the youth population are considered at risk as their prime descriptor. One's internal capacities, familial, and environmental indicators create challenges and opportunities. The at-risk label not only negates capacity, but defines youth exclusively by their potential deficits.

The dimension of resiliency as recovery is described as the internal process where one can maintain a sense of personal competence even when challenged by crisis (Gilgun, 1999). When adversity is acute and prolonged, resilience speaks to recovery once danger dissipates (Masten, Best, & Garmezy, 1990). Agaibi and Wilson's (2005) model of resilience provides a continuum of adaptation and resilience. Low resilience is associated with minimal coping, acute long-term negative adaptation, and risk for post-traumatic stress disorder (PTSD) and other types of psychopathology. This model highlights personality variables (protective factors), such as locus of control, self-esteem, and ego resilience as factors for healthy coping and adaptation. The trauma literature identifies post-traumatic recovery (PTR) at the opposite end of the PTSD spectrum. PTR encompasses the capacity for renewed functioning and positive change after facing adversity (Calhoun & Tedeshi, 2006; Mallow et al., 2011) and is associated with high resilience, optimal coping, and long-term positive adaptation (Agaibi & Wilson, 2005).

Richardson (2002) synthesizes the research on resilience as three waves of inquiry: resilient qualities (i.e., protective factors), resiliency process (how the coping and reintegration occurs with the use of protective factors), and innate resilience ("what and where is the energy source or motivation, to reintegrate resiliently," p. 313). Thus, resilience can be conceptualized as the relationship between risk and protective factors as illustrated in Fig. 14.1, the resiliency paradigm. Risks are stresses and vulnerabilities that can be (a) internally driven, as SUD and co-occurring mental health challenges; (b) originate in one's family, such as domestic violence or a parent with SUD; and (c) social environment, as in poverty, community violence, and access to drugs on the street. Protective factors inform one's resiliency potential that are derived from: (a) individual resources that are internal, such as insight, or external adaptations, such as academic achievement; (b) family dynamics that support well-being are effective parenting, support from extended family; and (c) the social environment, including integration and interrelationships with social institutions, and community safety (Friedman, 2006; Kaplan et al., 1996: Mallow et al., 2011).

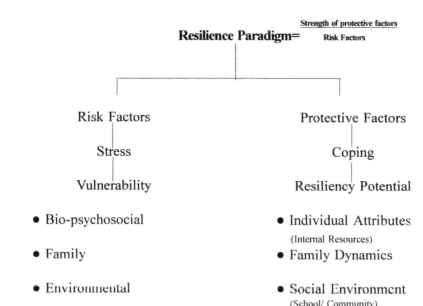

Fig. 14.1   Resiliency paradigm: the relationship between risk and protective factors

Individual Protective Factors

Individual attributes facilitate coping and contribute to resiliency potential in conjunction with, or in the absence of, family support and an embracing community. These protective factors or attributes can be considered in six categories clustered by type or relationship as illustrated below in Table 14.1: individual protective factor clustered.

Self-isms include internal locus of control, defined as the ability to be self-directed, take power and responsibility for one's decisions and life (Valentine & Feinauer, 1993). Self-efficacy is "confidence that one's internal and external worlds are predictable, controllable and hopeful" (Kaplan et al., 1996, p. 159). Cognitive processing allows one to problem solve, acquire and strengthen skills, and remove challenges and opportunities (Friedman, 2006). Use of one's self in the world encompasses being pro-active, use of cultural literacy and skills such as pro-social rituals to enhance well-being; civic activity is an example (DeNeve & Cooper, 1998; Kelly, 2008; Park, 2004; Williams-Gray, 1999).

Within the personality cluster, temperament is significant in facilitating human relatedness and our capacity to connect to others. Skills are the talents that make individuals unique, interests that motivate activity, and creativity that fosters expression. Often these traits provide respite, hobbies, entertainment, the means of self-expression, and shared experiences. Values highlight faith, or spirituality, is noted consistently in the literature of factors fostering resiliency in that faith (religious

Table 14.1 Individual protective factor clustered

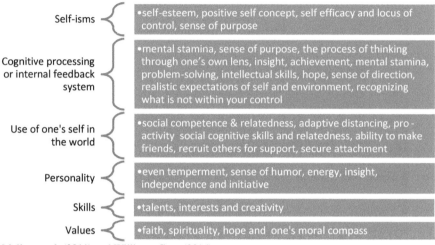

Self-isms	•self-esteem, positive self concept, self efficacy and locus of control, sense of purpose
Cognitive processing or internal feedback system	•mental stamina, sense of purpose, the process of thinking through one's own lens, insight, achievement, mental stamina, problem-solving, intellectual skills, hope, sense of direction, realistic expectations of self and environment, recognizing what is not within your control
Use of one's self in the world	•social competence & relatedness, adaptive distancing, pro-activity social cognitive skills and relatedness, ability to make friends, recruit others for support, secure attachment
Personality	•even temperment, sense of humor, energy, insight, independence and initiative
Skills	•talents, interests and creativity
Values	•faith, spirituality, hope and one's moral compass

Mallow et al. (2011) and Williams-Gray (2016)

faith, spiritual faith, moral beliefs, and internalizations) and supports one's morale compass and desire to understand the meaning and purpose of life (Brenda & Belcher, 2006; Fontana & Rosenheck, 2004; Mallow et al., 2011).

Practice Skills: The Use of Resiliency in Assessment and Engagement

Protective factors can promote well-being, psychosocial strength, and resiliency in adolescents with SUD and mental health challenges if social workers understand how to identify what protective factors an adolescent or young adult may have, such as humor, adaptive distancing, hope, and a sense of purpose. How can social workers and other mental health professionals assess resiliency potential and utilize the protective factors as part of treatment? The guidance offered here is consistent with sound social work practice skills and values.

1. Assessment – ask and listen: A sound assessment synthesizing the case information guides the treatment formulation and informs the contracting process and intervention methods. This requires asking strategic questions that help to uncover protective factors for inclusion in the assessment, to facilitate goal planning and to support treatment interventions. Some questions are meant to be asked directly; however, often, it is in describing a lived experience and the reflection about it that can provide the worker with insights into the young person's individual's protective factors. Table 14.2 is a list of assessment questions

Table 14.2 Assessment questions and statements to identify protective factors

I believe in my capacity to control my actions	I can recover from disappointment
I motivate myself to achieve what is important to me	I have a good sense of humor
	I believe that positive change will occur
I can laugh at myself	I am passionate about my beliefs
I have the energy I need to accomplish daily activities	I am resourceful
I can assess a situation and solve problems with others	I am flexible
	I like challenges
	I take the initiative with tasks
I think before acting when I under stress	I believe that I deserve to feel good
I consider the views of others	I look forward to each day
I can stand firm to my beliefs and opinions	I can end relationships that are emotionally toxic
I am honest with myself about my strengths and limitations	I have learned life lessons from challenging times
I make healthy choices for myself	
I am a doer	I define myself by my looks
I am a planner.	I define myself by my accomplishments
I can assess a situation and solve problems with others	I define myself in my role as_____
I can control my emotions	I define myself by school/work/career
I can forgive myself	I believe that I have character and integrity
	I feel responsible to help others in crisis
I can let go of shame	I volunteer in my community.
I can adapt to changing situations	I protect myself from abusive persons and situations
I can manage disappointment	
I believe in a power greater than myself	I have three friends
One thing I enjoy alone or with others is__	I can be counted on in an emergency
	I have three persons that I can count on in an emergency

or statements to ascertain one's protective factor inventory. A useful approach is to utilize the questions or statements to initiate dialogue and promote reflection from the client's lived experience and thoughts. The questions are not intended to be used all at once, and the social worker and other mental health professionals must think of the utility of each question on knowledge of the client. Some may find it more useful to take a Likert scale approach for standardized responses, such as often, sometimes, seldom, or never. The purpose is to inform the assessment process on the strength of the protective factors that can be called into play to create healthy outcomes.

2. Observe: When working with adolescents and young adults in congregate care settings, such as schools, day treatment, substance abuse programs, residential treatment, and psychiatric settings, there is an additional opportunity to observe the youth outside of the one-to-one treatment context. This provides chances to bear witness to their interactions in a less formal setting. Is there a talent in art? Is he/she a problem solver? Does he/she have the ability to distance one's self from trouble? Is there a relatability that is not seen during sessions?

3. Space: Make safe space for the young person's story. If you cannot tolerate their narrative, you become unsafe for their pain and authentic interactions.

4. Strengths: Being strength oriented does not meant to imply that problems are to be ignored or that accountability is not important. Adolescents and young adults with SUD's and co-occurring mental and behavioral health issues have layers of problems and need consistency and boundaries. However, supporting their capacities, ego functions, and strengths can create hopefulness, sustain motivation, and strengthen the therapeutic process. A strength perspective reinforces that behaviors, not adolescents or young adults, are at risk.
5. Coping: Give attention creative strategies in coping. Adolescents and young adults have their own vernacular, music, and technology that may be part of their coping skill set. Inquire and learn.
6. Environment: Don't ignore cultural, socio-eco-political issues that impact behaviors, substance use, or trauma. What may be maladaptive in some circumstances may be smart survival techniques in a different reality. Labeling as a deficit what the worker does not understand may be a missed opportunity.

Utilizing a resiliency perspective is consistent with theories that guide social work and mental and behavioral health interventions. Ego psychology and object relations theories both focus on ego sustaining techniques to enhance insight, self-identity, and ego strengths for youth with SUD. Cognitive coping and reframing seeks adaptive distancing from unhealthy distortions that impact thinking and behavior. Narrative theory puts the young person's story at the core of intervention (Walsh, 2014). Likewise, evidence-based practice (EBP) models are congruent with a resiliency perspective. For instance, motivational interviewing, functional, and multidimensional family therapy models are specifically designed for treatment of SUD with adolescents and young adults (Liddle, 2010; Waldron & Brody, 2010; Walsh, 2014). However, Marsiglia and Booth (2015) warn that successful EBP models require cultural adaptation, as studies that test for the model's efficacy often do not include diverse populations. Thus, the tension between model fidelity and cultural adaption exists. Working with adolescents and young adults with SUD and co-occurring mental health issues necessitates that social workers are knowledgeable about best practices and have a foundation of resiliency-based practice and that they are culturally responsive to the clients in their care. These are not mutually exclusive premises; resiliency-based practice and culturally responsive practice are interconnected.

Culturally Responsive Practice: The Move from Competence to Informed and Relevant

Culturally informed, relevant practice is responsive to the unique needs of diverse urban populations and requires social workers to be open to learning about the unique worldview of others and willing to be in a position of not knowing. For social work to be able to move from cultural competence as the standard, and shift toward culturally responsive practice, there are several assumptions that are useful.

First, self-awareness and cultural awareness are necessary for culturally informed and responsive social interactions. Self-awareness refers to insight into one's identity with attention to race, ethnicity, gender, socioeconomic status, sexual orientation, religion, and abilities (Mallow, 2010; Williams-Gray, 2014). Cultural awareness is the ability to appreciate other cultures and worldviews (Bender et al., 2010; Williams-Gray, 2014). The significance of the worker's use of self and self-awareness with young clients and their family cannot be overstated. The absence of cultural awareness can lead practitioners to erroneously label adolescents and young adults as resistant or unmotivated, or stereotyping, when it is the worker's misuse of self that has created a cultural of miscommunication. Boyd-Franklin's (1989) concept of "healthy cultural paranoia" speaks to the need of Black families to self-protection and hold back in the treatment relationship until they feel safe with the worker. This occurs only after the worker has demonstrated credibility, authenticity, and attunement. Working with youth who have SUD and co-occurring mental health issues requires that workers not only look at the presenting problem and symptoms, as consideration to relationship building is paramount. This requires understanding the meaning attached to substance abuse and mental health issues in the family. What appears to be resistance can be shame, fear of "crazy" or labeling, worries that medication will lead to drug dependency, and/or mistrust in the helping profession based on historic and current inequities.

Social workers and other mental health professionals can tune into intra- and inter-ethno-cultural transference and countertransference, which addresses transference themes associated with clients who work with professionals who have similar and dissimilar backgrounds and countertransference themes for workers working with clients from similar and dissimilar backgrounds (Comas Diaz & Jacobson, 1991). The following case example illustrates inter-ethno-cultural transference and countertransference. The 50-year-old middle class African- American parents may not trust that the young Caucasian worker is hearing their worries that the psychotropic medication prescribed to their 17-year-old daughter may be addictive or later be found to have horrific side effects. They don't want their daughter used as a guinea pig to test medication. The worker views them as paranoid and resistant. Their denial of their daughter's mental health issues masks their genuine fear about her losing her college scholarship and becoming a "full-fledged" drug addict like those they left behind when they moved to the suburbs.

Likewise, intra-ethno-cultural countertransference is illustrated by a social worker happy to provide services to the 20-year-old young man who is an immigrant from his (the worker's) country of origin; the client is relieved that his worker is Spanish speaking. However, the worker has difficulty managing his own expectations and anger when the young man expects the worker not to report that he is selling his antidepressants and sneaking out of the program to get high.

Second, understanding the social environment and the lived impact that it has on adolescents and young adults is critical. Working with an adolescent with SUD is a challenge. There are layers of current environmental realities facing young diverse persons in urban settings: a young person living in fear of immigration issues or deportation of family, fear based on recent police shootings of young Black men, changes in health coverage, and blatant racism against persons believed to be Muslim. These examples are relevant in the current sociopolitical climate and can adversely impact the person seeking treatment. Theories that support culturally responsive practice include knowledge of critical race theory (CRT) and an understanding of intersectionality.

CRT addresses the notion that race and racism are social constructs interwoven into all aspects of society creating power and privilege for the dominant racial group and exclusion from opportunities for other racial ethnic groups. Furthermore, a stance of color blindness negates the lived realities of those oppressed, whose experiences must be heard and validated (Abrams & Moio, 2009; Delgado & Stefanic, 2001; Warde, 2016). Intersectionality, first identified by Crenshaw (1991), addresses the interrelationship of race, ethnicity, gender, class, religion, sexual identity, and socioeconomic and immigration status, factors that are interconnected in one's identity and in the ways in which oppression occurs (Mallow, 2010; Warde, 2016). When working with diverse youth, adolescents, and their families already facing stigma about substance use and co-occurring mental health issues, it becomes critical for practitioners to be cognizant of policy and social work practices that can perpetuate discrimination and bias.

The aforementioned example of the 17-year-old whose parents fear psychotropic medication use for their daughter and are in denial about her mental health issues points to the intersectionality of race, age, and class. The social worker is not tuned into to their awareness of historic drug experimentation performed on Black Americans (race) and the generational gap (age) causing a disconnect between the parents and worker, which the worker views as paranoia. Finally, the worker has not accounted for the role of class in the parents priorities, specifically, not wanting their daughter to be viewed as a drug addict and the focus on education.

Finally, understanding the complexities of including culture in treatment is critical for work with diverse youth with SUD and co-occurring mental health issues. Sinclair and Davis Smith (2016) summarize levels of change designed to address the gaps of omitting culture from treatment interventions and best practices. Cultural attunement involves adding cultural themes to treatment; tailoring is designed to make changes for individual clients; and adaptation addresses the macro-systems dilemma infusing culturally appropriate modifications to intervention protocols. They further describe surface changes as adjustments to treatment materials, while deeper adaptations necessitate a fuller understanding of the group's norms. It is necessary to be aware of intersectionality, since people are more than their race, age, class, gender, sexual orientation, religion, occupation, and experiences which shape worldviews. Thus, there is no cookie cutter approach. Additionally, meanings that youth, young adults, and families attach to SUD and mental health can be subtle, culturally defined, and complex. Active listening, skilled use of self, awareness about culture, and genuineness in learning who the client is are the skills necessary to engage in culturally grounded practice.

Marsiglia and Booth (2015) describe culturally grounded social work:

> Culturally grounded social work challenges practitioners to see themselves as *the other*…
> A culturally grounded approach starts with assessing the appropriateness   of exist-
> ing evidence-based interventions and adapting when necessary, so that they are   more rel-
> evant and engaging to clients from diverse cultural backgrounds, without compromising
> their effectiveness. This process of assessment, refinement, and adaptation of interventions
> will lead to a more equitable and productive helping relationship. (Marsiglia & Booth,
> 2015, 423–424)

Implications for Practice and Education

Expanding the spectrum from cultural competence to culturally responsive practice
requires the continuous learning, openness, and empathy of others to be culturally
informed and attunement through the grounding of treatment protocols to provide
culturally relevant practice. How can social workers and other mental health professionals expand their culturally relevant capacity to support a productive worker-
client relationship? First, acknowledge discomfort in addressing race, class, culture,
and bias. Workers may need to seek support from peers, in supervision, or training
to explore their intra-ethnic and inter-ethnic stance. Workers can go through their
social work education with academic discussions about race without experiencing
an emersion into their own beliefs, values, and upbringing or exposure to others;
these factors can impact one's ability to practice with cultural clarity. A cultural
immersion and experiential exercise such as ethnic sharing can provide opportunity
for workers to explore their own and hear about others' worldview in undergraduate
and graduate social work courses (Williams-Gray, 2014).

Second, creating a safe space and verbal boundaries is necessary for the worker
and young person. This requires the worker to make decisions on what is permissi-
ble or not. For example, violence is always a no, but reenacting a scenario that
describes violence may be necessary. Language requires workers to understand the
vernacular, current music, and age- based contemporary issues, without a parental
stance. The worker has to be willing to share power and understand that they bring
expertise but that they are not the expert about the young person. They must be able
to ask questions about cultural norms with interest while avoiding assumptions,
stereotypes, and micro-aggressions. There is no checklist about all African-
American, Latino, Caucasian, and other ethnic groups in urban environments
because all neighborhoods are different; socioeconomic class, education levels, and
resources vary. Urban is not a code word for poor, inner-city minority. Substance
use issues cross geographic, socioeconomic boundaries and necessitate that workers
explore the variety and intersectionality of populations within each community.
Allowing the client story to unfold gives voice to adolescents or young adults to tell
their story from their worldview and concurrently expose the social worker to alternative and shared perspectives.

The connection between resiliency and culturally responsive practice is the orientation to a strength approach, the congruence of both perspectives to the social work Code of Ethics and professional values, the complementary nature of both perspectives with EBP models, a respect for the client's expertise in who they are, the commitment to the client's narrative as meaningful for engagement and assessment, and an outcome perspective that utilizes the client's inner resources and cultural perspective as the source for successful intervention. This case example will illustrate the integration of the resiliency and culturally responsive practice perspectives

Eli is an 18-year-old young man who was referred for an assessment at a mental health clinic following an incident at a school social event. The students admitted to marijuana and alcohol use, but became frightened when Eli seemed disoriented and incoherent. They reported that he was talking to objects as if they were humans. Since Eli is usually sullen and depressed, his friends were glad that he agreed to join them for "one last hurrah" before graduation. Eli is planning to attend a community college, has a part-time job, and has never been in any type of trouble. He reportedly is a talented artist, although much of his work had dark themes. He lives in a northeastern city in a working-class neighborhood with his parents and his two younger siblings. His family has strong ties to the community. His mother is a nurse who is Puerto Rican and his father is African-American and the supervisor/manager for the apartment building they live in.

Eli presents as depressed and moody. While in the waiting area, he alternated between texting on his phone and drawing cartoon-like figures on a small pad. Mr. Jones, the social worker, sat adjacent to Eli, introduced himself, and commented on the lifelike expressions of the characters in Eli's drawings. He reluctantly followed Mr. Jones to the meeting room and made it clear that he had nothing to say and that his friends were rats and had no business reporting him. Mr. Jones inquired about Eli's characters; Eli remarked that it was just junk and that only his younger sister and art teacher liked his work. He further offered that his mother is afraid that the scary images he creates make him look crazy; his father wants him to grow up and "get serious." Mr. Jones invited Eli to describe the feelings and stories of the characters, and his affect changed; he became animated. Mr. Jones noted how realistic the themes of loss, fear, and alienation were expressed by the characters. He reframes Eli's friends as heroes who were willing to get in trouble for drug use because his life was more important to them then the consequences for their actions. In subsequent sessions, Mr. Jones was able to engage Eli in a substance/use/misuse assessment and explore Eli's mental health issues and history gathering the developmental, familial, and ego function elements to understand Eli's current functioning while continuing to employ a resiliency-based, culturally relevant framework.

In a session with his parents, Mr. Jones explored their worries and wants for their son. Eli's mother was worried that the antidepressants prescribed were responsible for Eli's "crazy" drawings and others would think he was crazy and treat him like he was "loco." Her ambivalent messages to Eli contributed to his inconsistent use of the medication. Eli's father was worried that the medication would make him addicted and his experience seeing young people waste their lives and become a statistic was not happening to Eli. Plus, he didn't want anyone experimenting with his son. Eli's parents want him to be healthy and "make something of himself". They see education as the key for a better life and don't want him to "mess it up" with his crazy art and drugs and lose his small scholarship.

Mr. Jones arranged for the team's psychiatrist to meet with Eli's parents and hear their real fears about the psychotropic medication. He reframed their worries as authentic and supported that they were good parents in need of a real discussion about the side effects of the medication and clarity about their son's symptoms. He also recommended a support group with other parents with family members who have mental health and substance use issues. Mr. Jones supported Eli in explaining the viability of his dreams of being a visual artist. He demonstrated his ability to create apps and how his cartooning is a real work that he hopes to expand his skills in technology and media in college.

In this brief case scenario, Mr. Jones wisely slows down the assessment process to ensure engagement with Eli. He is able to see Eli's resiliency potential in his protective factors – use of one's self in the world, i.e., social competence and relatedness through strong relationships/friendships; cognitive processing, i.e., sense of direction; and talent. He also understood that Eli's parents' mistrust of the psychotropic medication and worries about a mental health label was not resistance, but genuine fear based on historic incidents and cultural perceptions. Educating and supporting them can facilitate their ability to be supportive of Eli's needs and challenges in addressing his co-occurring.

Adolescents and young adults with co-occurring substance abuse and mental health challenges require practitioners to fine-tune their use of self so as to maximize interventions that promote resiliency and are culturally relevant to lived experiences of the young people they serve.

References

Abrams, L. S., & Moio, J. A. (2009). Critical race theory and the cultural competence dilemma in social work education. *Journal of Social Work Education, 45*, 245–261.

Agaibi, C., & Wilson, J. (2005). Trauma, PTSD, and resilience. *Trauma, Violence & Abuse, 6*(3), 195–216.

Anthony, E. K., Alter, C. F., & Jenson, J. M. (2009). Development of risk and resilience – Based out-of- school time program for children and youths. *Social Work, 54*(1), 153–168.

Bender, K., Neigi, N., & Fowler, D. (2010). Exploring the relationship between self- awareness and student commitment and understanding of culturally responsive social work practice. *Journal of Ethnic and Cultural Diversity in Social Work, 19*(1), 34–53.

Bonanno, G. (2004). Loss, trauma, and human resilience: Have we underestimated the human capacity to thrive after extremely adverse events. *American Psychologist, 59*(1), 20–28.

Boyd-Franklin, N. (1989). *Black families in therapy: A multisystems approach.* New York: Guilford Press.

Brenda, B., & Belcher, J. (2006). Alcohol and other drug problems among homeless veterans: A life course theory of forgiveness. *Alcoholism Treatment Quarterly, 24*(1/2), 147–170.

Calhoun, L. G., & Tedeshi, R. G. (2006). *Handbook of posttraumatic growth: Research and practice*. Mahwah, NJ: Lawrence Erlbaum Associates.

Clark, T. T., Belgrave, F. Z., & Nasim, A. (2008). Risk and protective factors for substance use among urban African American adolescents considered high-risk. *Journal of Ethnicity in Substance Abuse, 7*(3), 292–303.

Comas Diaz, L., & Jacobson, F. (1991). Ethno-cultural transference and countertransference in the therapeutic dyad. *American Journal of Orthopsychiatry, 61*(3), 391–401.

Crenshaw, K. (1991). Mapping the margins: Intersectionality, identity politics, and violence against women of color. *Stanford Review, 43*(6), 1241–1299.

Delgado, R., & Stefanic, J. (2001). *Critical race theory: An introduction*. New York: New York University Press.

DeNeve, K. M., & Cooper, H. (1998). The happy personality: A meta-analysis of 137 personality traits and subjective well-being. *Psychological Bulletin, 124*(2), 197–229.

Fontana, A., & Rosenheck, R. (2004). Trauma, change in strength of religious faith, and mental health service use among veterans treated for PTSD. *The Journal of Nervous and Mental Disease, 192*(9), 579–584.

Friedman, M. J. (2006). Posttraumatic stress disorder among military returnees from Afghanistan and Iraq. *American Journal of Psychiatry, 163*(4), 586–594.

Garbarino, J., Dubrow, W., Kostelny, K., & Pardo, C. (1992). *Children in danger, coping with the consequences of community violence*. San Francisco: Jossey-Bass.

Gilgun, J. F. (1999). Mapping resilience as process among adults with childhood adversities. In H. I. McCubbin, E. A. Thompson, A. I. Thompson, & J. A. Futrell (Eds.), *The dynamics of resilient families* (pp. 41–70). Thousand Oaks, CA: Sage.

Herman, J. (1997). *Trauma and recovery*. New York: Basic Books.

Johnston, L., O'Malley, P., Miech, R., Backman, J., & Schulenberg, J. (2016). *Monitoring the future national survey results on drug use, 1975–2015: Overview, key findings on adolescent drug use*. Ann Arbor, MI: Institute for Social Research, The University of Michigan. Retrieved from http://monitoringthefuture.org/pubs/monographs/mtf-overview2015.pdf.

Kaplan, C., Turner, S., Norman, E., & Stillson, K. (1996). Promoting resilience strategies: A modified consultation model. *Social Work in Education, 18*(3), 158–166.

Kelly, D. (2008). In preparation for adulthood: Exploring civic participation and social trust among young minorities. *Youth & Society, 40*(4), 526–540.

Lam, J., & Grossman, F. (1997). Resiliency and adult adaptation in women with and with-out self-reported histories of childhood sexual abuse. *The Journal of Traumatic Stress, 10*(2), 175–196.

Liddle, H. (2010). Treating adolescent substance abuse using multidimensional family therapy. In J. Weisz & A. Kazdin (Eds.), *Evidence-based psychotherapies for children and adolescents* (2nd ed., pp. 416–432). New York: Guilford Press.

Mallow, A. (2010). Diversity management in substance abuse organizations: Improving the relationship between the organization and its workforce. *Administration in Social Work, 34*(3), 275–285.

Mallow, A., Williams-Gray, B., Cameron Kelly, D., & Alex, J. (2011). Living beyond the intersection of war theatre and home. In D. Cameron Kelly, S. Howe-Barksdale, & D. Gitelson (Eds.), *Treating young veterans: Promoting resilience through practice and advocacy*. New York: Springer Publishing.

Marsiglia, F. F. (2016). Youth substance use prevention interventions: Opportunities and challenges. *Revista Internacional de Investigación en Adicciones, 2*(2), 1–2.

Marsiglia, F. F., & Booth, J. (2015). Cultural adaptation of interventions in real practice settings. *Research on Social Work Practice, 25*(4), 423–432.

Masten, A. S. (2001). Ordinary magic: Resilience processes in development. *American Psychologist, 56*(3), 227–238.

Masten, A. S., Best, K. M., & Garmezy, N. (1990). Resilience and development: Contributions from the study of children who overcame adversity. *Developmental Psychology, 2*, 425–443.

Park, N. (2004). The role of subjective well-being in positive youth development. *Annals of the American Academy of Political and Social Science, 591*, 25–39.

Richardson, G. (2002). The metatheory of resilience and resiliency. *Journal of Clinical Psychology, 58*(3), 307–321.

Robbins, R. N., & Bryan, A. (2004). Relationships between future orientation, impulsive sensation seeking, and risk behavior among adjudicated adolescents. *Journal of Adolescent Research, 19*(4), 428–445.

Saleeby, D. (2013). *The strengths perspective in social work practice* (6th ed.). Boston: Allyn & Bacon.

SAMHSA: Lipari, R., Williams, M., Copello, E., & Pemberton, M. (2016). *Risk and protective factors and estimated of substance use initiation: Results from the 2015 National Survey on Drug Use and Health. NSDUH Data Review.* Retrieved from http://www.samhsa.gov/data/

Search Institute. (2017). *Developmental assets.* www.searchinstitute.com

Sinclair, M., & Davis Smith, B. (2016). Engaging urban African American adolescents in treatment. In R. Wells-Wilbon, A. McPhatter, & H. Ofahengaue Vakalahi (Eds.), *Social work practice with African Americans in urban environments* (pp. 55–75). New York: Springer.

Straussner, S. L. A., & Fridman, E. (2016). Substance use by urban children. In N. K. Phillips & S. L. A. Straussner (Eds.), *Children in the urban environment* (3rd ed., pp. 223, Charles C Thomas Publisher, Ltd–250). Springfield, IL.

Valentine, L., & Feinauer, L. (1993). Resilience factors associated with female survivors of childhood sexual abuse. *The American Journal of Family Therapy, 21*(3), 216–223.

Waldron, H., & Brody, J. (2010). Functional family therapy for adolescents substance use disorders. In J. Weisz & A. Kazdin (Eds.), *Evidence-based psychotherapies for children and adolescents* (2nd ed., pp. 401–415). New York: Guilford Press.

Walsh, J. (2014). *Theories for direct social work practice* (3rd ed.). Belmont, CA: Wadsworth/Cengage.

Warde, B. (2016). *Inequality in U.S. social policy: An historical analysis.* New York: Routledge.

Webb, N. B. (2007). *Play therapy with children in crisis* (3rd ed.). New York: Guilford Press.

Werner, E. (1993). Risk, resilience and recovery: Perspectives from the Kauai longitudinal study. *Development and Psychopathology, 5*, 503–515.

Williams-Gray, B. (1999). International consultation and intervention on behalf of children affected by war. In N. Boyd Webb (Ed.), *Play therapy with children in crisis.* New York: Guilford Press.

Williams-Gray, B. (2014). Ethnic sharing: Laying the foundation for culturally-informed BSW social work practice. *Journal of Baccalaureate Social Work, 19*, 151–159.

Williams-Gray, B. (2016). Teaching students effective practice with returning military personnel: A strength-based resiliency framework. *Journal of Baccalaureate Social Work, 21*, 1–11.

Yanovitzky, I. (2005). Sensation seeking and adolescent drug use: The mediating role of association with deviant peers and pro-drug discussions. *Health Communication, 17*(1), 67–89.

Chapter 15
Practice, Advocacy, and Outreach: Perspectives on Addiction Services

Rosalind October-Edun

This chapter addresses the concepts of practice, advocacy, and outreach as they pertain to addiction and/or substance abuse. There are many different ways that each of these concepts can be viewed. For the purpose of this chapter, definitions for each concept are provided to explain of how each is viewed. The terms addiction, substance dependence, and substance abuse are used interchangeably, as are substance abuse care and substance abuse treatment and client(s), patient(s), and individual(s) with an addiction.

Addiction is defined as a chronic brain disease because the structure of the brain changes with its use (National Institute for Drug Abuse [NIDA], 2016). The changes of the brain as a result of drug abuse lead an individual to make poor choices that affect his or her life. Therefore, a medical model is adapted when addressing addiction to substances. American Society of Addiction Medicine (ASAM), (2016a) notes, "Addiction is characterized by inability to consistently abstain, impairment in behavioral control, craving, diminished recognition of significant problems with one's behaviors and interpersonal relationships, and a dysfunctional emotional response" (para. 2). Understanding these elements of addiction as defined, gives clarity to how assessments are conducted, how treatment is administered, and how the recovery process unfolds. The goal of this chapter is to provide an overview of the aforementioned concepts that are integral when focusing on the perspectives of addiction services.

R. October-Edun (✉)
SUNY Empire State College, Human Services, Saratoga Springs, NY, USA
e-mail: Rosalind.October-Edun@esc.edu

© Springer International Publishing AG 2018
T. MacMillan, A. Sisselman-Borgia (eds.), *New Directions in Treatment, Education, and Outreach for Mental Health and Addiction*, Advances in Mental Health and Addiction, https://doi.org/10.1007/978-3-319-72778-3_15

Practice

Simply defined, practice has to do with the way a practitioner engages when providing treatment, care, or service. According to the National Association of Social Workers (NASW) (2017), the definition of practice involves the application of values, principles, and techniques whereby assisting others with achieving services; counseling individuals, families, and groups; and improving services within communities. Substance abuse practice is particularly directed at how substance abuse treatment is administered. Khoury and Rodriguez del Barrio (2015) specifically look at recovery-oriented practice that involves the focus on the client as a whole person from a strength-based perspective, with the understanding that the client has a right to be an active participant in the decision-making process. This emphasizes the importance of the client-practitioner relationship.

There are many systems to be considered and precautions to be aware of when engaging in practice in the addiction arena. In essence, one must be knowledgeable about the types and levels of substance abuse care being administered. For instance, types of substance abuse care ranging from cognitive behavioral therapy (CBT), to contingency management (CM), to motivational enhancement therapy (MET), to 12-step facilitation are commonly utilized when treating substance use disorders (Substance Abuse and Mental Health Services Administration [SAMHSA], 2016a, para. 6). When determining levels of care, there are some critical questions to be answered. For example, does the result of the assessment warrant detoxification, outpatient, inpatient, or residential substance abuse care? Is the care being administered for alcohol and other drugs (AOD) inclusive of nicotine? Is the level of care non-intensive or intensive? These considerations are integral when offering care, given the importance of screening and assessment in determining the type and level of care for the individual with an addiction. Ladson, Kornegay, and Lesane (2014) advise practitioners about the need to use appropriate screening tools that lend to the proper symptom identification and treatment of addictions and other disorders.

The client's self-responsibility is especially questioned when there are two and three substances. This is not to say that being addicted to one substance is better than being addicted to two or three substances. The important message is that addiction is detrimental. For instance, if a client's first substance of choice is cocaine, the second is alcohol, and the third is nicotine, the possibility exists that the client may not see a problem with substance substitution. This means, the client might have some difficulty in understanding that stopping the use of cocaine while continuing to use alcohol and/or smoking cigarettes is not considered the best behavior when working on recovery. According to Staiger, Richardson, Long, Carr, and Harlatt (2013), alcohol has the potential to become a substitution addiction (p. 1188). The abstinence from use of all substances is recommended for clients who are serious about the recovery process.

While in substance abuse treatment, it has to become a common practice that clients receive education about the various drugs and effects and improved quality of life that comes with sobriety and recovery. The smoking of cigarettes has been receiving more attention than usual due to its connection with addiction. A large number of individuals who use alcohol, also smoke cigarettes (Van Wormer & Davis, 2014). According to Cupertino et al. (2013), giving up smoking helps with both health and treatment outcomes for individuals who are engaged in substance abuse treatment. In recognition of nicotine addiction, many substance abuse treatment programs are offering interventions to address cigarette-smoking behavior (SAMHSA, 2010a). Essentially, educating clients about substances is likely to give them self-tools to better understand sobriety and recovery issues relative to the substitution of substances.

Levels of Care

Levels of care include and are not limited to inpatient treatment that involves detoxification and/or residential care, as well as outpatient patient treatment. On one hand, inpatient treatment is temporarily living at a treatment facility for a varied duration based on the outcome of a substance abuse assessment. On the other hand, outpatient substance abuse treatment is also considered ambulatory treatment.

Inpatient Substance Abuse Care

Inpatient substance abuse care varies depending on the type(s) of substance(s) used, the extent of substance abuse history, the level of care sought, and in some cases, the duration of treatment as determined by health insurance companies. According to NIDA (2016), inpatient or residential facilities provide structured 24-h care, comprising a safe living environment with medical care while using a variety of therapeutic approaches.

During inpatient treatment (detox or residential), the client does not get the opportunity to leave the facility and return to the community until the time scheduled and contracted for treatment has been completed. When clients are involved in this level of care, treatment is strategized to optimize clients' recovery. In other words, clients' engagement in individual and group activities is specific to time management, while the clients' sense of responsibility is being enhanced.

Detoxification care Detoxification care, a type of inpatient treatment, commonly known as detox or detox treatment, is usually done on a brief inpatient basis. The detoxification process is the body ridding itself of substances (NIDA, 2016), with treatment usually lasting 3–7 days (ASAM, 2009) depending on the results of the assessment, the client's response to treatment, and/or the client's type of health insurance coverage. An individual with an addiction is in need of detoxification care when there is dependence on a substance and the presence of withdrawal symptoms from the use of substances such as alcohol and/or heroin.

It is important to acknowledge that addiction to alcohol, heroin, and prescribed medications, such as OxyContin, Percocet, and Vicodin, are a few substances that require detoxification treatment. A searing problem for the public health industry is the use and misuse of prescribed opiates (Coplan, Kale, Sandstom, Landau, & Chilcoat, 2013) and the alarming high use of heroin (Buer, Southard, & Kummerow, 2017). ASAM (2016b) discloses teaming up with other institutions to form a coalition that recognizes that the use and overdose of opioids are public health issues for the United States of America (para. 2). Similarly, SAMHSA (2016b) highlights that Americans' health is affected by the misuse and abuse of alcohol, "over-the-counter medications," illicit drugs, and tobacco. Noteworthy, alcohol and opiate dependence pose life-threatening situations when the individual with an addiction is experiencing withdrawal symptoms. Physical dependence and withdrawal symptoms associated with opioid dependence are unpleasant for individuals with a history of chronic use (Bauer, Southard, & Kummerow, 2017), hence the importance of detox treatment.

Treatment facilities make referrals when unable to provide the assessed level of care (NYS OASAS, 2016a). The administration of detoxification treatment is usually done under the supervision of a medical team. SAMHSA (2015) briefly addressed ASAM's five levels of detoxification care: the first two are without and with "extended onsite monitoring," respectively, the third is "clinical managed medical care," the fourth is "medically monitored inpatient detoxification," and the last "medically managed intensive inpatient detoxification" (p. xvi). Additionally, SAMHSA (2015) warns that facilities offering detoxification services must be appropriately staffed to adequately address the medical and psychological issues that may be presented by patients during care.

Most times, upon completion of detox treatment, the facility that referred the patient to detox may be the facility to which the patient is returned for outpatient treatment. If the patient was not referred to detox by an outpatient or other facility, then the detox treatment personnel will refer the patient to an outpatient substance abuse treatment program for continued care. Unfortunately, many individuals do not follow up with needed treatment that enables them to achieve long-term abstinence and only 15% of those admitted to detoxification care through emergency rooms go on to receive treatment (SAMHSA, 2015).

In order to clearly understand the impact of AOD relative to treatment, it is noted that in New York, more than 158,800 referrals have been made to both detox and substance abuse treatment facilities (NYS OASAS, 2016a), with the annual budget that addresses unhealthy substance use being US$185 billion for alcohol and US$181 for other drugs (Holt et al., 2013). This significant amount of referrals coupled with the billions of dollars invested, speak to the seriousness of addiction and treatment as a public health issue.

Residential substance abuse or rehab care Residential care is another type of inpatient care that lasts for over a month. According to SAMHSA (2016a), inpatient or residential care can be provided at hospitals with specialized units. These therapeutic communities are highly "structured programs" where clients live for "6 to 12 months" (NIDA, 2016, para. 24; SAMHSA, 2016a). According to Buck (2011) residential programs have an average capacity of 32 beds with treatment being 30 or more days. When involved in this level of care, individuals with an addiction reside at the substance abuse facility based on the assessment outcome and the kind of care administered by the facility. Like inpatient treatment, patients are required to adhere to specific daily responsibilities as part of treatment compliance. At the end of treatment, the individual with an addiction is usually referred to an outpatient facility for the continuum of substance abuse care.

Outpatient Substance Abuse Care

The focus on this level of care is a client's scheduled visit to a "traditional" substance treatment facility, one to a few times weekly for a few hours where there is a structure of activities to be followed by both the client and practitioner. This level of care varies from non-intensive to intensive. Non-intensive means the client attends 1–2 days a week, for 45 min to an hour each day. Intensive means the client attends treatment three to five times, for a few hours each day (NIDA, 2016). The level of outpatient care is dependent on the outcome of an assessment which determines the duration of treatment engagement. Outpatient substance abuse care ranges from Methadone Maintenance Programs (MMP), to ambulatory visits to a qualified medical doctor's office for buprenorphine treatment, to traditional substance abuse treatment programs. The Drug Addiction Treatment Act of 2000 (DATA 2000) made provision for physicians with broad certification in addiction medicine, and psychiatry, and those who completed an approved course, to administer buprenorphine for as many as 30 patients at any given time (Stein et al., 2015).

Outpatient substance abuse treatment is also considered ambulatory care, whereby the client visits the facility based on scheduled appointments. MMPs are common examples of outpatient substance abuse care. Although all programs are medically supervised, there are various ways in which care is administered in outpatient treatment. For instance, a client who abuses heroin may be treated by a medical doctor who is qualified to administer buprenorphine in the office. A study conducted by Liebshultz et al. (2014) revealed that connecting patients with buprenorphine treatment in medical facilities proved effective in the reduction of illicit use of substances 6 months after hospitalization. In another scenario, an individual with an addiction may agree to a treatment schedule for a few times per week for a few hours, where the focus is on individual, group, and/or family counseling, with emphases on psychoeducation.

This level of care comprises many areas of treatment including but not limited to individual and group counseling, psychoeducational sessions, alcohol and drug monitoring, case management, and vocational and educational services (SAMHSA. 2007, pp. 16–17). The scope of outpatient substance abuse services must be recognized because it enables the practitioner to adapt eclectic approaches to treatment, based on the clients' presenting issues. In addition, there are various interventions that can be used in outpatient treatment.

The Impact on Health Insurance in Substance Abuse Treatment

Health insurance coverage, whether private or public, is critical for many clients seeking substance abuse care. According to McCabe and Wahler (2016), many individuals with addictions have trouble in becoming and maintaining employed in a manner that allows them to secure health insurance. As of the 1990s, with the birth of Managed Care, health insurance companies have begun playing a more intense and pivotal role in decisions made regarding addiction treatment. In many states, government-funded Medicaid health insurance can be found under managed care plans that have been privatized (Van Wormer & Davis, 2014). This shift in how public health is used highlights the deliberate link between clients' treatment and payment for care.

While Galanter, Keller, Mematis, and Egelko (2000) noted there has been a connection in the decline in duration and frequency of inpatient treatment, Fisher and Harrison (2013) pinpoint many helping professionals are either employed or contracted by managed care or "health maintenance organizations." Health insurance companies have a tendency to dictate the level of care by indicating to treatment facilities the duration of addiction treatment. This policy has the potential to negatively affect inpatient care. "Although the scope of coverage and applicable reimbursement rates are determined by individual states" (Rifenbark & Waltz, 2016, p. 20), the interference by health insurance companies presents many challenges mainly for the client, in that the duration of recommended care is shortened, thus threatening the client's recovery. The negative impact of health insurance companies determining the duration of a client's care also has the potential to create hardship for the client in maintaining sobriety.

The Affordable Care Act

According to Laudet and Humphreys (2013), substance abuse treatment is considered necessary for individuals who are covered by Medicaid and other state health insurances. Although treatment may be necessary, individuals who hold public health insurance are placed in situations where there are limitations on treatment. Some limitations include the choice of providers because many facilities do not accept public health insurance. Another limitation is the duration of treatment stipulated by those who manage the public health insurance companies.

The implementation of the Affordable Care Act (ACA) in 2010 changed the business and the relationship between substance abuse treatment facilities and clients, in this case, holders of Medicaid. This Act included that the requirement of finance and limitations of treatment cannot be restrictive than those that are surgically or medically beneficial (Buck, 2011). Clearly, since the Act, substance abuse issues have been recognized on the same level as medical issues. The Act has a requirement for insurance policies to offer health care coverage that include services for substance use disorders (Rifenbark & Waltz, 2016).

This Act was instrumental at a pivotal point in the arena of addictions, as it directly addressed the relevance of substance abuse care. There were many other changes directed to substance abuse treatment, including how reimbursement for services would be handled. Furthermore, treatment facilities are no longer allowed to bill for peer counseling, but only for counseling offered by qualified practitioners (Buck, 2011).

The Practitioner

A practitioner is someone who is actively engaged in the provision of care on some level. As a practitioner, the focus of treatment should not be through the practitioner's tunnel vision, but instead through a structured strategy that proposes holistic treatment where the clients' issues are addressed from various angles. According to Adedoyin, Burns, Jackson, and Franklin (2014), the concept of holism emphasizes the person as a whole while looking at the interrelatedness of other aspects of the person's life. Some of these aspects include the various aspects of the client's life such as work, school, family, living arrangements, intimate and other kinds of relationships, use of one or more substances, and history of substance abuse treatment, to list a few.

There are many issues and behaviors that contribute and lead to an individual's substance abuse and contribute to the continued abuse of substance dependence. The utilization of holistic practice is relevant when addressing clients' self-improvement and lifestyle changes during recovery (Adedoyin et al., 2014). An effective practitioner is one who is able to assess those contributory factors to a client's addiction, the client's struggles with sobriety, and issues of recovery. It is important to note that there is a difference between sobriety and recovery processes. SAMHSA (2016c) defines recovery as a change process that results in one's improvement of health and wellness, the living a life that is self-directed, and striving to reach one's full potential. When an individual with an addiction is in recovery, he or she is sober or abstains from use of substances and maintains sobriety. Explicably, in the initial stages of treatment and during the recovery process, a client is able to work on improving different areas of his or her life with the guidance of the practitioner. Once treatment is completed, the expectation is that the client is able to continue using the tools of recovery learned during the treatment experience(s) to foster positive changes in leading a sober lifestyle.

Roles of the practitioner The practitioner plays many critical roles as a treatment provider. These roles include being a broker, case manager, educator, organizer, facilitator, manager, and advocate (Chadron State College, 2016). Here, the role of the advocate is emphasized. One way of looking at an advocate is that of an individual who serves as a voice to the voiceless and is considered a leader. Disraeli (2015) notes that the greatness of respectable leadership is the ability to hold one and others accountable. Many practitioners in leadership roles are also able to effectively use their positions to advocate on behalf of clients. Social workers are professionals who hold positions to lend their voices on behalf of low-income clients with addictions and ensure that the results of changes positively influence the clients' needs (McCabe & Wahler, 2016).

Professional Awareness of Beliefs and Attitudes

Individuals in the field of social work can be of assistance to clients by becoming educated on ACA (McCabe & Wahler, 2016). For both budding professional helpers and the professional helpers, it is important to understand that someone who is struggling with addiction does not fit a distinct description. The individual struggling with addiction can range from a homeless person to the most affluent person. The treatment professional's beliefs and attitudes about the person who is struck with addiction have a tendency to impact the quality of care (Fisher & Harrison, 2013), if administered by a professional with limited and/or biased knowledge of addictions. At the core of one's knowledge is the comprehension that there is a place for cultural awareness and competency in providing addiction treatment and that addiction does not belong to someone's race, ethnicity, or socioeconomic background. As warned by Connors, DiClemente, Velasquez, and Donovan (2012), substance abuse crosses many classes of people, and there is no such person as a "typical substance abuser." Additionally, Senreich and Straussner (2013) encouraged that graduate social work students receive an education that bridges health and behavioral health in both the course-room and internship experiences, as this conveys knowledge about relevant skills required in the emerging field.

Cultural Sensitivity and Cultural Competency

In addressing substance abuse prevention and mental illness as related to cultural awareness and competency, SAMHSA (2016d) mentions that in order to bring forth enhanced changes, practitioners must understand the communities' culture and language and possess the willingness and skillset to work within the cultural and linguistic contexts. It is difficult to ignore the diversity that exists in America, let alone, the diverse groups of clients attending treatment programs. The recognition of this awareness is very critical for individuals who are new to the helping field, especially in the area of substance abuse treatment. Maiter, Allagia, and Trocmé (2004) posited that those treatment professionals who exhibit responsiveness to clients' cultural diversity (cultural sensitivity) most often tend to show cultural competence.

According to SAMHSA (2006), cultural competence involves practitioners' enhanced "knowledge of cultural differences," their recognition of personal "assumptions and biases," and their willingness to alter "thoughts and behavior to address those biases" (p. 53). It is critical to how education and knowledge with experience could play a role in the development of a professional. The ability to enhance education allows for substance abuse practitioners to better understand cultural competence when engaging in practice. SAMHSA (2006) noted that most helping professionals are different from the clients they serve and have different experiences. "Patient advocacy, selflessness and willingness to suspend judgment are hallmarks of compassionate care" (Bauer, Southard, & Kummerow, 2017, p. 234). Therefore, it is relevant that professionals are aware to take ownership and address personal biases in an effort to administer effective, sensitive, and competent substance abuse care. Furthermore, enhanced knowledge places the helping professional in a position where awareness is heightened, thus the potentiality of positively impacting treatment that is culturally sensitive and competent.

Advocacy

According to NASW (2016b), advocacy is standing up for the equality of resources and opportunities for others, in order to meet their basic needs in life. Working directly with a particular population or in a specific environment exposes advocates to critical issues that need visibility. For instance, social workers practicing in states that lack the expansion of Medicaid have the chance to assist many clients with addictions by advocating for Medicaid program expansion to include clients with low-level income (McCabe & Wahler, 2016). Additionally, advocates are individuals who have been directly or indirectly impacted by a situation either through personal experience or by knowledge of someone else's experience. Cargill, Weaver, and Patterson's (2012) study looked at four types of advocacy: formal, informal, peer-led, and ad hoc. A critical component of advocacy is the presence of passion involved in working toward change or for a cause.

Practitioners as Advocates

There are various ways that advocates work. The grassroots or local level in the community is one way, while going through legislature of the government, and/or working with an international agency is considered a global level. It is instrumental that practitioners are knowledgeable about the currency of policies in their perspective residential state (McCabe & Wahler, 2016). At the grassroots level, it could be as simple as filling a gap in service in a particular community. At the legislative level, it could be consistently contacting and/or working along with Senators and legislators to fill a gap in needed services for a specific population. For instance, the purpose of NASW's Public Policy Department is to advocate on behalf of the Association by addressing Congress members (NASW, 2016b) for changes to be made that would allow the Association to continue to work on addressing injustices faced by individuals.

As mentioned earlier, there are values and principles that guide practice. In addition to these values and principles, there are six standards of the NASW. Two critical standards that address advocacy are the first and the sixth. The first standard focuses on the social workers' commitment to clients in that the promotion of clients' well-being is the most important responsibility for social workers, while the sixth, looks at the social workers' responsibilities to the broader communities, in that it is integral that they are involved in the promotion of society's general welfare along with advocacy for policy and legislation changes for the improvement that meets human (NASW, 2016a). These are just a few of the parts of the NASW's Code of Ethics that specifically address the roles of social workers as an advocate.

Practitioners advocate for individuals with an addiction who face many issues. Some of these issues include and are not limited to the inadequate duration of substance abuse treatment as determined by health insurance companies, lacking coverage of medications for individuals with co-occurring disorders, and eligibility for types of health insurances. Many individuals with addictions face "prejudice from society, family, and providers" because of the stigma involved when diagnosed with co-occurring disorders (Bauer, Southard, & Kummerow, 2017), and advocacy helps with the reduction of stigmatization (Fomil & Weaver, 2008). In situations where health insurance companies dictate inadequate duration of a client's substance abuse treatment, and/or fail to cover needed medications, it is ethical that the practitioner advocates on behalf of the client. The existence of written policies that are standardized, along with medication agreements, provides practitioners a forum to be more effective as advocates for individuals with addictions (Fomil & Weaver, 2008). The presence of standardized materials has the potential to erase questions from insurance companies that may delay and/or hamper the administration of treatment.

Advocacy and Ethics

Generally, there are many professionals who provide addictions treatment. The list includes but is not limited to social workers, Credentialed Alcoholism and Substance Abuse Counselors (CASACs), mental health counselors, case managers, and psychologists. Aside from those who are certified as CASACs, the other professionals may have certifications in their respective fields along with the CASAC and or substance abuse education. These practitioners can advocate for individuals with addictions on the individual patient level and governmental level (Fomil & Weaver, 2008).

In the Code of Ethics of National Association of Social Workers (NASW), currency of education is specifically noted (NASW, 2016a). Maintenance of education currency is also a mandate in other professions, in order to attain certification renewal. It is worthy to note that these professionals' work is guided by ethical standards that involve the role of an advocate, both covert and overtly.

One way in which a professional covertly advocates for clients with an addiction is by empowering clients to speak up on their own behalf, while the professional is silently supportive as the resolution process unfolds in favor of the client. For instance, a client's insurance policy may present limitations on treatment services.

In this situation, the practitioner may guide the client about the required documents needed to process for the type of insurance that would allow for the receipt of enhanced care. As noted by McCabe and Wahler (2016), the move toward insurance coverage for a large number of individuals is one of the most publicly known aspects of the ACA. It is relative to highlight the practitioner also functions in many different roles and, in most situations, is ready to step in on behalf of the client, if resolution becomes a challenge for the client.

On the other hand, professionals commonly do overt advocacy. A client may be suffering with chronic physical pain due to an accident and need pain medication. According to Fomil and Weaver (2008), practitioners and other professionals are consistently responsible for balancing the administration of controlled substances for individuals who need them, along with harm reduction from abuse of controlled substances. This involves speaking on behalf of the client who may experience some challenges in being heard, and/or lobbying for changes to be made for the betterment of substance abuse treatment for clients. Practitioners who advocate for clients struggling with both addictions and pain assist with the promotion of effective care and the reduction of stigmatization (Fomil & Weaver, 2008). More importantly, many professionals and even politicians have advocated for the extension of substance abuse treatment and for payment to be covered by health insurance companies (Van Wormer & Davis, 2014). In these situations, overt advocacy has been effective and changes were made benefitting clients.

NASW Code of Ethics For social workers who work in the area of substance abuse, the NASW's Code of Ethics governs their work. In addressing the ethical principles of social work, social justice is listed as a value, with the principle being that "social workers challenge social injustice" (NASW, 2016a). In essence, this value and principle speak to the role of the practitioner as an advocate, whereby if a social worker is privy to a client facing any form of injustice, then it is imperative that the social worker becomes active in taking steps on behalf of the client to make a positive change.

CASAC (Canon of Ethical Principles) For practitioners with CASAC certification, the Canon of Ethical Principles governs how they work. There are 20 principles that have been adapted from the National Association of Drug Abuse Counselors. The last principle that speaks to advocacy includes information that the "CASAC must adopt a personal and professional stance which promotes the well-being of the recovery community" (NYS OASAS, 2016c). This means that the role of an advocate is embedded in the work of a CASAC.

Advocacy in the Field of Addiction

Yip et al. (2012) emphasized the importance of discussions that are unrestricted and direct about the values of a community, and the changes of policies and legislations. Like the social worker, the CASAC and other professionals working with clients in the field of addiction have responsibilities to fulfill in advocacy.

At the core of advocacy are the professionals' actualization of their responsibilities in making sure that changes are made that positively impact clients' lives. The duration within which change can be seen and felt varies, depending on the nature of the issues being addressed and the stakeholders involved in the process of change. Fomil and Weaver (2008) point out that organizations with professional specialty can utilize the combination of groups of professionals' voices as an advocacy strategy for enhanced care for individuals with addictions by not only educating other practitioners but also the public about critical issues faced in the field of addictions.

There is a wide scope of issues which impact successful advocacy. Many of these issues are directly related to clients. According to Laudet and Humphreys (2013), there is usefulness in the examination of expectations and experiences of clients with respect to the delivery of substance abuse treatment. In essence, although sometimes vague, clients' disclosure of negative treatment experiences lends to advocacy attention. An example of a negative treatment experience is the client's involvement in treatment that prematurely ended because the health insurance company refused to continue paying for treatment and the client is unable to afford to pay for the remainder of recommended treatment. With the challenge of maintaining employment self-payment for treatment is a hardship for clients. In such a situation, the practitioner has the opportunity, as well as the moral and professional responsibility to advocate on behalf of the client. The practitioner's knowledge of the ACA as it relates to Medicaid coverage of substance abuse treatment (Rifenbark & Waltz, 2016) is important in making sure that clients in need are owners of this type of insurance policy.

The practitioner could do a few things, and here is an example. After the client and practitioner sign the necessary releases/consent forms, the practitioner could request to speak directly with the personnel of the insurance company and ask that consideration is given to the client's unique situation. The practitioner may emphasize the dire emergency of the client's substance abuse on the client's impeded functioning, and inability to afford the self-payment for treatment. McCabe and Wahler (2016) posit that social workers in the field of addictions have advocacy skills and knowledge of the addictions and are obligated to work on behalf of clients with addictions. It is critical that practitioners lend their voices when clients go unheard by systems that should be catering to clients' needs.

Noteworthy, clients diagnosed with both an addiction and mental health disorders, such as depression and/or anxiety (co-occurring disorder) (SAMHSA, 2010b) are in most need of advocacy. Practitioners may need to advocate on behalf of a client with a co-occurring disorder by educating personnel from whom the client receives other services, about the impact of substance abuse and a mental health disorder. Historically, there has been a disconnection between behavioral and physical health care providers in primary care settings, as evident in treatment outcomes (Crowley & Kirschner, 2015); however, this dilemma could be remedied by the cross-training of these providers who work with individuals with addictions (Bauer, Southard, & Kummerow, 2017). In reality, while struggling with his or her substance abuse behavior, the client may also find it challenging to understand what it means to suffer with depression. In this situation, the counselor is expected to educate the client about the importance of following through with assessment and treatment of the mental health disorder, as well as encourage compliance with substance abuse treatment. CBT and relapse prevention are two models that are highly recommended when treating co-occurring disorders (SAMHSA, 2010b). Initially addressing the mental health disorder helps to rule out other issues that may impact the substance abuse and/or mental health diagnoses. It is expected that the client's compliance with treatment for co-occurring disorders may not minimize the counselor's role as an advocate.

Outreach

According to DeChiara, Unruh, Wolff, and Rosen (2001), community outreach is needed in order to provide accessibility to medical and social resources that benefit individuals, the family unit, and the community as a whole. The activities of outreach encompass showing concern, offering assistance/care, and/or working on behalf of someone or a group of people (population). When outreach is in effect, it is in support of a particular cause. These activities reveal the need for attention and visibility to be given to certain issues. Outreach activities done on behalf of an individual struggling with addiction who is transitioning from one level of substance abuse care to another is an important aspect of this individual's recovery (Carter et al., 2001). Outreach is also seen as a form of advocacy in the substance abuse treatment arena.

Types of Outreach in the Substance Abuse Treatment Arena

In targeting outreach strategies (Dugas et al., 2015) emphasized that outreach is most effective when community and peer workers work together, resulting in knowledge and behavioral enhancement. Outreach in the addiction community has quite a few layers. These layers range from the types of substance abuse services offered in communities to the additional ancillary care offered in substance abuse treatment. For instance, there are the syringe exchange programs in New York State (NYS). Additionally, there are outreach programs that promote the practice of safe sex by distributing condoms in treatment programs and at health fairs. Another example of outreach is where individuals with many years in recovery serve as sponsors to many who struggle with sobriety in 12-step fellowship. Outreach is also exemplified by individuals who have been incarcerated and rehabilitated and have become guest speakers/presenters at substance abuse treatment programs where there is a high rate of members who might have had encounters with the law or have a tendency to get involved in the law because of the presence or history of substance abuse.

Syringe Exchange Programs (SEPs)   The SEPs are also known as needle exchange programs (NEPs) that address harm reduction, with 17 in existence in New York State, to date (NYS OASAS, 2016a). The first program of such in the United States was an illegal or underground one founded in 1986 in Portland, Oregon (Heimer, 1998), while the American government was trying to figure out how to best handle the spread of diseases as a result of drug use with needles. As of March 2009, a total of 184 SEPs was operational "in 36 states and the District of Columbia" (Center for Disease Control and Prevention [CDCP], 2010, para. 1). These programs were the answer to the rise in the intravenous heroin use and the increase of individuals who were becoming infected with blood-borne diseases (SAMHSA, 2016d), due to sharing and/or using dirty syringes, also referred to as "works." Arguably, SEPs attribute to the reduction of blood-borne diseases related to heroin abuse (NYS OASAS, 2016a). These diseases include human immunodeficiency virus (HIV) and hepatitis B and C. The core of these programs is the safety of the individual with an addiction who would exchange used syringes for new ones, thus promoting a safe way of using heroin and decreasing diseases related to syringe-sharing behavior.

Another layer of the SEP is the Expanded Syringe Access Program (ESAP) that allows an individual with an addiction who are 18 years and older to not only safely dispose of used syringes but also receive a limit of 10 syringes without a prescription (NYS OASAS, 2016a). In order to offer care in this program, medical practitioners must be registered with NYS Department of Health in order to write a prescription for syringes. This program that began on January 1, 2001 (Fuller et al., 2007) is beneficial to individuals with an addiction who seek out syringe exchange services, given the legality and qualifications of the providers.

Views of SEPs

There are various arguments regarding SEPs, with viable conversations contributed by both opponents and proponents of this program. Generally, the commonality and costliness of unhealthy substance use is noted (Holt et al., 2013). On one hand, opponents of SEPs argue that the distribution of syringes is a way of allowing undeserving individuals to feel privileged; condoning substance abuse behavior; and encouraging the indulgence of crimes. The opponents argued that someone who is using substances, especially with the use of syringes, is not deserving of any attention. Additionally, the distribution of syringes was viewed as giving permission to individuals struggling with addiction to use illicit substances (Des Jarlais et al., 2006), hence being an accomplice to illegal behavior. Furthermore, it was speculated that an individual with an addiction under the influence is more likely to commit crimes. For these reasons and more, the opponents spoke against SEPs.

On the other hand, proponents of SEPs argued that syringe distribution is a way of saving lives of individuals with an addiction. From this stance, it is recognized that if a client is not ready for sobriety and/or recovery, whether by choice or due to fear of physical and medical discomfort, the individual with an addiction has a safe place, the SEP. Worthy of noting is that SEPs in NYS are part of a treatment model that is comprehensive with services ranging from outreach and education to the provision of support (NYS OASAS, 2016a). Accordingly, individuals with an addiction are granted the opportunity to use substances in a responsible way by visiting SEPs that provide clean works for the use of substances.

Condom distribution It is known that most clients in substance abuse treatment programs would have dealt with disempowerment in their lives, thus their struggle with addiction. One area in which this occurs is in sexual relationships. As a result, substance abuse treatment programs recognized the connection between addiction and sex, in that when someone is under the influence of substances, he or she is more likely to indulge in unsafe sexual practices. In promoting the importance of health and wellness as it relates to recovery, it is highlighted that individuals and families in recovery are empowered to develop a plan to optimize both physical and mental health (NYS OASAS, 2016b). Being in treatment and gaining enhanced education and awareness of the connection between one's self and health, clients are better able to make informed choices about health issues such as the use of protection during sexual practices. According CDCP (2015), the effectiveness of condom distribution programs has the potential to alter the way members of communities deal with the engagement of safe sex practices. This outreach activity not only targets the client's self empowerment but also equips clients with knowledge about self-care.

Sponsorship in 12-step fellowship Twelve-step fellowships include Alcoholics Anonymous and Narcotics Anonymous, known as self-help groups promoting abstinence (DiGangi et al., 2014). Sponsorship is a standard aspect of the 12-step process. This means that a member of a 12-step fellowship could be a sponsor or is sponsored (Cloud, Ziegler, & Blondell, 2004). As a way of giving back to the substance abuse community, individuals with an addiction who have many years in recovery become deeply involved in 12-step fellowship. Most take on the role of a sponsor whereby providing a supportive connection or mentorship for a member or "sponsee" in a particular fellowship. Most of the support comes from acknowledging the importance of spirituality connected to the 12 steps (DiGangi et al., 2014). Traditionally, the sponsor-sponsee relationship is gender specific, meaning that males sponsor males and females sponsor females. This is a very important relationship that warrants trust, openness, honesty, and willingness. In this relationship, the sponsor is available to provide general support to the sponsee, assists with the attainment and preservation of sobriety, and encourages the sponsee's self-work that is pertinent in recovery.

Individuals with an addiction, who are serious about recovery and have utilized 12-step fellowship in the process, value the combination of traditional substance abuse treatment and 12-step fellowship. The experience of being involved in both support systems has proven fruitful. Those who have been successful using both substance abuse treatment and 12-step fellowship understand that at the end of substance abuse treatment, ongoing support is needed. One of the supportive mechanisms is the relationship an individual with an addiction has with a sponsor. According to The Sponsor's Aide (2008), a sponsor is someone who is experienced in recovery, plays the role of a mentor, and works with the individual with an addiction or "sponsee" in actualizing the 12 steps of recovery. In this relationship, being a part of the 12-step fellowship is especially valued because of the unique and individual support given by the sponsor to the "sponsee."

Sobriety is referred to an individual's abstinence from using substances, while recovery is an extension of sobriety that warrants major self-work. Recovery involves but is not limited to individuals with an addiction owning his or her responsibility, gaining the needed self-tools through treatment for making positive changes that result in a visible altered lifestyle. In describing recovery, NYS OASAS (2016d) notes that the start of recovery is marked when an individual begins to make enhanced choices that positively impact "his or her physical, mental, and spiritual health" (para. 1). Recognizably, there is a place for the role of the sponsor for individuals with an addiction involved in 12-step fellowship.

Guest Speaking/Presenting There are many individuals with an addiction who have had encounters with the law, thus the link between being under the influence of substances and making choices that are detrimental to one's life. Some individuals, who have had experience with incarceration and rehabilitative care, find a way to give back and make a difference in the lives of others. For instance, some become guest speakers, and even motivational speakers with a renewed purpose of sharing personal experiences to encourage others to think about positive ways to change current lifestyles.

Cicchetti and Johnson (2015) describe the role of someone in recovery who is giving support to the substance abuse community as engagement in mutual aid. As guest speakers, these individuals outreach to substance abuse treatment programs and 12-step fellowships, while the recipients of encouragement are able to acknowledge their gratitude for such exposure. This type of outreach is effective in substance abuse treatment because the guest speaker is able to make a direct connection by sharing similar experiences with those in attendance to the forum. This gesture promotes motivation, decreases denial, and encourages change of behavior (Cicchetti & Johnson, 2015).

In addition to substance abuse treatment programs and 12-step fellowships, some guest speakers visit jails and prisons. This outreach is effective in preparing individuals with an addiction in these systems for reentry to society. Latkin (1998) noted that a workable approach is making a connection between leaders and organizations with similar goals. When listening to a guest speaker who has been in recovery, the individual with an addiction who is incarcerated is given an opportunity to reflect on possible positive lifestyle changes upon reentry to his or her respective community.

Activities of outreach ultimately assist with the rehabilitation of clients. These activities are culturally sensitive and competent in nature because they directly address the needs of a marginalized population – individuals who struggle with addiction. More importantly, these activities support positive lifestyle changes and reward society with individuals who no longer are addicted to substances, who have rehabilitated and become recognizable contributors to the development of respective communities. In essence, outreach is not only important in the personal rehabilitation of the client but also in community development. According to SAMHSA (2006), culturally competent care involves being sensitive to clients' first language; "understanding the cultural nuances of the client population," using "treatment methods that reflect culture-specific values and needs of clients," and including clients in "program policy- and decision-making" (p. 54).

In a nutshell, substance abuse does not occur in a vacuum because there are circumstances in life that leads someone to use a substance in the first place, let alone become addicted. This also means that substance abuse treatment cannot be administered in a vacuum. OASAS, the governing body of addiction treatment service in New York State is the gatekeeper, with specific functions as related to substance abuse care and regulations.

Conclusion

The concepts of practice, advocacy, and outreach with subtopics were discussed as related to addiction. In addressing the concept of practice, many levels of care were highlighted. Health insurance and the involvement of the Affordable Care Act were noted as pivotal in substance abuse treatment. The professional awareness of the practitioner, with some attention given to cultural sensitivity and cultural competency were also addressed. Ethical codes that are specific to social workers and CASACs were discussed as they relate to substance abuse practice. Ethical issues as linked to advocacy in the field of addiction were illuminated. The last concept of outreach activities, SEPs, condom distribution, sponsorship in 12-step fellowship, and guest speaking/presenting were acknowledged as relevant. These four concepts have given the perspectives of addiction services.

References

Adedoyin, C., Burns, N., Jackson, H. M., & Franklin, S. (2014). Revisiting holistic interventions in substance abuse treatment. *Journal of Human Behavior in the Social Environment, 24*, 538–546.

American Society of Addiction Medicine. (2009). *Public policy statement on managed care, addiction medicine and parity: Supplement for physicians and others.* Retrieved from https://www.asam.org/docs/default-source/public-policy-statements/1man-care-supplement-3-09.pdf?sfvrsn=d3fcdf24_0#search=%22levels%20of%20detox%22

American Society of Addiction Medicine. (2016a). *Definition of addiction.* Retrieved from http://www.asam.org/quality-practice/definition-of-addiction

American Society of Addiction Medicine. (2016b). *Coalition to stop opioid overdose.* Retrieved from http://www.asam.org/advocacy

Buck, J. A. (2011). The looming expansion and transformation of public substance abuse treatment under the Affordable Care Act. *Health Affairs, 30*(8), 1402–1410.

Buer, R. N., Southard, E. P., & Kummerow, A. M. (2017). Heroin abuse: Nurses confronting a growing trend. *Medsurg Nursing, 26*(4), 231–241.

Cargill, T., Weaver, T. D., & Patterson, S. (2012). The commissioning and provision of advocacy for problem drug users in English DATS: A cross-sectional survey. *Drugs: Education, Prevention, and Policy, 19*(2), 163–170.

Carter, R. E., Haynes, L. F., Back, S. E., Herrin, A. E., Brady, K. T., Leimberger, J. D., Sonne, S. D., Hubbard, R. L., & Liepman, M. R. (2001). Improving the transition from residential to outpatient addiction treatment: Gender differences in response to supportive phone calls. *American Journal of Drug & Alcohol Abuse, 34*(1), 47–59.

Center for Disease Control and Prevention. (2010). *Syringe exchange programs – United States 2008*. Retrieved from https://www.cdc.gov/mmwr/preview/mmwrhtml/mm5945a4.htm/ Syringe-Exchange-Programs-United-States-2008

Center for Disease Control and Prevention. (2015). *Effective interventions: HIV prevention that works*. Retrieved from https://effectiveinterventions.cdc.gov/en/HighImpactPrevention/ StructuralInterventions/CondomDistribution.aspx

Chadron State College. (2016). *Social work: Roles of social workers*. Retrieved from http://www.csc.edu/cpsw/sw/careers/roles.csc

Cicchetti, A., & Johnson, D. (2015). Recovery groups: Membership has its rewards. *Journal of Groups in Addiction & Recovery, 10*(2), 99–101.

Cloud, R. N., Ziegler, C. H., & Blondell, R. D. (2004). What is alcoholics anonymous affiliation? *Substance Use & Misuse, 39*(7), 117–136.

Connors, G. J., DiClemente, C. C., Velasquez, M. M., & Donovan, D. M. (2012). *Substance abuse treatment and the stages of change: Selecting and planning interventions* (2nd ed.). New York: Guilford.

Coplan, P. M., Kale, H., Sandstrom, L., Landau, C., & Chilcoat, H. D. (2013). Changes in oxyco-done and heroin exposures in the national Poison Data System after introduction of extended – Release oxycodone with abuse-deterrent characteristics. *Pharmacoepidemology and Drug Safety, 22*(12), 1274–1282.

Crowley, R. P., & Kirschner, N. (2015). The integration of care for mental health, substance abuse, and other behavioral health conditions into primary care. *Annals of Internal Medicine, 163*(4), 298–299.

Cupertino, A. P., Hunt, J. J., Gajewski, B. J., Marquis, J., Friedmann, P. D., Engleman, K. K., & Richter, K. P. (2013). The index of tobacco treatment quality: Development of a tool to assess evidence-based treatment in a national sample of drug facilities. *Substance Abuse Prevention and Policy, 8*(1), 1.

DeChiara, M., Unruh, E., Wolff, T., & Rosen, A. (2001). *Outreach works: Strategies for expanding health access in communities*. Amherst, MA: Merrimack Valley Area Health Education Center/ Community Partners.

Des Jarlais, D. C., Sloboda, Z., Friedman, S. R., Templaski, B., McKnight, C., & Braine, N. (2006). Diffusion of D.A.R.E. and syringe exchange programs. *American Journal of Public Health, 96*(8), 1354–1358.

DiGangi, J. A., Majer, J. M., Mendoza, L., Droege, J. R., Jason, L. A., & Contreras, R. (2014). What promotes wisdom in 12-step recovery? *Journal of Groups in Addiction & Recovery, 9*(1), 31–39.

Disraeli, B. (2015). Responsive leadership: From supervision to inspiration. In S. DeGroot (Ed.), *Responsive leadership in social services: A practical approach for optimizing engagement and performance* (pp. 26–49). New York: Sage.

Dugas, M., Bédard, W., Batona, G., Kpatchavi, A. C., Guédou, F. A., Dubé, E., & Alary, M. (2015). Outreach strategies for the promotion of HIV testing and care: Closing the gap between health services and female sex workers in Benin. *Journal of Acquired Immune Deficiency Syndromes, 68*, S198–S205.

Fisher, G. L., & Harrison, T. C. (2013). *Substance abuse: Information for school counselors, social workers, therapists, and counselors* (5th ed.). Upper Saddle River, NJ: Pearson Education.

Fomil, K., & Weaver, M. (2008). Pain and addiction. *Journal of Addictions Nursing, 19*, 213–216.

Fuller, C. M., Galea, S., Caceres, W., Blaney, S., Sisco, S., & Vlahov, D. (2007). Multilevel community-based intervention to increase access to sterile syringes among injection drug users through pharmacy sales in New York City. *American Journal of Public Health, 97*(1), 117–124.

Galanter, M., Keller, D. S., Dematis, H., & Egelko, S. (2000). The impact of managed care on substance abuse treatment. *Journal of Addiction Diseases, 19*(3), 13–34.

Heimer, R. (1998). Syringe exchange programs: Lowering the transmission of syringe borne dis-eases and beyond. *Public Health Reports, 113*(1), 67–74.

Holt, S. R., Ramos, J., Harma, M., Cabrera, F., Louis-Ashby, C., Dinh, A., Fiellin, D. A., & Tetrault, J. M. (2013). Physician detection of unhealthy substance use on inpatient teaching and hospitalist medical services. *American Journal of Drug & Alcohol Abuse, 39*(2), 121–129.

Khoury, E., & Rodriguez del Barrio, L. (2015). Recovery-oriented mental health practice: A social work perspective. *British Journal of Social Work, 45*(1), i27–i44.

Ladson, D., Kornegay, B., & Lesane, S. (2014). The early detection and proper treatment of bipolar disorder: Implications for social work practice with substance-abusing clients. *Journal of Human Behavior in the Social Work Environment, 24*, 547–556.

Latkin, C. A. (1998). Outreach in natural settings: The use of peer leaders for HIV prevention among injecting drug users' networks. *Public Health Reports, 113*(1), 151–159.

Laudet, A. B., & Humphreys, K. (2013). Promoting recovery in an evolving policy context: What do we know and what do we need to know about recovery support services? *Journal of Substance Abuse Treatment, 45*(1), 126–133.

Liebshultz, J. M., Crooks, D., Herman, D., Anderson, B., Tsui, J., Meshesha, L. Z., & Stein, M. (2014). Buprenorphine treatment for hospitalized, opioid dependent patients: A randomized clinical trial. *JAMA Internal Medicine, 174*(8), 1369–1376.

Maiter, S., Allagia, R., & Trocmé, N. (2004). Perceptions of child maltreatment by parents from the Indian subcontinent: Challenging myths about culturally based abusive parenting practice. *Child Maltreatment, 9*(3), 309–324.

McCabe, H. A., & Wahler, E. A. (2016). The Affordable Care Act, substance abuse disorders, and low-income implication for social work. *Journal of Social Work Education, 61*(3), 227–223.

National Association of Social Workers. (2016a). *Code of ethics of the National Association of Social Workers*. Retrieved from http://socialworkers.org/pubs/code/code.asp

National Association of Social Workers. (2016b). *Advocacy.*. Retrieved from http://socialworkers.org/advocacy/default.asp

National Association of Social Workers. (2017). *Practice & professional development: Practice.*. Retrieved from Retrieved from http://socialworkers.org/practice/default.asp

National Institute for Drug Abuse. (2016). *Treatment approaches for drug addiction.* Retrieved from https://www.drugabuse.gov/publications/drugfacts/treatment-approaches-drug-addiction

New York State Office of Alcoholism and Substance Abuse Services. (2016a). *OASAS/DOH health advisory: Interventions to prevent opioid overdose.*. Retrieved from https://www.oasas.ny.gov/AdMed/meds/oasdasdohodadvisory.cfm

New York State Office of Alcoholism and Substance Abuse Services. (2016b). *OASAS recovery projects.*. Retrieved from https://www.oasas.ny.gov/recovery/RecoveryProjects.cfm

New York State Office of Alcoholism and Substance Abuse Services. (2016c). *Credentialed Alcoholism and Substance Abuse Counselor (CASAC) Canon of Principles.*. Retrieved from https://www.oasas.ny.gov/sqa/credentialing/casac_canon.cfm

New York State Office of Alcoholism and Substance Abuse Services. (2016d). *OASAS overview.* Retrieved from https://oasas.ny.gov/pio/oasas.cfm

Rifenbark, R., & Waltz, J. A. (2016). Beyond the 12 steps: Key legal issues for substance use disorder treatment facilities. *Journal of Health Care compliance, 18*(6), 15–20.

Senreich, E., & Straussner, S. L. A. (2013). The effect of MSW education on students' knowledge and attitudes regarding substance abusing clients. *Journal of Social Work Education, 49*, 321–336.

Staiger, P. K., Richardson, B., Long, C. M., Carr, V., & Harlatt, G. A. (2013). Overlooked and underestimated? Problematic alcohol use in clients recovering from drug dependence. *Addiction, 108*(7), 1188–1193.

Stein, B. D., Pacula, R. L., Gordon, A. J., Burns, R. M., Leslie, D. S., Sonbero, M. J., Bauhoff, S., Mandell, T. W., & Dick, A. W. (2015). Where is buprenorphine dispensed to treat opioid disorders? The role of private offices, opioid treatment programs, and substance abuse treatment facilities in urban and rural counties. *The Milbank Quarterly, 93*(3), 561–583.

Substance Abuse and Mental Health Services Administration .(2006). *Substance abuse: Administrative issues in outpatient treatment. A treatment improvement protocol (TIP) 46.* Retrieved from https://www.ncbi.nlm.nih.gov/books/NBK64075/pdf/Bookshelf_NBK64075.pdf

Substance Abuse and Mental Health Services Administration. (2007). *Clinical issues in intensive outpatient treatment: Quick guide for clinicians based on TIP 47.* Retrieved from https://store.samhsa.gov/shin/content//SMA07-4233/SMA07-4233.pdf

Substance Abuse and Mental Health Services Administration. (2010a). *More substance abuse treatment centers are providing nicotine replacement therapy to help patients quip tobacco use.* Retrieved from https://www.samhsa.gov/newsroom/press-announcements/201011180500-0

Substance Abuse and Mental Health Services Administration. (2010b). *Substance abuse treatment for persons with co-occurring disorders. Quick guide for mental health professionals. Based on TIP 42.* Retrieved from https://store.samhsa.gov/shin/content//SMA10-4531/SMA10-4531.pdf

Substance Abuse and Mental Health Services Administration. (2015). *Detoxification and substance abuse treatment. A treatment improvement protocol (TIP) 45..* Retrieved from https://store.samhsa.gov/shin/content//SMA15-4131/SMA15-4131.pdf

Substance Abuse and Mental Health Services Administration. (2016a). *Treatment of substance use disorders..* Retrieved from https://www.samhsa.gov/treatment/substance-use-disorders

Substance Abuse and Mental Health Services Administration. (2016b). *Alcohol, tobacco, and other drugs.* Retrieved from http://www.samhsa.gov/atod

Substance Abuse and Mental Health Services Administration. (2016c). *Recovery and recovery support.* Retrieved from https://www.samhsa.gov/recovery

Substance Abuse and Mental Health Services Administration. (2016d). *Opioids.* Retrieved from https://www.samhsa.gov/atod/opioids., https://www.samhsa.gov/prevention

The Sponsor's Aide. (2008). *What is a sponsor?* Retrieved from http://thesponsorsaide.org/WhatIsASponsor.htm

Van Wormer, K., & Davis, D. E. (2014). *Addiction treatment: A strengths perspective* (4th ed.). Boston: Cengage.

Yip, P. S. F., Caine, E., Yousuf, S., Chang, S., Wu, K., & Chen, Y. (2012). Means restriction for suicide prevention. *The Lancet, 379,* 2393–2399.

Chapter 16
Preventing Substance Abuse and Addiction

A. Jordan Wright and Rachel Henes

Beyond the obvious social benefits of preventing substance abuse among teenagers, studies have shown that substance abuse costs America hundreds of billions of dollars per year (Harwood, 2000), and implementing effective prevention programs would save an estimated $18 to the nation for every dollar spent on prevention programming (SAMHSA Center for Substance Abuse Prevention, 2008). Adolescence is the developmental period that can be clearly identified as the most "sensitive period" for the onset of experimentation with drugs and alcohol, as well as the risk for transition from use to problematic use to dependence (Jordan & Andersen, 2016). Studies have found that by 12th grade, and certainly by college, many adolescents report binge drinking and using marijuana (Degenhardt et al., 2008; Johnston, O'Malley, Bachman, & Schulenberg, 2010). The earlier this binge drinking, often considered alcohol abuse in the literature, and drunkenness occurs in life, the more likely these individuals are to develop significant functional (such as behavioral) problems and alcohol-related disorders, a finding that has been replicated in many different countries (Kuntsche et al., 2013; Lee & DiClemente, 1985; Parrella & Filstead, 1988). While there are many risk factors for developing substance-related problems, including genetic, personality, attachment, and environmental (e.g., Meyers & Dick, 2010; Ormel et al., 2012; Schindler & Bröning, 2015), much research (both brain research and longitudinal research) has supported the fact that delaying the onset of experimenting with substances, including cigarettes, alcohol, drugs, and concurrent use of multiple substances, is the most effective strategy for preventing both problems and addiction later in life (Buchmann et al.,

A. J. Wright (✉)
Department of Applied Psychology, Steinhardt School of Culture, Education, and Human Development, New York University, New York, NY, USA
e-mail: ajordanwright@nyu.edu

R. Henes
Freedom Institute, Hallways, New York, NY, USA

© Springer International Publishing AG 2018
T. MacMillan, A. Sisselman-Borgia (eds.), *New Directions in Treatment, Education, and Outreach for Mental Health and Addiction*, Advances in Mental Health and Addiction, https://doi.org/10.1007/978-3-319-72778-3_16

2013; Gillespie, Neale, & Kendler, 2009; Grant, Stinson, & Hartford, 2001; Hingson, Heeren, & Winter, 2006; Lisdahl, Gilbart, Wright, & Shollenbarger, 2013; Moss, Chen, & Yi, 2014). In fact, Bukstein and Kaminer (2015) found that when the use of substances was controlled at age 18, there was no significant link between major risk factors and either the rate/intensity of use in adulthood or the negative consequences of use in adulthood. Thus, targeting adolescent substance use (and abuse) can effectively curtail problematic consequences and addiction later in life.

Theoretical Foundations of Prevention

The field of prevention science has been through a significant history of thought, trial, and error. Multiple theoretical models have emerged throughout the years, to varying success. Although some have been somewhat high-profile failures (such as the "Just Say No" campaign and D.A.R.E.'s early models; Paglia & Room, 1999; West & O'Neal, 2004), there is significant promise (and conceptual overlap) in many of the theoretical models widely used presently.

Information Dissemination

Early efforts to prevent substance abuse among youth were centered on increasing knowledge about the negative consequences of using drugs and alcohol. Disseminating information about both the proximal consequences (such as bad breath from cigarette smoking and poor decision making when using alcohol) and distal consequences (such as physical problems from alcohol and cigarette abuse and longer-term risk of addiction) and allowing students to ask questions to gain more in-depth knowledge about substance use and abuse were key components, with the theory that increased knowledge about the negative effects of substance abuse would necessarily deter adolescents' use. Much early research revealed that information dissemination was inadequate for the reduction of substance use in adolescence (for several examples, see Harmon, 1993; Kinder, Pape, & Walfish, 1980; Malvin, Moskowitz, Schaps, & Schaeffer, 1985; and Unlu, Sahin, & Wan, 2014). In fact, some found that increasing knowledge about substances and substance use actually increased rates of use (Botvin, Baker, Dusenbury, Tortu, & Botvin, 1990). While there is no clear evidence for reasons (and research in this area ceased when information dissemination programs stopped being developed and utilized), some have theorized that increasing knowledge also stimulated curiosity about using the substances. In all, information dissemination has fallen out of favor as a stand-alone technique based on the heavily negative empirical evaluation of it.

Fear Arousal

In an intuitive prevention strategy, a theory emerged that if an adolescent's fear about using substances were increased, he or she would be significantly less likely to actually use those substances. Techniques employed in these methods (which are often paired with information dissemination) include scaring adolescents from using tobacco, alcohol, and other drugs, based on dramatizing negative consequences (such as showing blackened lungs from cigarette smoking) or emphasizing worst-case scenarios (such as deaths from drunk driving). Although fear arousal techniques have been found to generate reactions in their audience, and may even contribute to some attitude change in some adolescents, overall they seem not to have any long-term deterring effects (Thrul, Buhler, & Herth, 2014). Even if they do increase adolescents' appraisal of the risk of using substances, this does not seem to affect their behavior in a positive way on its own (Sheeran, Harris, & Epton, 2014). As such, fear arousal techniques, like information dissemination as a stand-alone technique, have fallen out of favor.

Social Influence Models

In a first and groundbreaking break from the information dissemination and fear arousal models (which do not seem to work well, if at all), Evans (1976) pioneered a shift in focus from drug facts to psychosocial factors that contribute to substance use and abuse. He focused on an inoculation model, premised on the hypothesis that persuasive messages (from peers, the media, etc.) played a pivotal role in adolescents choosing to engage in substance use. The theory held that by exposing adolescents to "low doses" of persuasive messages, they could build up "antibodies," in the form of anti-drug attitudes, beliefs, and normative expectations, that would protect them in the future from exposure to further "doses" (which would naturally come from their environments in the forms of peer pressure, cultural exposure, media, etc.). Evans' model of preventing (or at least delaying) substance use was replicated and studied multiple times, with positive outcomes (e.g., Flay, 1985; Sussman et al., 1995), and many of the techniques developed in the social influence model are utilized in current, evidence-based comprehensive programs.

Ecological and Liability Models

The newer "wave" of prevention theories are much more comprehensive and based in cross-disciplinary theory and research. Specifically, they focus on the complex interplay between individual and context. Ecological models are based in the seminal work of Bronfenbrenner (1977) and subsequent work by Belsky (1993) focused on the multiple, interconnected systems that influence an individual's behavior. Beyond just internal, individual factors (like genetics, personality/traits, etc.), many different levels of influence are at play, such as peer relationships, parent relationships, neighborhoods, schools, broader culture, and, perhaps most importantly, the interplay between all of these. The liability model (Tarter & Vanyukov, 1994) focuses on the interaction between individual vulnerability to addiction (which increases use and problems in adolescence) and environmental factors that contribute to the vulnerability being "triggered" into actual problem (versus those environmental factors that interrupt the vulnerability). Both models focus on the interplay between individual, personal characteristics (or vulnerabilities) and contextual and environmental factors. The ecological models focus on risk and protective factors at every level/system, as well as how they interact, strengthen, or mitigate each other, while the liability model focuses on how environmental and contextual factors either propel or reverse the trajectory from personal risk to actual addiction. Some examples of these contextual factors include deviant peers and low parental monitoring (Blackson, Tarter, Loeber, Ammerman, & Windle, 1996), but there are many personal and contextual/environmental factors that have been implicated. While more comprehensive prevention efforts should interact with all the systems, as well as both the personal and contextual/environmental factors associated with risk and protection, multiple models of prevention have emerged from these broader umbrellas, including risk and protective factor models, skills training models, normative education, and competence-enhancement models.

Risk and Protective Factors

The focus on risk and protective factors has permeated the theoretical and practical literature on prevention programming, as it has yielded some of the most positive and promising results. While some risks are genetic (Meyers & Dick, 2010) and not so amenable to psychosocial intervention, many are personal and either teachable or remediable (such as specific social and life skills), social, or cultural. Understanding those factors that pose risks for problems and those factors which protect youth against them directly informs prevention programming. A section of this chapter below will be dedicated to the discussion of risk and protective factors at these different levels.

Skills Training

Hearkening back to the work of Evans (1976), the primary tenet of skills training models for prevention is that early use of drugs and alcohol is dependent primarily on social influences, such as peers and media. The major skills that have been the focus of these models of prevention relate to resisting peer influence to use substances and resisting media influence that promote substance use (Hansen, 1992). The premise of these programs is that an increase in skills (seen as a protective factor) will decrease individuals' susceptibility to negative influences, and this premise has fared well in the research literature (Sheeran et al., 2014). Many programs are built around skills training, and many comprehensive programs include skills development as a primary component.

Normative Education

It was observed fairly early that when asked, adolescents tend to significantly overestimate the prevalence of substance use among their peers (Evans, Hansen, & Mittlemark, 1977). This has been somewhat refuted more recently in the literature (Henry, Kobus, & Schoeny, 2011; Pape, 2012; Simons-Morton & Kuntsche, 2012); it has been found that those adolescents who are using substances tend to overestimate peer use, while those who are not using substances actually tend to underestimate. Regardless, the theory holds that youth should challenge any misconceptions about prevalence of use so as not to believe that it is more normative than it is. Adolescents should not believe that using substances is normative, harmless, or socially acceptable (or worse, a way to "fit in"), and normative education programs are based on ensuring that they learn about actual rates of use (along with some consequences of use).

Competence Enhancement

The competence-enhancement approach to prevention incorporates components of many of the above models, comprehensively addressing substance use as a socially learned and reinforced behavior (based on the work of Bandura (1977) and Jessor & Jessor (1977)), with those individuals with lower personal and social competence (operationalized most often as self-management and social skills) at highest risk for maladaptive coping strategies (Botvin, 2000). The theory posits that adolescents with better cognitive, affective, and behavioral coping skills to manage their everyday challenges are more likely to do so in a healthy manner, rather than turning to substance use to cope (which then becomes reinforced as it helps mitigate negative emotions). These goals are aligned with positive youth development, and increased personal and social competence has many benefits. However, to affect substance use specifically, these programs need to have substance-use-specific information, such as peer pressure resistance skills, normative education, and media resistance skills, such as those developed in the social influence model (Caplan et al., 1992).

Levels of Prevention

In 1994, the Institute of Medicine (Mrazek & Haggerty, 1994) proposed three levels of prevention, which they defined specifically as interventions that occur before the onset of a specific disorder (such as a substance use disorder). *Universal prevention* is the broadest form of prevention and is aimed at an entire population of individuals, regardless of level of risk, "red flag" indicators of problems or potential problems, or any other distinguishing factor. These types of prevention efforts may be more aligned with public health initiatives, such as anti-drug mass media campaigns, which reach everyone equally. They may also take the form of broad educational initiatives, such as school-based prevention programs (like teaching general life skills) that are offered to entire schools, without singling any specific children out for different programming. These universal prevention efforts have been shown to be effective at improving multiple factors, especially at reducing cigarette use for those who receive the programs, and on a broader population level, they have been linked with lower rates of use of both cigarettes and marijuana (Shamblen & Derzon, 2009). Universal prevention has been shown to be most effective for those individuals who are at low baseline risk, having low risk factors, and not yet using any substances.

Selective prevention represents programs and initiatives aimed at subsections of populations, specifically those who are seen as being at higher risk for problems, such as substance abuse. Those youth with multiple individual risk factors (see section on risk factors later in the chapter) present, for example, could be separated out and provided with specific interventions targeting those risk factors (or increasing protective factors, etc.). While some selective preventions may look similar to universal prevention, aiming at increasing protective factors and mitigating risk factors, techniques that have been found to be effective for selective prevention include motivational interviewing with a harm-reduction framework (Catalano, Haggerty, Hawkins, & Elgin, 2011).

Indicated prevention is targeted toward individuals who are either already engaging in some high-risk behaviors, such as experimentation with substances, or who are showing warning signs of danger, such as dramatic change in behavior (these are considered "indicators" of potential imminent problems). Not yet meeting criteria for a specific disorder (such as a substance use disorder), these individuals need significant intervention to change the course of their problematic trajectory. Interventions for indicated prevention are much less general than universal prevention and even selective prevention, both which often focus on skill development. Interventions for indicated prevention are much more heavily focused on the problem indicators themselves, antecedents to those indicators, and outcomes that reinforce the negative behaviors. Both selective and indicated prevention efforts have been shown to be effective, most of all with problematic alcohol use (Shamblen & Derzon, 2009).

Strategic Prevention Framework

SAMHSA has developed a model for prevention work called the Strategic Prevention Framework (SPF; http://www.samhsa.gov/capt/applying-strategic-prevention-framework). This framework is especially important as it balances the use of evidence-based prevention science approaches to preventing problems (including substance-related ones) with the understanding of several limitations to the prevention literature. First, much of the literature on prevention programs focuses on faithful implementation of specific programs by trained professionals leading to positive outcomes. While this is an ideal circumstance, most often in the real world, there are not enough resources to implement these programs in the same ways that they were developed and tested. Second, and perhaps more importantly, many of the prevention efforts were developed for and tested on populations that were seen to be high-need (if not high-risk) populations, such as school-based prevention programs tested in urban, high-minority schools. While many of the findings are likely to transfer somewhat easily to other populations, this assumption may not be entirely sound. In fact, one dimension of this, cultural adaptation of programs and interventions, has been found to be absolutely key in programs' success (Kucukuysal & Beyhan, 2011). Strategic prevention aims to balance the use of evidence-based techniques with the acknowledgement that implementing preventative interventions in a fully evidence-based way is not entirely possible.

The Strategic Prevention Framework involves five steps. First, a comprehensive assessment of the needs of the community/population is necessary. This assessment can include multiple methodologies toward better understanding the potential problem to be addressed, the risk and protective factors present within the community or population, and epidemiological trends within the community. Second, the framework requires the increasing of prevention capacity within the community/population itself. This step acknowledges that many situations will not allow for fully trained "experts" to come in and implement prevention programming in perpetuity. Capacity for making preventative efforts themselves must be built into the process with communities. Third, strategic plans for addressing the needs must be developed. These plans can be a collaboration between a prevention team and community/population members themselves, again working to address the needs that emerged from the assessment in as evidence-based a way as possible, with the acknowledgement that evidence-based programs and techniques may not fully apply to the population at hand. That is, tweaks (such as culturally-driven alterations) may need to be made in order to make programming most effective for the specific community. Fourth, the actual preventative interventions are implemented. These may include direct services (such as school-based workshops for adolescents), changes in policies and practices through consultation, and other interventions. Finally, fifth, the SPF requires the evaluation of outcomes, to ensure the effectiveness of the process as a whole, which then informs future prevention programming. The overarching guiding principles that are integrated throughout the SPF process are sustainability (the second step is especially important for this) and cultural competence (steps one and four lean most heavily on this). Strategic preventions have been shown to be quite effective, from small-scale programs within single schools all the way up to entire communities (for several examples, see Anderson-Carpenter, Watson-Thompson, Chaney, & Jones, 2016; Eddy et al., 2012).

Risk and Protective Factors

Much of the emphasis in the prevention science literature is on risk and protective factors related to the development of problems, such as substance abuse and substance use disorders. While some risk factors are difficult to assess and are invisible, such as genetic risk factors (Meyers & Dick, 2010), others are easier to evaluate and perceive, such as some temperamental factors (Ormel et al., 2012), interpersonal factors (Schindler & Broning, 2015), social and other life skills, and social, cultural, and environmental factors.

Periods of Risk

Periods within individuals' lives that are marked by transition have a long-standing place in the literature as periods in which these individuals are at higher risk for problems emerging (Griffin, 2010). During transitions, such as the transition from high school to college, the transition into parenthood, and getting married, individuals' coping skills are tested and challenged. Moving into significantly different environments (such as a switch of school or moving away for college), facing dramatically different responsibilities (such as parenthood), or having a significant change in support or life circumstances (such as after the loss of a spouse) requires individuals to manage more than usual amounts of stress, monitor and self-regulate their emotions and behaviors, and cope with things they are not used to, and these requirements place them at higher risk for maladaptive coping or being overwhelmed. For example, the transition to college can be quite a difficult one. Alcohol may offer several "benefits" to new college students: some may find socializing and making new friends easier with some alcohol in their system; others may feel they need to drink alcohol in order to "fit in" with new college peers; still others may simply be overwhelmed by stress, anxiety, and other emotions, and alcohol can serve to relieve some of the immediate symptoms of these. The traditional move to college from high school is a transition that brings with it social demands, emotional demands (often missing parents and certainly old friends and other social supports), and environmental demands (often new autonomy and the need to manage personal time and responsibilities significantly differently than before). Other transitions in life bring with them different demands, but all transitions come with some demands.

Adolescence represents one of these major transition periods, full of navigating new situations (including social situations, biological/hormonal situations, educational, behavioral, independence-related, identity development-related, and others) and extreme demands on the coping skills of individuals. Steinberg (2008) has done quite a bit of research on brain development through adolescence and early adulthood, which consistently finds development ongoing (thus not fully completed) in areas of the brain related to impulse control, emotion regulation, and behavioral regulation. New forms of social interaction, limit testing, searching for identity

(Marcia, 1966), and particular psychological phenomena unique to adolescents (such as feeling uniquely invulnerable to problems (Hill, Duggan, & Lapsley, 2012)) characterize this period as particularly transitional, and as stated previously, this is a period of particular risk for the onset of problematic substance use that can develop into substance abuse or a substance use disorder.

Individual Risk and Protective Factors

Many of the primary risk and protective factors that are the focus of prevention efforts are characteristics inherent to individuals, such as genetic factors, attitudinal and personality factors, developmental factors, and emotional factors (Swadi, 1999). Some examples include attitudes about drug use and expectancies, including level of knowledge about the risk of use and how normative individuals believe it is (Kandel, Kessler, & Margulies, 1978; Krosnick & Judd, 1982; Smith & Fogg, 1978). These are important cognitive factors that have been found to be associated with substance abuse risk, especially as they are easily addressed through psycho-educational means. More complex emotional and skill-related factors that have been implicated in substance abuse and addiction risk include capacity to regulate emotions and behaviors (Khantzian, 1997); to cope with stress, distress, and negative situations (Berkowitz & Begun, 2003; Botvin, 2000); and to resist social influence and be assertiveness (Berkowitz & Begun, 2003; Botvin, 2000). Importantly, more ingrained personality factors have been found to be related to risk for substance misuse, as well as to motivation for using and how reinforcing, and thus self-sustaining, substances themselves are (Comeau, Stewart, & Loba, 2001; Conrod, Peterson, Pihl, & Mankowski, 1997; Conrod, Pihl, Stewart, & Dongier, 2000; Conrod, Pihl, & Vassileva, 1998; Cooper, Frone, Russell, & Mudar, 1995; Woicik, Stewart, Pihl, & Conrod, 2009). While some have discovered personality trait links to substance abuse such as those related to self-esteem and risk for depression, anxiety, and antisocial behaviors (Armstrong & Costello, 2002; Cerda, Sagdeo, & Galea, 2008), Conrod and colleagues have found four specific characteristics extremely predictive of substance abuse and problem use: hopelessness, anxiety sensitivity, impulsivity, and sensation seeking (Conrod, Castellanos-Ryan, & Mackie, 2011; Conrod, Stewart, Comeau, & Maclean, 2006; O'Leary-Barrett, Mackie, Castellanos-Ryan, Al-Khudhairy, & Conrod, 2010). While understanding the genetic and biological risk factors may ultimately be useful in assessment and identification of individuals at risk, knowing these individual characteristics that are more amenable to intervention can not only aid in identification but also in understanding how best to intervene with individuals at risk.

Family, Peer, School, and Neighborhood Risk and Protective Factors

The direct contexts in which individuals operate have a strong influence on potential problems. Bronfenbrenner (1977) emphasized the importance of these *microsystems* in personal adaptation, noting just how important one's family, peers, school, and neighborhood are at any given moment. Indeed research has borne out many interactional factors that are related to substance abuse, particularly in youth. For example, Lochman and van den Steenhoven (2002) enumerate many of the family factors that seem to affect risk for substance use problems, including some directly related to substances, like direct modeling of use and family attitudes toward substance use, but also some more general family factors, like the harshness of disciplinary practices, the level of monitoring and limit-setting parents provide their children, levels of family bonding and open communication, and the general level of conflict within the family. Similarly, peer use and peer attitudes about use have been correlated with substance abuse behaviors (Mason, Mennis, Linker, Bares, & Zaharakis, 2014; Monahan, Rhew, Hawkins, & Brown, 2014), as have more general social factors like peer rejection (Cairns, Cairns, Neckerman, Gest, & Gariepy, 1988; Coie, 1990).

Multiple school-related variables have been implicated in risk and protection for problematic substance use. Included in these are attitudes that are affected by individuals, families, peers, and schools themselves, such as level of feeling engaged with school and how committed one is to school and academics (Fletcher, Bonell, & Hargreaves, 2008). Obviously many of these factors are multiply determined, such that personality characteristics, family values, the quality of school, and many other contextual variables will affect them. Ultimately, in addition to these emotional and attitudinal school variables, actual success or failure at school has been linked to risk for developing problematic substance use (Jessor, 1976; Smith & Fogg, 1978).

Community and neighborhood factors have also been implicated as influencing risk for problematic substance use. As would be expected, major problems in neighborhoods are related to higher risk for substance abuse and dependence. Included are a lack of safety, community disorganization, extreme population density and overcrowding, and physical infrastructure deterioration, as well as the more internalized feeling of being disengaged from one's local community (Hays, Hays, & Mulhall, 2003; Murray, 1983; Simcha-Fagan & Schwartz, 1986). The physical and emotional environment in which one lives can serve as a risk or protective factor, in addition to the social environment.

Sociocultural Risk and Protective Factors

Culture and broader societal factors, what Bronfenbrenner (1977) termed the *exosystem*, also have a significant role in risk and protection for substance-related problems. Some social factors that are more concrete have been found to be related to rates of substance abuse, including taxation of substances (Cook & Tauchen, 1982; Saffer & Grossman, 1987) and laws regulating substances and substance use, such as drinking age laws (Cook & Tauchen, 1982; Krieg, 1982; Saffer & Grossman, 1987). Related to laws and regulations is simply the availability of substances, another major factor implicated in rates of use and abuse (Gottfredson, 1987). Finally, major societal problems also play a role, such as extreme poverty and economic deprivation (Murray, Richards, Luepker, & Johnson, 1987; Robins & Ratcliff, 1978; Zucker & Harford, 1983).

In addition to concrete societal factors, "softer" cultural factors also play a role in risk of and protection from substance use and abuse. For example, more exposure to advertisements promoting alcohol use has been linked to higher rates of actual use (Atkin, Hocking, & Block, 1984). Ultimately, culture significantly affects attitudes, values, and expectations about what individuals can expect if they use substances (Abbott & Chase, 2008). Both structural and "softer" sociocultural factors play central roles in how at risk individuals are for using substances, using them early, and developing problems as a result.

Prevention Programs

Many prevention programs have been developed, and many have shown promise or even extremely good results. While this may sound exciting, a review of the landscape of actual practice in the real world revealed that the overwhelming majority of programs being implemented outside of controlled research protocols were not one of these evidence-based programs, or, if they were, very few were implemented faithfully or sustained over time (Ennett et al., 2003; Ringwalt et al., 2002; Spoth, Greenberg, & Turrisi, 2008). Clearly, there is a disconnect between research and practice in the field, and while practitioners need to understand the empirically-driven basis for successful programs, researchers need to understand the practical limitations to implementing programs outside of highly structured (and often grant-funded) research protocols. This section provides a brief review of many of the programs that have proven successful in research, and the following section presents principles that have emerged from these successful programs that may be more easily integrated into actual prevention programming in the real world, when and if entirely faithful implementation of one of the evidence-based, empirically-proven programs is not feasible.

School-Based Prevention Programs

The literature and development of prevention science have focused quite a bit on schools as a primary and appropriate setting for programming, as they occupy a great deal of adolescents' waking lives, as well as having the explicit mission of educating youth, which is in direct opposition to substance use (and certainly problematic use and abuse). Additionally, there are many common goals of prevention programs and educational institutions, such as improving decision-making skills and impulse control in general, at which substance abuse prevention programs have proven extremely successful (Pokhrel et al., 2013).

Many school-based programs have been developed, and many have been found to have beneficial effects on children. Across many meta-analyses, it appears those programs that teach social competence, including resistance to social influence and other social skills both generally and substance-use-specific, are the most effective at preventing taking up smoking cigarettes (Hwang, Yeagley, & Petosa, 2004; Thomas, McLellan, & Perera, 2013), though there is not much evidence for long-term effectiveness of any school-based programs (Wiehe, Garrison, Christakis, Ebel, & Rivara, 2005). These findings are consistent with school-based skill-building programs being most effective at reducing both marijuana and other illicit drug use (Faggiano et al., 2008). Information-based and affective programs have not had the same success (Faggiano et al., 2008; Thomas et al., 2013). When it comes to alcohol prevention, although stated goals are often to delay the onset of use, school-based programs are much better at decreasing rates of heavy use, such as drunkenness and binge drinking, though many have been shown to be effective at improving alcohol attitudes, expectancies, and use (Foxcroft & Tsertsvadze, 2011). Importantly, while there is some evidence of brief school-based interventions, especially based on motivational enhancement techniques (Hennessy & Tanner-Smith, 2015), there is no evidence to suggest that these brief interventions are effective if administered in group formats (which is primarily the case in school-based prevention programming), and there is much more evidence that longer programs (more than a year) and those with booster sessions in following years are more effective (La Torre, Chiaradia, & Ricciardi, 2005; Thomas et al., 2013). Programs that target multiple theoretical factors hypothesized to impact the onset of substance use seem to be the most effective, as well (Porath-Waller, Beasley, & Beirness, 2010). Some newer research is supporting the use of school-based computer or internet-implemented prevention programs, with some showing decreases in alcohol and drug use and increases in knowledge and intentions not to use in the future (Champion, Newton, Barrett, & Teesson, 2013; Champion, Newton, Stapinski, & Teesson, 2016).

Family-Based Prevention Programs

While, theoretically, family-based interventions for the prevention of substance use and abuse make intuitive sense, the actual findings on program effectiveness has not been as promising. Most programs aimed at families attempt to improve parenting practices, including increasing parental monitoring of children, improving behavior management techniques and clarity of boundaries, and increasing support, nurturance, and family cohesion. Studies have found some positive effects of these programs in the short- and medium-term, but these effects tend to be extremely small and may not actually influence initiation of using substances (Foxcroft & Tsertsvadze, 2012; Kuntsche & Kuntsche, 2016). Similarly, some benefits were found in programs focused on parental involvement and explicit parental disapproval of substance use, though some programs that targeted only parent behavior actually saw increases in adolescents' substance use (Petrie, Bunn, & Byrne, 2007). Youth- and individually-focused programs, even if focused on improving family interactions, seem to be much more effective at curbing problematic substance use, especially over time (Tripodi, Bender, Litschge, & Vaughn, 2010; Van Ryzin, Roseth, Fosco, Lee, & Chen, 2016). It is important to note that a major hurdle in family-based prevention efforts is that those families who are at the highest risk and have the most need are the least likely to participate in these kinds of programs (Diaz et al., 2006).

Workplace Prevention Programs

The workplace is in many ways an ideal place to implement universal prevention efforts to attempt to reduce alcohol and drug misuse, as workplaces can reach an extremely broad audience (many of whom may not be reached by other methods) and reducing alcohol and drug misuse benefits both the employer and the employees. Workplace prevention can include the use of work policies that attempt to change attitudes toward alcohol and other drug use (Liira et al., 2016), including strict policies and limiting access to alcohol (Ames & Bennett, 2011), which have been shown to be promising tactics, as have larger social norm-targeting campaigns (Frone & Brown, 2010). Most, though, focus on general health promotion and healthy lifestyle education (Bennett & Lehman, 2003; Cook & Schlenger, 2002). It should be noted that the field of workplace prevention programs is quite young, and while studies have found some workplace prevention efforts to be successful, there are no long-standing and well-established (and thus thoroughly studied) programs, so even promising results are quite tentative. The most promising to date seem to be programs that integrate alcohol interventions with health promotion, combining education, assessment, and brief interventions (Ames & Bennett, 2011). An intensive, 2-day intervention aimed at promoting healthy behaviors (including information about alcohol and cigarette use) and even a brief, targeted intervention focused on making healthy life choices and encouraging seeking professional help seem promising for reducing alcohol use (though not cigarette smoking; Reynolds & Bennett, 2015; Spicer & Miller, 2016).

In addition to universal prevention in the workplace, programs often focus on screening and selective and indicated prevention efforts in order to curb the escalation of problematic substance use (Liira et al., 2016). For example, the Alcohol Screening and Brief Intervention (ASBI) model, which has been applied extremely successfully (and cost-effectively) in primary healthcare settings to reduce harmful and hazardous alcohol use (O'Donnell et al., 2014), has been applied in workplace settings, with varied success (Schulte et al., 2014). It is likely that the varied success has to do with the extreme heterogeneity of cultures and contexts in the workplace, as opposed to the relative homogeneity of the primary healthcare setting. Additionally, although theoretically an online approach to workplace prevention makes sense, to increase privacy and mitigate the potential effects of stigma, research has not provided much evidence of the effectiveness of online prevention programs administered at work (Khadjesari, Freemantle, Linke, Hunter, & Murray, 2014).

Community-Based Prevention Programs

Of all the different types of prevention programs, community-based programs are the most difficult to study, as most of them include multiple varied components, often including family- and school-based ones. The most promising community-based prevention programs seem to incorporate a coordinated, targeted "message" across all of their different components. Some program components have included education for primary care physicians and community partners, community activation and coalition building, collecting and monitoring of data, policy work, mass media campaigns, and public relations work, among others (Albert et al., 2011; Clark, Wilder, & Winstanley, 2014; Gripenberg Abdon, Wallin, & Andreasson, 2011). It should be noted that these multicomponent, community-based preventative interventions are often quite cost- and labor-intensive.

Specific multimodal, community-based prevention programs have shown promise for discouraging the sale of alcohol to intoxicated individuals, which included law enforcement efforts, skills training, information campaigns, and policy work (Warpenius, Holmila, & Mustonen, 2010), and lowering rates of uptake of cigarette smoking in children and adolescents (Sowden & Stead, 2003). Some of the most effective and promising community-based prevention programs help guide communities through a specific and explicit process of identifying needs and resources, selecting community leaders, creating an action plan with clear goals and objectives, and selecting evidence-based programs and policies (Hawkins et al., 2012). In all, however, large-scale community-based prevention efforts are difficult to evaluate as a single construct, as they are so heterogeneous and often have many varied components.

Prevention Science-Based Principles

As stated previously, it is often the case that, in practice, prevention programming cannot adhere faithfully to the models that have proven effective in the research literature, for a variety of logistical reasons. As such, it is important to extract some of the most salient and important "lessons" learned from evidence-based prevention programming, to guide practitioners in what is most likely to be effective in the real world.

Goals of Prevention

Prevention programs seem most effective when they are well coordinated and take aim at specific, evidence-based goals. As information dissemination and fear arousal tactics have been found to be ineffective (and worse, potentially harmful), programs should focus on enhancing social and psychological (coping) competencies, mitigating risk factors, and improving protective factors (including family cohesion and school connection) in youth. Because cost is often a primary factor in the decision-making process, the Strategic Prevention Framework paradigm can be particularly useful in assessing the *greatest* needs (competencies, etc.), as well as the easiest-to-target goals for a particular population. While conducting a comprehensive needs assessment may seem costly, targeted interventions that emerge from the assessment provide a more-bang-for-your-buck alternative to comprehensive programming, which is time-, cost-, and labor-intensive. If an evaluation reveals that a specific population's greatest risk factor lies in disconnection from school, decision makers can use evidence-based models for improving school connectedness in adolescents, rather than creating comprehensive programming to address all social and psychological skills and competencies. Comprehensive, long-term programming seems to be the most effective overall, but pragmatic limitations preclude many communities from delivering this kind of prevention effort.

Developmental, Cultural, and Contextual Appropriateness

Because there are different risks for different problems at different ages, it is important to understand developmental factors related to prevention programming. It is unlikely that the uptake of alcohol, cigarette, or drug use will happen early in the elementary school years. Therefore, programming at this age should be universal and target the known *eventual* risk factors for the initiation of problem behaviors, such as improving social competencies. Later in adolescence and the high school years, though, it may be more appropriate to evaluate groups of individuals for potential selective intervention and focus more on substance-specific skills, such as normative education and peer refusal skills. It is important to be deliberate about the risks, protective factors, and competencies that are being targeted at different developmental levels.

Similarly, multiple researchers have found that adapting programs is necessary for contextual appropriateness (Colby et al., 2013). Different cultures respond to different interventions in specific ways, in addition to potentially having different risk and protective factors (see, e.g., Castro et al., 2006). Researchers have found that, at the very least, culturally-specific adaptation of prevention programs tends to lead to more satisfaction with the programs and more personal meaning and identification with the content of them, and for some that translates into greater effectiveness (Springer et al., 2005). Adapting programs successfully should take into consideration both surface-level changes, such as names used in examples, and deep-level changes, such as truly understanding and addressing the culture-specific normative attitudes and beliefs or motivations of a specific group (Gewin & Hoffman, 2016).

Targeting Risk and Protective Factors

It is clear that the most promising programs for deterring onset of substance use and problematic misuse focus on risks and protective factors, including building competencies. In fact, the most successful programs seem to target multiple different risk and protective factors, from genetic to sociocultural factors (Scheier, 2010). Whenever possible, programs should evaluate and target the factors that are likely to provide the greatest support for the individuals involved (at least as much as is possible). Comprehensive and multicomponent programs seem to hold the most promise for "tackling" the most different factors, though of course these programs are often cost-, time-, or labor-prohibitive. Building competencies and protective factors and mitigating any salient risk factors, though, should make some impact on the population being targeted.

Practical Issues in Prevention Programming

A number of pragmatic issues can improve (or derail) the effectiveness of prevention programs. One of the most common ones to be investigated is fidelity, how faithfully and precisely an evidence-based program is delivered in real life. If a program has been proven to be effective in a specific format, that format should be respected and replicated as closely as possible, in order to maximize the likelihood of replicating its effects (Botvin, Baker, Dusenbury, Botvin, & Diaz, 1995; Durlak & DuPre, 2008). Failure of a poorly replicated program to produce positive effects cannot easily be linked to program ineffectiveness, poor fit with the population, or any other explanatory model, simply because the program is not the same program that was evaluated in the research literature. This principle is not meant to preclude the deliberate adaptation of programs for specific purposes, but it warns against sloppiness and poor attention to detail in the delivery of programs.

Some specific practical application issues have emerged as potentially extremely useful in prevention programming. For example, many have found that booster sessions in years after the main preventative intervention help the effects of the initial intervention last longer and be more effective (Resnicow & Botvin, 1993). Additionally, similar to general educational techniques, interventions that are specifically more interactive have proven more effective (Tobler & Stratton, 1997). Even when full program fidelity is not feasible in a given setting, some of these smaller, more practical aspects that have been shown to be more effective in prevention programming can be implemented for increased likelihood of program effectiveness.

Conclusion

There is a great deal known about prevention of substance use, substance abuse, and substance use disorders; however, there is often a disconnect between what is known and what is actually enacted in communities, agencies, and other practice settings. One major problem is the difficulty implementing evidence-based programs either in their entirety or faithfully, given pragmatic constraints. However, principles learned from prevention research can help actual programs increase the likelihood of effectiveness.

References

Abbott, P., & Chase, D. M. (2008). Culture and substance abuse impact of culture affects approach to treatment. *Psychiatric Times, 25*(1), 43–46.

Albert, S., Brason, I. I., Fred, W., Sanford, C. K., Dasgupta, N., Graham, J., et al. (2011). Project Lazarus: Community-based overdose prevention in rural North Carolina. *Pain Medicine, 12*(s2).

Ames, G. M., & Bennett, J. B. (2011). Prevention interventions of alcohol problems in the workplace: A review and guiding framework. *Alcohol Research and Health, 34*(2), 175–179.

Anderson-Carpenter, K. D., Watson-Thompson, J., Chaney, L., & Jones, M. (2016). Reducing binge drinking in adolescents through implementation of the strategic prevention framework. *American Journal of Community Psychology, 57*(1 2), 36–46.

Armstrong, T. D., & Costello, E. J. (2002). Community studies on adolescent substance use, abuse, or dependence and psychiatric comorbidity. *Journal of Consulting and Clinical Psychology, 70*(6), 1224–1239.

Atkin, C., Hocking, J., & Block, M. (1984). Teenage drinking: Does advertising make a difference? *Journal of Communication, 34*(2), 157–167.

Bandura, A. (1977). *Social learning theory*. Englewood Cliffs, NJ: Prentice Hall.

Belsky, J. (1993). Etiology of child maltreatment: A developmental ecological analysis. *Psychological Bulletin, 114*(3), 413–434.

Bennett, J. B., & Lehman, W. E. (2003). *Preventing workplace substance abuse: Beyond drug testing to wellness*. Washington, DC: American Psychological Association.

Berkowitz, M. W., & Begun, A. L. (2003). Designing prevention programs: The developmental perspective. In Z. Sloboda & W. J. Bukoski (Eds.), *Handbook of drug abuse prevention: Theory, science, and practice* (pp. 327–348). New York: Kluwer Academic/Plenum Publishers.

Blackson, T. C., Tarter, R. E., Loeber, R., Ammerman, R. T., & Windle, M. (1996). The influence of paternal substance abuse and difficult temperament in fathers and sons on sons' disengagement from family to deviant peers. *Journal of Youth and Adolescence, 25*(3), 389–411.

Botvin, G. J. (2000). Preventing drug abuse in schools: Social and competence enhancement approaches targeting individual-level etiologic factors. *Addictive Behaviors, 25*(6), 887–897.

Botvin, G. J., Baker, E., Dusenbury, L., Botvin, E. M., & Diaz, T. (1995). Long-term follow-up results of a randomized drug abuse prevention trial in a white middle-class population. *Journal of the American Medical Association, 273*(14), 1106–1112.

Botvin, G. J., Baker, E., Dusenbury, L., Tortu, S., & Botvin, E. M. (1990). Preventing adolescent drug abuse through a multimodal cognitive-behavioural approach: Results of a 3-year study. *Journal of Consulting and Clinical Psychology, 58*(4), 437–446.

Bronfenbrenner, U. (1977). Toward an experimental ecology of human development. *American Psychologist, 32*(7), 513–531.

Buchmann, A. F., Blomeyer, D., Jennen-Steinmetz, C., Schmidt, M. H., Esser, G., Banaschewski, T., et al. (2013). Early smoking onset may promise initial pleasurable sensations and later addiction. *Addiction Biology, 18*(6), 947–954.

Bukstein, O. G., & Kaminer, Y. (2015). Adolescent substance use disorders: Transition to substance abuse, prevention, and treatment. In M. Galanter, H. D. Kleber, & K. T. Brady (Eds.), *The American psychiatric publishing textbook of substance abuse treatment* (5th ed., pp. 641–650). Washington, DC: American Psychiatric Publishing.

Cairns, R. B., Cairns, B. D., Neckerman, H. J., Gest, S. D., & Gariepy, J. L. (1988). Social networks and aggressive behavior: Peer support or peer rejection? *Developmental Psychology, 24*(6), 815–823.

Caplan, M., Weissberg, R. P., Grober, J. S., Sivo, P. J., Grady, K., & Jacoby, C. (1992). Social competence promotion with inner-city and suburban young adolescents: Effects on social adjustment and alcohol use. *Journal of Consulting and Clinical Psychology, 60*(1), 56–63.

Castro, F. G., Barrera, M., Pantin, H., Martinez, C., Felix-Ortiz, M., Rios, R., et al. (2006). Substance abuse prevention intervention research with Hispanic populations. *Drug and Alcohol Dependence, 84*, S29–S42.

Catalano, R. F., Haggerty, K. P., Hawkins, J. D., & Elgin, J. (2011). Prevention of substance use and substance use disorders: The role of risk and protective factors. In Y. Kaminer & K. C. Winters (Eds.), *Clinical manual of adolescent substance abuse treatment* (pp. 25–63). Washington, DC: American Psychiatric Publishing.

Cerdá, M., Sagdeo, A., & Galea, S. (2008). Comorbid forms of psychopathology: Key patterns and future research directions. *Epidemiologic Reviews, 30*(1), 155–177.

Champion, K. E., Newton, N. C., Barrett, E. L., & Teesson, M. (2013). A systematic review of school-based alcohol and other drug prevention programs facilitated by computers or the internet. *Drug and Alcohol Review, 32*(2), 115–123.

Champion, K. E., Newton, N. C., Stapinski, L. A., & Teesson, M. (2016). Effectiveness of a universal internet-based prevention program for ecstasy and new psychoactive substances: A cluster randomized controlled trial. *Addiction, 111*(8), 1396–1405.

Clark, A. K., Wilder, C. M., & Winstanley, E. L. (2014). A systematic review of community opioid overdose prevention and naloxone distribution programs. *Journal of Addiction Medicine, 8*(3), 153–163.

Coie, J. D. (1990). Toward a theory of peer rejection. In S. R. Asher & J. D. Coie (Eds.), *Peer rejection in childhood* (pp. 365–402). Cambridge, UK: Cambridge University Press.

Colby, M., Hecht, M. L., Miller-Day, M., Krieger, J. L., Syvertsen, A. K., Graham, J. W., et al. (2013). Adapting school-based substance use prevention curriculum through cultural grounding: A review and exemplar of adaptation processes for rural schools. *American Journal of Community Psychology, 51*(1–2), 190–205.

Comeau, N., Stewart, S. H., & Loba, P. (2001). The relations of trait anxiety, anxiety sensitivity, and sensation seeking to adolescents' motivations for alcohol, cigarette, and marijuana use. *Addictive Behaviors, 26*(6), 803–825.

Conrod, P. J., Castellanos-Ryan, N., & Mackie, C. (2011). Long-term effects of a personality-targeted intervention to reduce alcohol use in adolescents. *Journal of Consulting and Clinical Psychology, 79*(3), 296–306.

Conrod, P. J., Peterson, J. B., Pihl, R. O., & Mankowski, S. (1997). Biphasic effects of alcohol on heart rate are influenced by alcoholic family history and rate of alcohol ingestion. *Alcoholism: Clinical and Experimental Research, 21*(1), 140–149.

Conrod, P. J., Pihl, R. O., Stewart, S. H., & Dongier, M. (2000). Validation of a system of classifying female substance abusers on the basis of personality and motivational risk factors for substance abuse. *Psychology of Addictive Behaviors, 14*(3), 243–256.

Conrod, P. J., Pihl, R. O., & Vassileva, J. (1998). Differential sensitivity to alcohol reinforcement in groups of men at risk for distinct alcoholism subtypes. *Alcoholism: Clinical and Experimental Research, 22*(3), 585–597.

Conrod, P. J., Stewart, S. H., Comeau, N., & Maclean, A. M. (2006). Efficacy of cognitive–behavioral interventions targeting personality risk factors for youth alcohol misuse. *Journal of Clinical Child and Adolescent Psychology, 35*(4), 550–563.

Cook, P. J., & Tauchen, G. (1982). The effect of liquor taxes on heavy drinking. *The Bell Journal of Economics, 13*(2), 379–390.

Cook, R., & Schlenger, W. (2002). Prevention of substance abuse in the workplace: Review of research on the delivery of services. *The Journal of Primary Prevention, 23*(1), 115–142.

Cooper, M. L., Frone, M. R., Russell, M., & Mudar, P. (1995). Drinking to regulate positive and negative emotions: A motivational model of alcohol use. *Journal of Personality and Social Psychology, 69*(5), 990–1005.

Degenhardt, L., Chiu, W. T., Sampson, N., Kessler, R. C., Anthony, J. C., Angermeyer, M., et al. (2008). Toward a global view of alcohol, tobacco, cannabis, and cocaine use: Findings from the WHO World Mental Health Surveys. *PLoS Medicine, 5*(7), e141.

Díaz, S. A. H., Secades-Villa, R., Errasti Pérez, J. M., Fernández-Hermida, J. R., García-Rodríguez, O., & Carballo Crespo, J. L. (2006). Family predictors of parent participation in an adolescent drug abuse prevention program. *Drug and Alcohol Review, 25*(4), 327–331.

Durlak, J. A., & DuPre, E. P. (2008). Implementation matters: A review of research on the influence of implementation on program outcomes and the factors affecting implementation. *American Journal of Community Psychology, 41*(3–4), 327.

Eddy, J. J., Gideonsen, M. D., McClaflin, R. R., O'Halloran, P., Peardon, F. A., Radcliffe, P. L., et al. (2012). Reducing alcohol use in youth aged 12–17 years using the strategic prevention framework. *Journal of Community Psychology, 40*(5), 607–620.

Ennett, S. T., Ringwalt, C. L., Thorne, J., Rohrbach, L. A., Vincus, A., Simons-Rudolph, A., et al. (2003). A comparison of current practice in school-based substance use prevention programs with meta-analysis findings. *Prevention Science, 4*(1), 1–14.

Evans, R. I. (1976). Smoking in children: Developing a social psychological strategy of deterrence. *Preventive Medicine, 5*(1), 122–127.

Evans, R. I., Hansen, W. B., & Mittelmark, M. B. (1977). Increasing the validity of self-reports of behavior in a smoking in children investigation. *Journal of Applied Psychology, 62*(4), 521–523.

Faggiano, F., Vigna-Taglianti, F. D., Versino, E., Zambon, A., Borraccino, A., & Lemma, P. (2008). School-based prevention for illicit drugs use: A systematic review. *Preventive Medicine, 46*(5), 385–396.

Flay, B. R. (1985). Psychosocial approaches to smoking prevention: A review of findings. *Health Psychology, 4*(5), 449–488.

Fletcher, A., Bonell, C., & Hargreaves, J. (2008). School effects on young people's drug use: A systematic review of intervention and observational studies. *Journal of Adolescent Health, 42*(3), 209–220.

Foxcroft, D. R., & Tsertsvadze, A. (2011). Universal multi-component prevention programs for alcohol misuse in young people. *Cochrane Database of Systematic Reviews, 9*, CD009307.

Foxcroft, D. R., & Tsertsvadze, A. (2012). Cochrane review: Universal school-based prevention programs for alcohol misuse in young people. *Evidence-Based Child Health: A Cochrane Review Journal, 7*(2), 450–575.

Frone, M. R., & Brown, A. L. (2010). Workplace substance-use norms as predictors of employee substance use and impairment: A survey of US workers. *Journal of Studies on Alcohol and Drugs, 71*(4), 526–534.

Gewin, A. M., & Hoffman, B. (2016). Introducing the cultural variables in school-based substance abuse prevention. *Drugs: Education, Prevention and Policy, 23*(1), 1–14.

Gillespie, N. A., Neale, M. C., & Kendler, K. S. (2009). Pathways to cannabis abuse: A multi-stage model from cannabis availability, cannabis initiation and progression to abuse. *Addiction, 104*, 430–438.

Gottfredson, D. C. (1987). An evaluation of an organization development approach to reducing school disorder. *Evaluation Review, 11*(6), 739–763.

Grant, B. F., Stinson, F. S., & Harford, T. C. (2001). Age at onset of alcohol use and DSM-IV alcohol abuse and dependence: A 12 year follow-up. *Journal of Substance Abuse, 13*, 493–504.

Griffin, K. W. (2010). The epidemiology of substance use among adolescents and young adults: A developmental perspective. In L. M. Scheier (Ed.), *Handbook of drug use etiology: Theory, methods, and empirical findings* (pp. 73–92). Washington, DC: American Psychological Association.

Gripenberg Abdon, J., Wallin, E., & Andréasson, S. (2011). Long-term effects of a community-based intervention: 5-year follow-up of 'Clubs against Drugs'. *Addiction, 106*(11), 1997–2004.

Hansen, W. B. (1992). School-based substance abuse prevention: A review of the state of the art in curriculum, 1980–1990. *Health Education Research, 7*(3), 403–430.

Harmon, M. A. (1993). Reducing the risk of drug involvement among early adolescents: An evaluation of Drug Abuse Resistance Education (DARE). *Evaluation Review, 17*(2), 221–239.

Harwood, H. (2000). *Updating estimates of the economic costs of alcohol abuse in the United States: Estimates, update methods, and data*. Washington, DC: National Institute on Alcohol Abuse and Alcoholism.

Hawkins, J. D., Oesterle, S., Brown, E. C., Monahan, K. C., Abbott, R. D., Arthur, M. W., et al. (2012). Sustained decreases in risk exposure and youth problem behaviors after installation of the Communities That Care prevention system in a randomized trial. *Archives of Pediatrics & Adolescent Medicine, 166*(2), 141–148.

Hays, S. P., Hays, C. E., & Mulhall, P. F. (2003). Community risk and protective factors and adolescent substance use. *Journal of Primary Prevention, 24*(2), 125–142.

Hennessy, E. A., & Tanner-Smith, E. E. (2015). Effectiveness of brief school-based interventions for adolescents: A meta-analysis of alcohol use prevention programs. *Prevention Science, 16*(3), 463–474.

Henry, D. B., Kobus, K., & Schoeny, M. E. (2011). Accuracy and bias in adolescents' perceptions of friends' substance use. *Psychology of Addictive Behaviors, 25*(1), 80–89.

Hill, P. L., Duggan, P. M., & Lapsley, D. K. (2012). Subjective invulnerability, risk behavior, and adjustment in early adolescence. *The Journal of Early Adolescence, 32*(4), 489–501.

Hingson, R. W., Heeren, T., & Winter, M. R. (2006). Age at drinking onset and alcohol dependence: Age at onset, duration, and severity. *Archives of Pediatrics & Adolescent Medicine, 160*(7), 739–746.

Hwang, M. S., Yeagley, K. L., & Petosa, R. (2004). A meta-analysis of adolescent psychosocial smoking prevention programs published between 1978 and 1997 in the United States. *Health Education & Behavior, 31*(6), 702–719.

Jessor, R. (1976). Predicting time of onset of marijuana use: A developmental study of high school youth. *Journal of Consulting and Clinical Psychology, 44*(1), 125–134.

Jessor, R., & Jessor, S. L. (1977). *Problem behavior and psychosocial development: A longitudinal study of youth*. New York: Academic Press.

Johnston, L. D., O'Malley, P. M., Bachman, J. G., & Schulenberg, J. E. (2010). *Monitoring the future national results on adolescent drug use: Overview of key findings, 2009 (NIH Publication No. 10–7583)*. Bethesda, MD: National Institute on Drug Abuse.

Jordan, C. J., & Andersen, S. L. (2016). Sensitive periods of substance abuse: Early risk for the transition to dependence. *Developmental Cognitive Neuroscience*. https://doi.org/10.1016/j.dcn.2016.10.004.

Kandel, D. B., Kessler, R. C., & Margulies, R. Z. (1978). Antecedents of adolescent initiation into stages of drug use: A developmental analysis. *Journal of Youth and Adolescence, 7*(1), 13–40.

Khadjesari, Z., Freemantle, N., Linke, S., Hunter, R., & Murray, E. (2014). Health on the web: Randomised controlled trial of online screening and brief alcohol intervention delivered in a workplace setting. *PLoS One, 9*(11), e112553.

Khantzian, E. J. (1997). The self-medication hypothesis of substance use disorders: A reconsideration and recent applications. *Harvard Review of Psychiatry, 4*(5), 231–244.

Kinder, B. N., Pape, N. E., & Walfish, S. (1980). Drug and alcohol education programs: A review of outcome studies. *International Journal of the Addictions, 15*(7), 1035–1054.

Krieg, T. L. (1982). Is raising the legal drinking age warranted? *Police Chief, 49*(HS-036 226), 32–34.

Krosnick, J. A., & Judd, C. M. (1982). Transitions in social influence at adolescence: Who induces cigarette smoking? *Developmental Psychology, 18*(3), 359–368.

Kucukuysal, B., & Beyhan, E. (2011). Contingency theory approach for effective community policing. *Süleyman Demirel Üniversitesi Fen-Edebiyat Fakültesi Sosyal Bilimler Dergisi, 2011*(23), 259–268.

Kuntsche, E., Rossow, I., Simons-Morton, B., Ter Bogt, T., Kokkevi, A., & Godeau, E. (2013). Not early drinking but early drunkenness is a risk factor for problem behaviors among adolescents from 38 European and North American countries. *Alcoholism: Clinical & Experimental Research, 37*(2), 308–314.

Kuntsche, S., & Kuntsche, E. (2016). Parent-based interventions for preventing or reducing adolescent substance use—A systematic literature review. *Clinical Psychology Review, 45*, 89–101.

La Torre, G., Chiaradia, G., & Ricciardi, G. (2005). School-based smoking prevention in children and adolescents: Review of the scientific literature. *Journal of Public Health, 13*(6), 285–290.

Lee, G. P., & DiClemente, C. C. (1985). Age of onset versus duration of problem drinking on the Alcohol Use Inventory. *Journal of Studies on Alcohol, 46*, 398–402.

Liira, H., Knight, A. P., Sim, M. G., Wilcox, H. M., Cheetham, S., & Aalto, M. T. (2016). Workplace interventions for preventing job loss and other work related outcomes in workers with alcohol misuse. *The Cochrane Library*.

Lisdahl, K. M., Gilbart, E. R., Wright, N. E., & Shollenbarger, S. (2013). Dare to delay? The impacts of adolescent alcohol and marijuana use onset on cognition, brain structure, and function. *Frontiers in Psychiatry, 4*, 25–43.

Lochman, J. E., & van den Steenhoven, A. (2002). Family-based approaches to substance abuse prevention. *Journal of Primary Prevention, 23*(1), 49–114.

Malvin, J. H., Moskowitz, J. M., Schaps, E., & Schaeffer, G. A. (1985). Evaluation of two school-based alternative programs. *Journal of Alcohol and Drug Education, 30*(3), 98–108.

Marcia, J. E. (1966). Development and validation of ego-identity status. *Journal of Personality and Social Psychology, 3*(5), 551–558.

Mason, M. J., Mennis, J., Linker, J., Bares, C., & Zaharakis, N. (2014). Peer attitudes effects on adolescent substance use: The moderating role of race and gender. *Prevention Science, 15*(1), 56–64.

Meyers, J. L., & Dick, D. M. (2010). Genetic and environmental risk factors for adolescent-onset substance use disorders. *Child and Adolescent Psychiatric Clinics of North America, 19*(3), 465–477.

Monahan, K. C., Rhew, I. C., Hawkins, J. D., & Brown, E. C. (2014). Adolescent pathways to co-occurring problem behavior: The effects of peer delinquency and peer substance use. *Journal of Research on Adolescence, 24*(4), 630–645.

Moss, H. B., Chen, C. M., & Yi, H. Y. (2014). Early adolescent patterns of alcohol, cigarettes, and marijuana polysubstance use and young adult substance use outcomes in a nationally representative sample. *Drug and Alcohol Dependence, 136*, 51–62.

Mrazek, P. J., & Haggerty, R. J. (1994). *Reducing risks for mental disorders: Frontiers for preventive intervention research.* Washington, DC: National Academic Press.

Murray, C. A. (1983). The physical environment and community control of crime. In J. Q. Wilson (Ed.), *Crime and public policy* (pp. 107–122). San Francisco: Institute for Contemporary Studies.

Murray, D. M., Richards, P. S., Luepker, R. V., & Johnson, C. A. (1987). The prevention of cigarette smoking in children: Two-and three-year follow-up comparisons of four prevention strategies. *Journal of Behavioral Medicine, 10*(6), 595–611.

O'Donnell, A., Anderson, P., Newbury-Birch, D., Schulte, B., Schmidt, C., Reimer, J., et al. (2014). The impact of brief alcohol interventions in primary healthcare: A systematic review of reviews. *Alcohol and Alcoholism, 49*(1), 66–78.

O'Leary-Barrett, M., Mackie, C. J., Castellanos-Ryan, N., Al-Khudhairy, N., & Conrod, P. J. (2010). Personality-targeted interventions delay uptake of drinking and decrease risk of alcohol-related problems when delivered by teachers. *Journal of the American Academy of Child & Adolescent Psychiatry, 49*(9), 954–963.

Ormel, J., Oldehinkel, A. J., Sijtsema, J., van Oort, F., Raven, D., Veenstra, R., et al. (2012). The TRacking Adolescents' Individual Lives Survey (TRAILS): Design, current status, and selected findings. *Journal of the American Academy of Child & Adolescent Psychiatry, 51*(10), 1020–1036.

Paglia, A., & Room, R. (1999). Preventing substance use problems among youth: A literature review and recommendations. *Journal of Primary Prevention, 20*(1), 3–50.

Parrella, D. P., & Filstead, W. J. (1988). Definition of onset in the development of onset-based alcoholism typologies. *Journal of Studies on Alcohol, 49*, 85–92.

Petrie, J., Bunn, F., & Byrne, G. (2007). Parenting programmes for preventing tobacco, alcohol or drugs misuse in children< 18: A systematic review. *Health Education Research, 22*(2), 177–191.

Pokhrel, P., Herzog, T. A., Black, D. S., Zaman, A., Riggs, N. R., & Sussman, S. (2013). Adolescent neurocognitive development, self-regulation, and school-based drug use prevention. *Prevention Science, 14*(3), 218–228.

Porath-Waller, A. J., Beasley, E., & Beirness, D. J. (2010). A meta-analytic review of school-based prevention for cannabis use. *Health Education & Behavior, 37*(5), 709–723.

Pape, H. (2012). Young people's overestimation of peer substance use: An exaggerated phenomenon?.Addiction, 107(5), 878–884.

Resnicow, K., & Botvin, G. (1993). School-based substance use prevention programs: Why do effects decay? *Preventive Medicine, 22*(4), 484–490.

Reynolds, G. S., & Bennett, J. B. (2015). A cluster randomized trial of alcohol prevention in small businesses: A cascade model of help seeking and risk reduction. *American Journal of Health Promotion, 29*(3), 182–191.

Ringwalt, C. L., Ennett, S., Vincus, A., Thorne, J., Rohrbach, L. A., & Simons-Rudolph, A. (2002). The prevalence of effective substance use prevention curricula in US middle schools. *Prevention Science, 3*(4), 257–265.

Robins, L. N., & Ratcliff, K. S. (1978). Risk factors in the continuation of childhood antisocial behavior into adulthood. *International Journal of Mental Health, 7*(3–4), 96–116.

Saffer, H., & Grossman, M. (1987). Beer taxes, the legal drinking age, and youth motor vehicle fatalities. *The Journal of Legal Studies, 16*(2), 351–374.

SAMHSA Center for Substance Abuse Prevention. (2008). *Substance abuse prevention dollars and cents: A cost-benefit analysis.* Retrieved from https://store.samhsa.gov/shin/content/SMA07-4298/SMA07-4298.pdf

Scheier, L. M. (Ed.). (2010). *Handbook of drug use etiology: Theory, methods, and empirical findings*. Washington, DC: American Psychological Association.

Schindler, A., & Bröning, S. (2015). A review on attachment and adolescent substance abuse: Empirical evidence and implications for prevention and treatment. *Substance Abuse, 36*(3), 304–313.

Schulte, B., O'Donnell, A. J., Kastner, S., Schmidt, C. S., Schäfer, I., & Reimer, J. (2014). Alcohol screening and brief intervention in workplace settings and social services: A comparison of literature. *Frontiers in Psychiatry, 5*, 131.

Shamblen, S. R., & Derzon, J. H. (2009). A preliminary study of the population-adjusted effectiveness of substance abuse prevention programming: Towards making IOM program types comparable. *The Journal of Primary Prevention, 30*(2), 89–107.

Sheeran, P., Harris, P. R., & Epton, T. (2014). Does heightening risk appraisals change people's intentions and behavior? A meta-analysis of experimental studies. *Psychological Bulletin, 140*(2), 511–543.

Simcha-Fagan, O. M., & Schwartz, J. E. (1986). Neighborhood and delinquency: An assessment of contextual effects. *Criminology, 24*(4), 667–699.

Simons-Morton, B., & Kuntsche, E. (2012). Adolescent estimation of peer substance use: Why it matters. *Addiction, 107*(5), 885–886.

Smith, G. M., & Fogg, C. P. (1978). Psychological predictors of early use, late use, and nonuse of marijuana among teenage students. In D. B. Kandel (Ed.), *Longitudinal research on drug use: Empirical findings and methodological issues* (pp. 101–113). Washington, DC: Hemisphere.

Sowden, A. J., & Stead, L. F. (2003). Community interventions for preventing smoking in young people. *The Cochrane Library*.

Spicer, R. S., & Miller, T. R. (2016). The evaluation of a workplace program to prevent substance abuse: Challenges and findings. *The Journal of Primary Prevention, 37*(4), 329–343.

Spoth, R., Greenberg, M., & Turrisi, R. (2008). Preventive interventions addressing underage drinking: State of the evidence and steps toward public health impact. *Pediatrics, 121*(Supplement 4), S311–S336.

Springer, J. F., Sale, E., Kasim, R., Winter, W., Sambrano, S., & Chipungu, S. (2005). Effectiveness of culturally specific approaches to substance abuse prevention: Findings from CSAP's national cross-site evaluation of high risk youth programs. *Journal of Ethnic and Cultural Diversity in Social Work, 13*(3), 1–23.

Steinberg, L. (2008). A social neuroscience perspective on adolescent risk-taking. *Developmental Review, 28*(1), 78–106.

Sussman, S., Dent, C. W., Simon, T. R., Stacy, A. W., Galaif, E. R., Moss, M. A., et al. (1995). Immediate impact of social influence-oriented substance abuse prevention curricula in traditional and continuation high schools. *Drugs & Society, 8*(3–4), 65–81.

Swadi, H. (1999). Individual risk factors for adolescent substance use. *Drug and Alcohol Dependence, 55*(3), 209–224.

Tarter, R. E., & Vanyukov, M. (1994). Alcoholism: A developmental disorder. *Journal of Consulting and Clinical Psychology, 62*(6), 1096–1107.

Thomas, R. E., McLellan, J., & Perera, R. (2013). School-based programmes for preventing smoking. *Evidence-Based Child Health: A Cochrane Review Journal, 8*(5), 1616–2040.

Thrul, J., Bühler, A., & Herth, F. J. (2014). Prevention of teenage smoking through negative information giving, a cluster randomized controlled trial. *Drugs: Education, Prevention and Policy, 21*(1), 35–42.

Tobler, N. S., & Stratton, H. H. (1997). Effectiveness of school-based drug prevention programs: A meta-analysis of the research. *Journal of Primary Prevention, 18*(1), 71–128.

Tripodi, S. J., Bender, K., Litschge, C., & Vaughn, M. G. (2010). Interventions for reducing adolescent alcohol abuse: A meta-analytic review. *Archives of Pediatrics & Adolescent Medicine, 164*(1), 85–91.

Unlu, A., Sahin, I., & Wan, T. T. (2014). Three dimensions of youth social capital and their impacts on substance use. *Journal of Child & Adolescent Substance Abuse, 23*(4), 230–241.

Van Ryzin, M. J., Roseth, C. J., Fosco, G. M., Lee, Y. K., & Chen, I. C. (2016). A component-centered metaanalysis of family-based prevention programs for adolescent substance use. *Clinical Psychology Review, 45*, 72–80.

Warpenius, K., Holmila, M., & Mustonen, H. (2010). Effects of a community intervention to reduce the serving of alcohol to intoxicated patrons. *Addiction, 105*(6), 1032–1040.

West, S. L., & O'Neal, K. K. (2004). Project DARE outcome effectiveness revisited. *American Journal of Public Health, 94*(6), 1027–1029.

Wiehe, S. E., Garrison, M. M., Christakis, D. A., Ebel, B. E., & Rivara, F. P. (2005). A systematic review of school-based smoking prevention trials with long-term follow-up. *Journal of Adolescent Health, 36*(3), 162–169.

Woicik, P. A., Stewart, S. H., Pihl, R. O., & Conrod, P. J. (2009). The substance use risk profile scale: A scale measuring traits linked to reinforcement-specific substance use profiles. *Addictive Behaviors, 34*(12), 1042–1055.

Zucker, R. A., & Harford, T. C. (1983). National study of the demography of adolescent drinking practices in 1980. *Journal of Studies on Alcohol, 44*(6), 974–985.

Part III
Education

Chapter 17
Creating Programs for Professional Development and Academic Programs: Integrating Previous Knowledge and Experience into the Educational Program

Amanda Sisselman-Borgia and Thalia MacMillan

Many would say that the portrait of the modern day college student is changing. No longer is the typical student between the ages of 18 and 22 years. Statistics indicate that 71% of college students are nontraditional; thus, these students might now be the new normal (Education Commission, 2017; Freed & Mollick, 2010). For the past 15 years, the number of nontraditional students has continued to rise steadily for a variety of reasons (Ross-Gordon, 2011). Albeit changes to the economic climate, social dynamic, or technological advances, an increased number of students over the age of 25 are returning to school (Pelletier, 2010). Many students may be attempting to further their careers, obtain a raise, and change careers due to layoffs, and as a result, they need or want a degree (Pelletier, 2010; Ross-Gordon, 2011).

There is a need to define or determine what a nontraditional student is and why this is important within higher education (Pelletier, 2010). As noted by the National Center for Education Statistics (2017), nontraditional students are defined as meeting at least one of the following characteristics: delayed enrollment into college from high school, attends college part time, works full time, is financially independent with respect to financial aid eligibility, has dependents other than a spouse, is a single parent, or does not have a high school diploma. Research demonstrates that when compared to traditional students, nontraditional students tend to be more motivated in their academic endeavors (Bye, Pushkar, & Conway, 2007).

While many colleges and universities are beginning to recognize the value of previous life experience, one limitation is that many do not know how to deal with the heterogeneous needs for this growing population. When it comes to academic program and support services, what works for the nontraditional student may not be

---

A. Sisselman-Borgia (✉)
Department of Social Work, CUNY Lehman College, Bronx, NY, USA
e-mail: Amanda.sisselman@lehman.cuny.edu

T. MacMillan
SUNY Empire State College, Community & Human Services, New York, NY, USA

© Springer International Publishing AG 2018
T. MacMillan, A. Sisselman-Borgia (eds.), *New Directions in Treatment, Education, and Outreach for Mental Health and Addiction*, Advances in Mental Health and Addiction, https://doi.org/10.1007/978-3-319-72778-3_17

what is present on the college campus. For example, academic programs may have specific required courses that are part of the degree. However, nontraditional students may have foundational or applied knowledge due to life or work experience; as a result, typically these students do not wish to "repeat" a course with existing knowledge or delay time to degree taking classes on knowledge that they already have.

As noted by Ebersole (2010), a degree may be comprised of several components. These include credits transferred from other institutions, through trainings by examination, standardized examination, assessment, or coursework (Ebersole, 2010; United States Department of Education, 2011). While many students typically have a combination of prior or current coursework, institutions may explore other options. These other options are presented briefly below:

- Credit from training: Training may be a result of prior military experiences, corporate training, or prior certifications. The American Council on Education (ACE) provides credit recommendations. These recommendations are based on a review of the training or experience.
- Credit by examination: Typically, these are standardized examinations on specific topics, such as general education topics. The College Board CLEP program and the Educational Testing Service DSST program are two such examples.
- Credit by assessment: Credits gained in this manner reflect forms of learning and competency assessment.

In order to empower students to complete their degree and provide the best effective service to students interested in mental health and addiction, there is a need to explore the above three options further (Freed & Mollick, 2010). Simply assuming that all students wish to take only coursework for their degree or only assessing skills obtained from employment is no longer enough for modern students (Travers, 2012). As higher education costs are increasing for each student, one way to offset this is by utilizing alternative means of credit (Merisotis, 2011; Travers, 2012). This chapter will discuss the various ways to include nontraditional or life experience credit in the academic program, what types of experiences the individual may have, and additional ways to recognize the experiences of students within the academic program, as they relate to comorbid substance use and mental health diagnoses.

Types of Experiences

Students bring a wealth of experiences with them to school, especially when they enroll later in life. Experiences can vary from student to student. This may include personal experiences, such as dealing with one's own sobriety or being a caretaker for a family member who has struggled with alcoholism; semiprofessional volunteer work, such as disaster relief or leading self-help groups; and paid employment in schools, hospitals, or human services organizations. Experiences have the potential to bring more than just a familiarity with a topic. The student may have knowledge that they have learned related to symptoms and relapse, as well as recovery process.

Helping students to sort out or assess their life experiences can at times be a tedious process but is often worth the extra effort. Part of the process is to determine or sort out experience only versus learning. This can provide students with alternative means to reach their end goal of a college degree and has potential to improve graduation and retention rates. Being able to utilize experiences toward a degree can be quite powerful for a student as it reduces time and money. For example, a student may also have years of experience as an emergency medical technician, either paid or volunteer, and possess knowledge about substance use in the community as well as details related to overdose. This student may also have knowledge about the ways in which mental health diagnoses present themselves in everyday life.

While firsthand/personal knowledge of substance abuse and recovery, as well as mental health diagnosis, could certainly mean knowledge on these topics, students should be cautioned to consider their own health and potential discomfort in bringing such personal material into a public arena. In order to ascertain knowledge and learning for an experience, an evaluator needs to assess the student's experiences and their learning as a result. For some, this may cause them to relive any potential trauma or uncomfortable issues that they may have experienced.

Credit by Training

As nontraditional students typically have knowledge garnered from vocational experiences, they may have received work- and non-work-sponsored training, military experience, continuing education, professional development opportunities, or self-directed learning. Many students wish to achieve credit for this (Freed & Mollick, 2010). The latest CAEL Report (2010) indicates that close to 70% of colleges accept transfer credits from other colleges or military credits. While these estimates reveal that some types of training are accepted, a greater range of diversity in training and professional development should be examined for their credit-bearing potential.

There is a need, however, to standardize local training or certifications. Professional certifications, such as the Certificate in Alcohol and Substance Abuse Counseling (CASAC), have clear guidelines and regulations associated with the certification process. For example, organizations or training programs that offer preparation for the CASAC are required to utilize a standardized curriculum. Within some organizations or agencies, in-service trainings or continuing education is provided on a regular basis. For example, each staff member may need to go to a formal 5-day training every year on casework. While this training may not follow a formal, standardized curriculum, it would behoove a college to partner with this organization as all staff members who apply to the college could potentially receive a fixed number of credits based on attendance at this training. In this way, schools of higher education and training institutions could partner with one another to maximize potential for transfer of credit and certifications.

Development of protocol and templates for common certificates or in-service trainings can be helpful for students and educators alike. Partnering with human services organizations and medical institutions can also maximize ease in developing templates for certifications and professional trainings. While these types of opportunities are helpful for students as their learning can be evaluated when they apply for admission to school, they should also be evaluated on a regular basis to determine that they are meeting current standards.

One example of this is the CASAC. Colleges and training programs must follow a standardized curriculum that is determined by the state Office of Alcoholism and Substance Abuse Services. As new information is gathered via evidence-based research, OASAS updates the CASAC training requirements accordingly. When changes are made to the curriculum, it is necessary to review the credits that would be awarded by the college.

Another example is first aid or basic life support training. Courses on basic life support, which include CPR, are provided by the American Heart Association. A standard curriculum is followed for all trainings, which includes an examination and an assessment of individual skills. A college can review this curriculum, an acceptable time frame for the training (i.e., if a student took the training last year versus 3 years ago), and determine how many credits will be awarded for this learning. In that way, all students who can provide documentation of this training will be awarded this credit.

Credit by Examination

CAEL (2006) estimates that 87% of colleges accept College-Level Examination Program (CLEP) or Dantes Subject Standardized Test (DSST) exams. While many students will utilize this to meet general education requirements, such as humanities or a foreign language, the question remains what types of standardized exams are appropriate for those interested in mental health and addiction. The college may wish to determine which exams are appropriate for the requisite knowledge. Some examples of this may include:

- CLEP – College Board

  - Human growth and development
  - Introductory psychology
  - Introductory sociology
  - Biology
  - Chemistry

Credit by Assessment: Prior Learning Assessment

Close to two-thirds of colleges have now begun to examine prior learning in various forms (CAEL, 2006). As noted by Starr-Glass (2002), the assessment of prior learning is grounded in the idea that learning is not limited to academic settings. However, a college or university must be willing to accept this alternate form of learning. Many institutions require that student's learning matches in some way to the outcomes of a current course at the institution (Popova-Gonci & Ruth Tobol, 2011). Others allow students to apply all types of learning to their degree. This one-size-fits-all approach may be problematic for a variety of reasons, including that it does not take into account the student's unique experiences (Popova-Gonci & Ruth Tobol, 2011).

Whitaker (1989), in a seminal piece, outlines the PLA process utilizing ten standards in order to achieve academic quality. As noted by Freed and Mollick (2010), these standards include the following:

- Credit should be awarded only for learning and not for experience.
- College credit should be awarded only for college-level learning.
- Credit should be awarded only for learning that has a balance of theory and practical application, as appropriate to the subject.
- Determination of competence levels and of credit awards must be made by appropriate subject matter experts.
- Credit should be appropriate to the academic context in which it is accepted.
- Credit awards and their transcript entries should be monitored to avoid giving credit twice for the same learning.
- Policies and procedures applied to assessment should be available.
- Fees charged for assessment should be based on the services performed in the process and not determined by the amount of credit awarded.
- All personnel involved in the assessment of learning should receive adequate training for the functions they perform, and there should be provisions for continued professional development.
- Assessment programs should be regularly monitored, reviewed, evaluated, and revised as needed to reflect changes in the assessment process.

Both negative and positive aspects of the evaluative process have been noted in the literature and are summarized in Table 17.1 (Hoffman, Travers, Evans, & Treadwell, 2009; Ross-Gordon, 2011; Travers, 2012).

The Student Experience

The student is never alone on their educational journey. In most cases, a mentor, advisor, or educator may work with students to guide selection of coursework and to determine prior learning. It can be helpful to have a collaborative relationship

Table 17.1 Pros and cons of PLA process

Positives of PLA	Negatives of PLA
More likely to earn a bachelor's degree within 7 years	Students don't understand what "learning" or "learned knowledge" is versus "experience"
More successful in achieving goals	Process can be cumbersome
Higher GPAs in coursework overall	Validity and reliability of the assessment can be quite subjective and qualitative
More engaged in courses	Context and the individual's assumptions, expectations, and language should be taken into account
Higher level of motivation	
Increased graduation rates – especially for Hispanic and African American students	

between the student and the educator; in this way, both can work together toward a common goal that is established by both through determining prior credit awards, possible assessment of learning, and courses that may be of interest to the student. The discussion of experiences or assessment of prior learning can be framed and examined within the boundaries of a collaborative relationship. In the anecdotal experience of both authors, students will typically share what they feel comfortable discussing. Through these discussions on experiences, bits of learned knowledge come through, and work with the student can begin in order to develop a document that demonstrates this learned knowledge.

Within coursework, an independent study can be a vehicle for this type of work, as it offers both the student and the faculty member credit for the time spent on these important discussions and tasks. While the student is exploring their experiences to determine where the learned knowledge is, it may also be appropriate to examine what other types of knowledge the student wishes to gain or what they would like to do next. This type of discussion is important, as the student's own self-direction can be used to increase motivation about goals and maintain engagement while improving degree completion and graduation (Ross-Gordon, 2011).

Within other types of coursework, the educator can also guide the student on how their experiences can best be reflected. Together, the types of standardized exams, assessments, or courses can be used to meet the student's goals. For example, if the student wishes to go forward to get their master's in social work degree, the student and educator can determine together what type of knowledge is needed for graduate work. If the student is interested in obtaining the CASAC, the discussion and exploration can focus on the number of clock hours that can be reduced with the bachelor's degree and how the courses can transfer to meet the needs of the standardized curriculum.

Case Example

Jan is 45 years old and spent 20 years working as a recreation aide at a residential substance abuse facility and enjoyed working with this population. Her children were nearing the end of high school and getting ready to apply for college, and she began to wonder about her own career and whether or not she would be able to advance at the facility where she worked. She frequently noticed that there was a distinct connection between difficult life circumstances that people endured and their first use of drugs or alcohol. She was very tuned into clients at the facility who so often also suffered from depression and anxiety, as well as bipolar disorder. She wanted to work more closely with the clients in a counseling role and help them find ways to cope differently. She saw major differences after they took up recreational activities in the arts or movement, such as dance. After talking with her supervisor, it seemed as if she would need to obtain a college degree and possibly a master's degree if she were going to advance her position professionally. Jan was at first hesitant because she felt she was already 45 years old and did not want to "waste" a number of years in school after working for so long in the field. Finally, at her supervisor's insistence, she signed up to visit an open house at a local college and learn more about going back to school. Much to her surprise, she learned that she could earn college credit for some of the experiences she had and the knowledge that she had gained over the years at her job.

In this case example, as a trained professional and educator, it would be important to ask the student about specific information that she learned during her time at this workplace. Her knowledge of particular symptoms and possible side effects of medications as well as socio-emotional ramifications of substance abuse and mental health diagnoses could be content worthy of prior learning credit. Descriptions of the experiences themselves, as the student has laid them out, while extremely valuable, will not alone be enough for credit. So, it might be the job of the educator to assist the student in finding the content and the learned knowledge through guided questions.

Conclusion

Students who are able to reduce their time to degree completion are more likely to finish a degree. Related, those who are able to receive credits through examinations, assessment, or standardized assessment are more likely to be motivated to finish their degree. As such, college programs may wish to explore ways to aid their students in degree completion. While many have begun to adopt credits outside of traditional coursework, additional exploration of various credit-bearing mechanisms to benefit students should be explored. Levels of engagement and motivation should also be explored regularly to determine their impact on receipt of alternative credits. Currently, there is a dearth of research on the impact of these different types of credit on the student's academic progress. Additional research should determine which type of credit is most beneficial for students, if there is a "right" amount of credits, and how the students can best use them to meet their academic needs.

References

Bye, D., Pushkar, D., & Conway, M. (2007). Motivation, interest, and positive affect in traditional and nontraditional undergraduate students. *Adult Education Quarterly, 57*(2), 141–158.

Council of Adult and Experiential Learning [CAEL]. (2010). Fueling the race to postsecondary success: A 48-institution study of prior learning assessment and adult student outcomes. [Executive Summary]. Chicago: CAEL.

Council for Adult and Experiential Learning [CAEL]. (2006). Serving adult learners in higher education. Chicago: CAEL.

Ebersole, J. (2010). Degree completion: Responding to a national priority. *Continuing Higher Education Review, 74*, 23–31.

Education Commission of the States. (2017). *27 is the new 18: Adult students on the rise*. Retrieved online at: https://www.ecs.org/27-is-the-new-18-adult-students-on-the-rise/

Freed, R., & Mollick, G. M. (2010). Using prior learning assessment in adult baccalaureate degrees in Texas. *Journal of Case Studies in Accreditation and Assessment, 1*, 1–14.

Hoffman, T., Travers, NI, Evans, M., & Treadwell, A. (2009, September). Researching critical factors impacting PLA programs: A multi-institutional study on best practices. *CAEL Forum and Notes*.

Merisotis, J. P. (2011). President's message. *Lumina Foundation Focus Summer*. Retrieved online at: https://focus.luminafoundation/org/summer2011

National Center for Education Statistics. (2017). *Definitions and statistics*. Retrieved online at: https://nces.ed.gov/fastfacts/display.asp?id=98

Pelletier, S. G. (Fall, 2010). Success for adult students. Public Purpose. American Association of State Colleges and Universities. Retrieved from: http://www.aascu.org/uploadedFiles/AASCU/Content/Root/MediaAndPublications/PublicPurposeMagazines/Issue/10fall_adultstudents.pdf

Popova-Gonci, V., & Ruth Tobol, A. (2011). PLA-based curriculum: Humanistic model of higher education. *Journal of Continuing Higher Education, 59*(3), 175–177.

Ross-Gordon, J. M. (2011). Research on adult learners: Supporting the needs of a student population that is no longer non-traditional. *Peer Review, 13*(1), 26–29.

Starr-Glass, D. (2002). Metaphor and totem: Exploring and evaluating prior experiential learning. *Assessment & Evaluation in Higher Education, 27*(3), 221–231.

Travers, N. L. (2012). Academic perspectives on college-level learning: Implications for workplace learning. *Journal of Workplace Learning, 24*(2), 105–118.

United States Department of Education. (2011). *College completion tool kit*. Retrieved online at: https://www.ed.gov/college-completion/governing-win

Whitaker, U. (1989). *Assessing learning: Standards, principles, and procedure for good practice*. Philadelphia: Council for Adult and Experiential Learning.

Chapter 18
Developing an SBIRT Curriculum in Advanced Practice

Jill Becker Feigeles

A social work intern at a community senior center is working with an older woman who is insistent that her doctor refills her pain medication prescription. The intern is unsure if her medication-seeking behavior signifies a substance abuse problem and is uncertain how to proceed to tease out what is going on.

The social work intern at a public elementary school is working with an 8-year old boy who lost his single mother last year. An adolescent aunt has legal custody. Coupled with the fact that the child is underperforming academically, the intern grows concerned about substance abuse when the client reveals some of what is taking place in the home.

Stephanie, an 18-year-old college freshman, arrives by ambulance to the hospital emergency room accompanied by her terrified roommate who reports the two were at a fraternity party playing "drinking games involving many rounds of shots" when Stephanie passed out.

Carolyn is 25 years old and is 4 months pregnant. She is visiting a comprehensive health clinic for prenatal care for the first time where she sits down with the social work intern for an intake interview. During the interview, she responds that she has "always" consumed one or two drinks, almost every day, when she comes home from work to unwind from the stress of her job. There are also regular social events with family and friends that typically involve some drinking.

From these and many other experiences reported by MSW students, it is evident that social work interns frequently encounter individuals where substance use becomes a concern. In addition, credentialed social workers feel underprepared or lack training to intervene or even bring up and explore issues related to substance use (Steenrod, 2014). Given that professional social workers practicing in the field feel unprepared, social work students engaged in field practicums are even less prepared. Extensive literature detailing the importance of teaching evidence-based

J. B. Feigeles (✉)
Wurzweiler School of Social Work, Yeshiva University & Lehman College/CUNY,
Livingston, NJ, USA
e-mail: JILL.FEIGELES@lehman.cuny.edu

© Springer International Publishing AG 2018
T. MacMillan, A. Sisselman-Borgia (eds.), *New Directions in Treatment, Education, and Outreach for Mental Health and Addiction*, Advances in Mental Health and Addiction, https://doi.org/10.1007/978-3-319-72778-3_18

practice in social work supports the integration of EBP into social work education (Gambrill, 2007; Grambrill, 2014; Gibbs & Gambrill, 2002; Mullen & Streiner, 2004; Thyer & Wodarski, 2007). Screening, brief intervention, and referral to treatment (SBIRT) is an evidence-based practice (EBP) model that can be incorporated into advanced practice curriculum to provide students with practical tools to explore risky substance use behaviors in their clients and is a meaningful addition to social work education.

The economic cost of substance use (i.e., alcohol and illegal drug use) in the USA is a staggering $426 billion per year (Substance Abuse and Mental Health Services Administration [SAMHSA], 2013; National Drug Intelligence Center, 2011). Statistics reveal that 8.2% of individuals aged 12 years and older in the USA have been diagnosed with a substance use disorder (Center for Behavioral Health Statistics and Quality [CBHSQ], 2013; SAMSHA, 2012). The use of alcohol and illicit substances contributes significantly to morbidity and mortality; it is deleterious to common medical conditions such as diabetes, blood pressure, and heart disease (Gordon & Alford, 2012). One in every four deaths in the USA is the result of alcohol, illegal drug, or tobacco use (National Institute of Drug Abuse, 2012). The literature indicates few health-care professionals, including social workers; routinely screen clients for substance misuse or offer intervention (Pringle, Kowalchuk, Meyers, & Seale, 2012; SAMHSA, 2011). In an effort to address this, the Office of National Drug Control Policy and SAMHSA have advanced an evidence-based model for substance abuse screening known as SBIRT. SAMHSA and the Council on Social Work Education (CSWE) encourage social workers to make use of the SBIRT model in their work with clients (SAMHSA, 2015).

SBIRT is a well-established evidence-based protocol for reducing problematic substance use (SAMHSA, 2015). It was originally developed as a public health model for universal screening, secondary prevention (detection of risky/hazardous use prior to abuse/dependence), early intervention, and treatment within primary health-care settings (Babor et al., 2007; Babor & Higgins-Biddle, 2001). The goal of the method is to mitigate and prevent related health consequences, disease, accidents, and injury (SAMHSA, 2015) with the additional prospect of reducing costs related to mental health and behavioral health care, crime and incarceration, and loss of productivity. The integration of SBIRT into social work classroom education and internship practice provides social work students with skills that become incorporated into a repertoire of clinical proficiencies.

The SBIRT Model

SBIRT is an evidence-based practice model rooted in motivational interviewing strategies. The three primary areas of this model are screening, brief intervention, and referral to treatment. Screening begins with a prescreen for alcohol and other substance use as part of the initial intake when a social work student first meets with a client. It can be worked into a routine intake or become part of the information gathered in the beginning phase of client-worker interaction. The SBIRT screening process is time limited, intended to identify clients who have a problem with alcohol, illicit drugs, and prescription drugs as well as identify the appropriate level of care for the client (Russett, 2015; Satre et al., 2012; Stanton et al., 2012). The prescreen is a universal method used with all clients in the population. It is similar to screenings like mammograms and colonoscopy, gestational diabetes screenings for pregnant woman, or cholesterol testing used to screen everyone for specific conditions (Steenrod, 2014). By screening all clients regardless of whether there has been an identified concern about substance use, workers have the opportunity to identify substance use issues that may not otherwise emerge.

One of the three outcomes is possible when administering the prescreen: no intervention, brief intervention, or referral to treatment. If the client response to the prescreen is negative, the SBIRT screen is completed, and no further action is taken. However, if the response is positive, the social worker (or other clinician) administers a standardized instrument, the results of which determine the direction of the brief intervention. Among the more common standardized tools are the AUDIT (Alcohol Use Disorders Identification Test) and the MAST (Michigan Alcohol Screening Test) for alcohol screening, the DAST (Drug Abuse Screening Test) for drug screening, and the ASSIST (Alcohol, Smoking, and Substance Involvement Screening Test), CAGE-AID (Cut down, Annoyed, Guilty, Eye opener), and the CRAFFT (Car, Relax, Alone, Forget, Friends, Trouble) for adolescents.

Brief intervention occurs if the client indicates moderate risk for substance use/abuse. The idea behind the intervention is to increase awareness in the client of their risk behavior and motivate them to make a change. One of the key aspects of brief interventions is educating the client about relevant safe drinking parameters, risks associated with substance use, and the consequences of alcohol and substance use. Brief intervention invites a treatment plan to either reduce or eliminate substance use and scheduled follow-up to hold the client accountable as well as provide an opportunity to recommend higher levels of treatment when necessary.

Referral to treatment is provided when a screening indicates a serious risk of dependence. In this case, a referral to a specialized substance abuse program is made using a "warm handoff." It is not enough to give the client a referral name, number, and address. Social workers need to contact the referral agency/program with the client present, make the appointment for the client, and follow up to be sure the client keeps the appointment. Where possible, physically "handing the client off" with an in-person introduction to the referral agency representative is preferable.

The Spirit of Motivational Interviewing and the Stages of Change Theory

Motivational interviewing (MI) is a clinical approach to client work consistent with social work values of empathy, respect, unconditional positive regard, and nonjudgment of clients. Social workers are trained to uphold the dignity and worth of every client while working toward positive change. The primary goal of motivational interviewing (MI) is to enhance client motivation by discussing and resolving their ambivalence toward change. This is principally achieved by helping the client develop a discrepancy between what she/he believes about where they are now and where they want to be in the future. Ideally, recognizing this would encourage a desire to change and a motivation to adhere to treatment (Miller & Rollnick, 2002). Given that the goal of SBIRT is to motivate clients toward changing their substance use behavior, motivational interviewing offers a useful method for working with clients to facilitate change and can enhance clinical skill sets.

The spirit of MI speaks to the importance of partnering with the client in an active collaboration between experts. The client is the expert on him/herself, while the social worker is a partner with knowledge to share and support to lend. The social worker seeks to create a positive interpersonal atmosphere conducive to change by not being coercive (Miller & Rollnick, 2013). In fact, the spirit of MI is consistent with social work values as it incorporates many of the same concepts around genuine acceptance of the client including *absolute worth* (i.e., unconditional positive regard), *accurate empathy* (i.e., empathic understanding), *autonomy support* (i.e., self-determination), *affirmation* (i.e., using the strengths perspective), and *compassion* (i.e., promoting the client's welfare). MI works from the strength-based premise that people already have much of what is needed to make change. It is the worker's task to evoke or call it forth (Miller & Rollnick, 2013). These concepts have a strong similarity to the core beliefs of Rogers' person-centered theory (Rogers, 1959).

The four basic principles of MI are also consistent with social work values. These principles are (1) express empathy, (2) develop discrepancy, (3) roll with resistance, and (4) support self-efficacy (i.e., client's belief they can make successful change). Expressing empathy in a manner that values the client experience is essential to building a helping relationship. In MI, this skill is directed toward recognizing ambivalence and expressing empathy with both sides of the struggle for change. The social worker uses skillful reflective listening and stays out of judgment. To develop discrepancy the client is encouraged to explore and articulate goals and values while identifying small steps toward reaching goals with a focus on what is healthy and feasible. When the topic of substance use emerges, MI offers an opportunity to explore the impact that such use has on reaching the client's expressed goals and/or the consistency of using substances in terms of the client's expressed values. The worker encourages the client to enumerate the pros/cons of using vs. quitting (always starting with the pros of using) allowing the client to make the argument for change. Rolling with resistance is a way to avoid argument. MI ascribes to the belief that people have an innate capacity for setting things right (a righting reflex). When the righting reflex collides with ambivalence, the client tends to defend the status quo. Therefore, if one becomes confrontational with a client about making change, the client will typically argue for staying the same, investing more in this position. When a worker encounters resistance, it is a signal to change strategies. Finally, support the client's self-efficacy. This refers to expressing optimism that change is possible, pointing out past successes, and using reflective listening, summaries, and affirmations. The worker can validate expressed frustrations while remaining optimistic about the possibility for change (Miller & Rollnick, 2013; Miller, Zweban, DiClemente, & Rychtarik, 1992).

MI uses four strategies familiar to social work practice to motivate clients toward change. Open-ended questions are used to gather descriptive information and facilitate dialogue. Affirmations support and validate the client's self-efficacy, acknowledge difficulties, validate feelings and experiences, and emphasize strengths and successes from their past experiences. Reflective listening demonstrates more than interest in what the client has to say; it shows a desire to really understand how the person sees things. Reflective listening begins with hypothesis testing, what you really think the client means. It can ultimately reflect a much deeper connection to the meaning behind what the client has shared. One can begin with a simple reflection of repeating, move to rephrasing, and paraphrasing and finally reflection of deeper feeling and meaning. Finally, summarizing reinforces what has been said and demonstrates the worker has been listening carefully. Seeds are then planted for the client to express talk of change, either through preparatory talk (expressing desire, ability, reasons for need for change) or implementing talk (commitment, activation, or taking steps) (Miller & Rollnick, 2013).

Recognition of change talk is essential, as this reveals where the client is situated in motivation for and commitment to change. Using MI, the worker seeks to guide the client to articulate change talk as a conduit to actual behavioral change (Miller & Rollnick, 2013). There is a clear correlation between statements made by the client about change and the outcome; the more client change talk that occurs, the more likely a change in behavior will result (Miller & Rollnick, 2013). Prochaska and DiClemente's (1984) stages of change offers social work students a framework to conceptualize the process of change that works in harmony with MI and SBIRT.

The theory is based on the notion that change takes place in stages of a circular nature. Starting with pre-contemplation, the individual moves to → contemplation → preparation → action → maintenance. Relapse is routine and possible at any point. Relapse is understood and accepted as an important part of the change process.

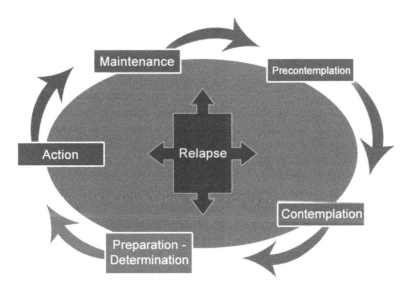

Prochaska & DiClemente (1984)

When MI is informed by the stages of change, the worker or student has the framework for evaluating where the client is situated in the change process, and they can make more effective use of their MI skills for screening, brief intervention, and referral. In the pre-contemplation stage, the client does not think there is problem therefore does not consider change. This is the time to build a trusting relationship, engage, explore, encourage, and acknowledge lack of readiness. At this stage the worker or student asks open-ended questions such as "you mentioned you enjoy a few drinks on a pretty regular basis, I'd like to talk more about that but before we do, tell me a little about how you spend your free time." Genuine interest in the client and their story along with validation of their experience is important to understanding the positive and negatives of substance use for the client. The student can return to the use of substances during later inquiry, for example, "so how and where does alcohol fit in for you? What are some of the good things and the not-so-good things about drinking?" As the client enumerates pros and cons, the student summarizes using a decisional balance approach such as "so on the one hand [positives]; and on the other hand you get [negatives], is that accurate?" Identifying the negatives second leaves the client to ponder the more problematic aspects of their substance use (Miller & Rollnick, 2013).

The brief intervention moves forward once the student has gathered and assessed information provided in discussion with the client as well as information garnered from applicable standardized instruments. Now the worker asks permission to discuss the screening findings and share information with the client with the aim to link substance use to known consequences. The information provided should be objective information pertinent to the client. Once the information is provided, the student elicits a response to the feedback. The process is elicit (permission) ➜ provide (information) ➜ elicit (feedback). For example, if the client indicates consumption of a high-risk amount of alcohol and has given permission (elicited) for the student to discuss the screen findings, the student proceeds to inform the client of the physical, social, and other risks associated with this level of consumption (provide). Once the client is informed of the risks, the student asks the client if they have any thoughts or reactions to the information (elicit). From here, the worker begins the process of building readiness to change. If client feedback is demonstrating an unwillingness to consider change, the student can continue to explore the meaning/role of substances in the client's life. If the client is intrigued and interested in more information, they are likely open to the idea of change.

In the contemplation stage, the client sees the possibility for change but is ambivalent and unsure of taking that step. The goal for the social worker is to help the client resolve this ambivalence and build motivation and confidence by focusing, exploring, and evaluating the pros and cons of making change without judging the client. It is at this point that further exploration about the pros and cons of actually making a change is discussed. *Rulers* are a useful tool for measuring the client's feeling about actually making change. Employing the *readiness ruler* can be a useful tool in building readiness to change. The idea is to inquire of the client how disposed they are toward making change on a scale of

0–10 (with 0 being the least ready and 10 the most ready). The worker always asks why the number is not lower as and reinforces motives for change. If the client says "I'm at a 5," the affirmation response might be "wow, it sounds like you are 50% of the way there!"

Readiness Ruler

Readiness Ruler

On the line below, mark where you are now on this line that measures your change in
_____.

Are you not prepared to change, already changing, or somewhere in the middle?

| 0 | 1 | 2 | 3 | 4 | 5 | 6 | 7 | 8 | 9 | 10 |

**Not Prepared
to Change**   **Already
Changing**

In the preparation stage, the client begins to make plans for change and to set some goals. The task for the social worker is to support self-efficacy and motivation, negotiate a plan, and facilitate decision-making. Sometimes the plan is for harm reduction; other times it can be followed up with specialty services. What is important is to develop a plan that reflects the client's wishes.

The action stage is distinguishable by the beginning of change implementation. The client takes specific action steps making behavioral changes. Here the social worker needs to support implementation as well as the client's follow through and self-efficacy. The SBIRT model refers the client to higher-level services when assessed as appropriate for the individual client. It is important for the social worker to be knowledgeable about various services and providers to whom referrals can be made when clients need a higher level of service.

Maintenance is identifiable by continued, sustained action. The social worker helps the client maintain change and identify strategies to prevent relapse. The relapse stage is a normal part of the change cycle, as people do not sustain change immediately. Often, they attempt to make change only to return to a previous behavior after a period of abstinence, at which time they may revert to an earlier stage such as contemplation. Clients can feel disheartened about change and temporarily averse to try the process again; however, clients do not necessarily abandon the commitment to change. It is important for the worker to recognize this and continue to accept the client unconditionally and continue to offer hope and belief in the client.

Experience with SBIRT Curricula in Medical Health-Care Training

The literature concerning integration of SBIRT into teaching curricula is overwhelmingly focused on medical health-care settings (Gordon & Alford, 2012; Childers et al., 2012; Cole et al., 2012; Hettema et al., 2012; Pringle et al., 2012; Tanner, Wilhelm, Rossie, & Metcalf, 2012). Although SBIRT was designed for implementation in health-care settings, there remains "suboptimal development and implementation of evidence-based training curricula for healthcare providers" (Hettema et al., 2012, p.241). One consequence has been the notoriously slow use of models such as SBIRT for patients who are at risk or abusing substances (Broyles & Gordon, 2010).

From the literature on developing curricula in medical health-care settings, we learn of the importance of initially training teaching faculty in SBIRT and the ongoing importance of modeling and reinforcement of developing skills from trained personnel (Childers et al., 2012). Curricula that yielded increased confidence in implementing SBIRT incorporated this approach across the board (Puskar, Mitchell, Kane, Hagle, & Talcott, 2014; Cole et al., 2012; Hettema et al., 2012; Pringle et al., 2012). Faculty buy-in was a key component identified in a study of nursing faculty who were trained to implement SBIRT into undergraduate nursing curricula (Puskar et al., 2014). Childers et al. (2012) point out that teaching faculty with limited prior training in SBIRT score low in measures of role adequacy and professional satisfaction when it comes to working with at-risk or abusing substance users. Despite the lack of EBP training, faculty score high on role legitimacy and motivation measures indicating, "they believe SBIRT is an important part of their job and that they are motivated to work with drinkers" (Childers et al., 2012, p.277). In 2014, slightly more than half (52.7%) of Americans of ages 12 and up reported being current drinkers of alcohol. Of those 176.6 million alcohol users, an estimated 17 million have an alcohol dependency disorder (ADU) (SAMSHA, 2014). It is clear there is a great need for more effective EBP training in models such as SBIRT as individuals are not being routinely screened for substance use in the USA (SAMSHA, 2011).

There is a dearth of literature regarding the use of SBIRT specifically in social work, where there is much opportunity to help move this EBP forward. Cochran and Field (2013) point out that "greater involvement in the SBI [Screening and Brief Intervention] field for the social work profession is a natural fit given the connection between SBI, social work practice and social work education" (p. 255). Social workers practice in settings where brief interventions are regularly employed, such as emergency rooms and trauma centers where social workers routinely provide mental and behavioral health services to patients (Cochran & Field, 2013). Social workers are a consistent presence in other settings where delivery of substance abuse screenings is easily translatable such as schools, senior centers, homecare agencies, after-school programs, and clinical agencies to name but a few. Integrating SBIRT training into advanced curriculum is a natural fit falling into place with humanistic theory and the strengths perspective and offering students an additional tool for assessment and intervention with at-risk substance-using clients.

SBIRT Curricula and Advanced Social Work Practice

Developing SBIRT curricula in advanced practice necessitates consideration of the intertwined nature of three stakeholders in social work education: faculty, students, and field instructors. Faculty play the lead role in teaching students the underlying concepts of motivational interviewing, stages of change, and the SBIRT model. Field instructors, and agencies, must also buy into the usefulness of SBIRT screening with their clients for the model and training to be useful.

Challenges for Faculty

The term *curriculum* comes from the Latin for "course," as in the course of a journey. The term denotes a process; one could say a means rather than an end. It signifies movement from a starting point to an end and provides a route. The Sherpa along that journey are the teaching faculty; they are the student's guides. Among the challenges students may encounter in learning SBIRT, one of the largest is having a faculty whom are not adequately trained in the techniques or protocols.

Training

Russett and Williams (2014) report there is a paucity of faculty trained in substance abuse resulting in limited social work education focused in this area of practice. Lack of faculty preparation and training is one of the several barriers to integrating new methods into Advanced Social Work Practice (Kognito, 2016). Skepticism of using new methods including lack of adequate training and preparation and inadequate time to learn new material along with unfamiliarity with substance abuse knowledge, skills, and educational resources was described as faculty barriers to embracing SBIRT in the curriculum (Kognito, 2016).

This highlights the importance of providing adequate training to faculty prior to the inclusion of SBIRT in the teaching curriculum. Ogden, Vinjamuri, and Kahn (2016) describe "a train the trainer approach used to disseminate SBIRT material and knowledge to the social work department faculty at a public urban college serving bachelor and master-level social work students" (p. 3–4), which included a SAMHSA (2013) toolkit and MI training from a national expert. In addition, Ogden et al. (2016) describe a step-by-step manual, PowerPoint slides, instructional videos, and role-play suggestions that were either created or provided by lead faculty members for use in the classroom as tools. Periodic workshops and trainings provided additional support to faculty throughout the academic year (Ogden et al., 2016). Even with training and ongoing support for faculty, there is always the possibility that new faculty, full time or adjunct, will join the teaching staff and need more intensive onboard training.

Challenges for Students

The student experience illustrates another set of barriers encountered in the implementation of SBIRT in advanced practice curricula. Students appeared to be more receptive to the SBIRT curriculum, found the skills useful, and felt that SBIRT fit with their professional identity (Ogden et al., 2016). Student internships provide practice experience across a broad spectrum of client populations. Some students were able to integrate the use of SBIRT seamlessly into their internship practice, while others struggled with whether or not the protocol was applicable to the population they worked with.

Obstacles faced by students in implementing SBIRT can be understood as struggles with diversity, stereotyping, and countertransference. Although SBIRT is taught as a universal screening, students often come with preconceived notions about substance abuse and those who engage in at-risk substance abuse and use.

Diversity and Stereotyping: Issues of Cultural Competence

Students were generally receptive and comfortable with the SBIRT material, but for some, stereotypes about substance-using clients created barriers (Ogden et al., 2016). Existing stereotypes about substance users can shape students likelihood of screening or not screening particular individuals that fall into the stereotyped category. For these students, SBIRT provided the tools with which to approach a subject that they may not have been comfortable asking about previously. It gave them permission to ask and empowered them see this as part of their professional role. There were students who were not comfortable with the idea of asking about substance use and were unable to find a fluid way to introduce the screening to clients. These students were more likely to begin by saying "I'm in school now and I have to do this as a project. . .is it ok if I ask you these questions about substance use?"

The issue of age was another area in which a number of students struggled with SBIRT. Many students working with the elderly mistakenly believed that there was no need to screen their clients for substance use. Their own preconceived notions about older adults and substance use coupled with their own cultural values prevented them from addressing substance use with elder clients believing it disrespectful to ask. "What we are learning in class doesn't apply to my clients since I am working with seniors." Social work students don't often consider that elders are at risk for substance abuse as well as medication overuse/misuse and abuse as illustrated in the vignette from the beginning of the chapter. Students have also shared their hesitation to address substance abuse with older clients believing they "should be allowed to do what they want, they're old and have lived a long life, they know what to do." Again, this speaks to age as a factor when young students are working with older adults.

On the other end of the spectrum, students working with children often believed using the SBIRT model was a waste of time, thinking young children could not be substance users. The fallacy of this is highlighted by a case mentioned in the introduction.

The student's internship was at a public elementary school in an urban environment. He was working with an 8-year-old boy, Jim, who had lost his single mother to illness within the prior year. He was living with his 19-year-old aunt, who had become his legal guardian, and her boyfriend. Jim's academic performance was suffering, and his behavior was challenging the teachers. His teachers became more and more concerned and finally requested counseling intervention from the school-based social workers. As Jim began to describe the environment he was living in, it became clear that he was self-medicating with sleeping pills and alcohol. Student assumptions about *who* might be at risk for substance uses can create barriers to using SBIRT. It is important to point out that SBIRT can also be a tool for exploring substance use in the homes of younger clients. It can be a way of opening up a dialogue and letting the client know it is safe to share such information with the social worker.

Other stereotypes about what substance-abusing clients *look like* created barriers. Students who have had experience working in the field of substance abuse have shared the belief they can tell who abuses substances by their appearance. One student stated, "I can tell physically, how they look. . .whether they have a history of some kind of use" (Ogden et al., 2016). The importance of stressing the universal use of SBIRT is illustrated by the examples provided above.

Countertransference

As much as social work educators stress the importance of remaining nonjudgmental with regard to clients, students may still struggle with actually staying out of judgment. Some of this can be understood as the student's countertransference, the student's inability to differentiate the client's cognitive/emotional experience from their own, and as a result, they respond subjectively. Process recordings are often where we see such student struggles illustrated. A student working with a client who is at risk for substance abuse tells the client what to do and is then puzzled when the client does not do it. Then there is the student who makes a statement such as "you know drugs are bad for you, why are you doing this?" Other students often short-circuit the amount of time spent exploring client behaviors around substance use. They are too quick to jump to the readiness ruler to ascertain the client commitment to behavior change. These are examples of responses that highlight the barriers countertransference can present for students when working with clients to make behavioral change.

Identification

Another issue students struggled with is the definition of the measure of *one drink* and what constitutes *at-risk* levels of alcohol use. For a good number of students, there was recognition that they, themselves or others they know personally, may engage in at-risk behavior with alcohol. When students are honest and comfortable talking about their own behavior, it presents rich material for role-play and discussion using MI, the theory of stages of change, and SBIRT. As noted previously, the use of role-play and simulation, regular feedback, and opportunity to practice are essential components of successful integration of SBIRT skills. Making use of student experiences in the classroom whether with clients, friends, family members, or themselves can enhance opportunities for practicing these skills.

Timing and Agency

The timing of SBIRT in the curriculum has the potential to present obstacles for students. When SBIRT is presented after students have developed a working relationship with clients, many found it offensive to clients and disruptive to their existing relationship (Ogden et al., 2016). This was particularly evident in substance use settings where students work with clients who have a known history of substance abuse. Students have internships at a myriad of agencies with a broad spectrum of populations and focus. Although SBIRT is a universal screening model, students are very conscious of the relative importance SBIRT has in their agencies (Ogden et al., 2016). Agencies with a concrete focus such as a welfare-to-work program, GED focus, etc. may view SBIRT as setting up a conflict for the agency. If a client, especially an adolescent, is referred out for substance use, it can directly impact the agency census.

Field Instructors

Fieldwork is the pedagogy of social work education and by that very nature must be an important part of the way curriculum is designed. The confidence of field instructors (FIs) in guiding and supporting student learning around SBIRT may depend on their own training in the model (Russett, 2015). Field educators should be offered, if not advanced training, simultaneous training to that received by their supervisees. SBIRT education opportunities are provided to field instructors with formal and informal training during annual and semiannual field education meetings (Russett, 2015). More formal training in SBIRT could include continuing education credits (CEUs) as incentive for field instructors to participate including full and half-day trainings. This provides FIs an opportunity to stay connected with the schools of social work as well as stay abreast of advances in the social work profession. Given what we know from the studies of SBIRT curricula in medical settings, modeling, feedback, and reinforcement of SBIRT skills are important aspects of supporting student learning and integration of practice skills. Field instructors are essential team members in the training of MSW students and therefore have a critical role in supporting the implementation of a SBIRT curriculum.

Misconceptions

FI's receptiveness to learning about SBIRT could be a barrier to student learning and opportunity to practice skills learned in SBIRT training. Similar to the issues some students had around stereotyping and diversity, FIs belief that SBIRT was not universally relevant to the agency population (Ogden et al., 2016) can present an obstacle in fieldwork settings. This emerged more consistently in agencies that served young children, for example, in elementary school settings. Several FIs showed reluctance to allow students to use SBIRT with their elementary-age clients citing the inappropriateness of the population and the need to get parental permission. Others pointed out that the population needing specialized treatment for substance use was not served by their agency. FIs may be constrained by agency protocols or have their own stereotypes about substance use and substance users. Ogden et al. (2016) cite one FI who stated, "As for speaking the language, I mean addicts have a different language. Try to pick up on that. So they can know what the client or person is talking about" (p.12). Stereotyping and judging are not reserved only for students; FIs struggle with these same issues. In all of the instances detailed, the field instructors failed to see the usefulness of the universal screening.

Conclusions

Ideally, SBIRT curricula would include uniform training to faculty and field instructors where they had the opportunity to learn, if not master, the material prior to the onset of student learning. Real-world experience makes this nearly impossible, as personnel are subject to eleventh-hour changes in both academic and agency settings. As well, field placements can be finalized at the last minute, can change mid-year, or may not be settled well enough in advance to facilitate consistent implementation of training for field instructors. Faculty and field instructor buy-in are vital to the successful student translation of academic learning to practice learning. Without support from both of these stakeholders, student learning and practice opportunity can be significantly limited. Attentiveness to timing of the SBIRT model in the curriculum is an important factor for student comfort in their professional role with clients. Introducing the model late in the semester creates discomfort for both students and, as they report, clients, once the relationship has been established. Other factors such as stereotyping, diversity issues, and countertransference can be addressed in both classroom and fieldwork settings when there has been adequate integration of SBIRT training for faculty and field instructors through classroom discussion, modeling, and ongoing feedback. Future exploration regarding integration of SBIRT into social work education that examines barriers and obstacles in various fields of practice could be helpful to developing more targeted training for students, faculty, and FIs. Other areas of social work education to be explored include a comparison of undergraduate- and graduate-level approaches to integrating and teaching SBIRT in the curriculum.

References

Babor, T. F., & Higgins-Biddle, J. C. (2000). Alcohol screening and brief intervention: Dissemination strategies for medical practice and public health. *Addiction, 95*, 677–686.

Babor, T. F., McRee, B. G., Kassebaum, P. A., Grimaldi, P. L., Ahmed, K., & Bray, J. (2007). Screening, Brief Intervention, and Referral to Treatment (SBIRT). *Substance Abuse, 28*(3), 7–30.

Broyles, L. M., & Gordon, A. J. (2010). SBIRT implementation: Moving beyond the interdisciplinary rhetoric. *Substance Abuse, 31*(4), 221–223.

Center for Behavioral Health Statistics and Quality. (2013). *Results from the 2012 national survey on drug use and health: Summary of national findings, HHS Publication No. SMA 13–4795, NSDUH Series H-46*. Rockville, MD: United States of America 2013.

Childers, J. W., Broyles, L. M., Hanusa, B. H., Kraemer, K. L., Conigliaro, J., Spagnoletti, C., et al. (2012). Teaching the teachers: Faculty preparedness and evaluation of a retreat in screening, brief intervention, and referral to treatment. *Substance Abuse, 33*(3), 272–277.

Cochran, G., & Field, C. (2013). Brief intervention and social work: A primer for practice and policy. *Social Work in Public Health, 28*, 248–263.

Cole, B., Clark, D. C., Seale, J. P., Shellenberger, S., Lyme, A., Johnson, J. A., et al. (2012). Reinventing the reel: An innovative approach to resident skill-building in motivational interviewing for brief intervention. *Substance Abuse, 33*(3), 278–281.

Gambrill, E. (2007). Transparency as the Route to Evidence-Informed Professional Education. *Research on Social Work Practice, 17*(5), 553–560.

Gambrill, E. (2014). Social work education and avoidable ignorance. *Journal of Social Work Education, 50*(3), 391–413.

Gibbs, L., & Gambrill, E. (2002). Evidence-based practice: Counter-arguments to objections. *Research on Social Work Practice, 12*, 452–476.

Gordon, A. J., & Alford, D. P. (2012). Screening, brief intervention, and referral to treatment (SBIRT) curricular innovations: Addressing a training gap. *Substance Abuse, 33*(3), 227–230.

Kognito. (2016, December). *Integrating adolescent SBIRT throughout social work and nursing education*. A Webinar Presentation Retrieved from http://go.kognito.com/rs/143-HCJ 270/images/Hel_Webinar_121316_SBIRTWebinar2016Presentation.pdf

Hettema, J. E., Ratanawongsa, N., Manuel, J. K., Ciccarone, D., Coffa, D., Jain, S., et al. (2012). A SBIRT curriculum for medical residents: Development of a performance feedback tool to build learner confidence. *Substance Abuse, 33*(3), 292–297.

Miller, W. R., & Rollnick, S. (2002). *Motivational interviewing: Preparing people for change* (2nd ed.). New York, NY: The Guilford Press.

Miller, W. R., & Rollnick, S. (2013). *Motivational interviewing: Helping people change*. New York: NY Guilford Press.

Miller, W. R., Zweban, A., DiClemente, C. C., & Rychtarik, R. G. (1992). *Motivational enhancement therapy manual: A clinical research guide for therapists treating individuals with alcohol abuse and dependence*. Rockville, MD: National Institute on Alcohol Abuse and Alcoholism.

Mullen, E. J., & Streiner, D. L. (2004). The evidence for and against evidence-based practice. *Brief Treatment and Crisis Intervention, 4*(2), 111–121.

National Drug Intelligence Center. (2011). *The impact of illicit drug use on American society*. Washington, DC: United States Department of Justice. Retrieved from http://www.justice.gov/ndic.

National Institute of Drug Abuse. (2012). *Medial consequences of drug abuse*. Retrieved from https://www.drugabuse.gov/related-topics/medical-consequences-drug-abuse/mortality

Ogden, L. P., Vinjamuri, M., & Kahn, J. M. (2016). A model for implementing and evidence-based practice in student fieldwork placements: Barriers and facilitators to the use of "SBIRT". *Journal of Social Service Research, 42*(4), 425–441.

Pringle, J. L., Kowalchuk, A., Meyers, J. A., & Seale, J. P. (2012). Equipping residents to address alcohol and drug use: The national SBIRT residency training project. *Journal of Graduate Medical Education, 4*(1), 58–63.

Pringle, J. L., Melczak, M., Johnjulio, W., Campopiano, M., Gordon, A. J., & Costlow, M. (2012). Pennsylvania SBIRT medical and residency training: Developing, implementing, and evaluating an evidence-based program. *Substance Abuse, 33*(3), 278–281.

Prochaska, J. O., & DiClemente, C. C. (1984). *The transtheoretical approach: Crossing the traditional boundaries of change.* Homewood, IL: Dow Jones Irwin.

Puskar, K., Mitchell, A. M., Kane, I., Hagle, H., & Talcott, K. S. (2014). Faculty buy-in to teach alcohol and drug use screening. *The Journal of Continuing Education in Nursing, 45*(9), 403–408.

Rogers, C. R. (1959). A theory of therapy, personality, and interpersonal relationships, as developed in the client-centered framework. In *Psychology: A study of a science.* New York: McGraw-Hill.

Russett, J. (2015). Changing systems: Integrating screening brief intervention and referral to treatment (SBIRT) in social work practice. *The Field Educator Practice Digest, 5*(2), 1–5.

Russett, J. L., & Williams, A. (2014). An exploration of substance abuse course offerings for students in counseling and social work programs. *Substance Abuse, 36*(1), 51–58.

Satre, D. D., McCance-Katz, E. F., Moreno-John, G., Julian, K. A., O'Sullivan, P. S., & Satterfeild, J. M. (2012). Using needs assessment to develop curricula for screening, brief intervention, and referral to treatment (SBIRT) in academic and community health settings. *Substance Abuse, 33*(3), 298–302.

Stanton, M. R., Atherton, W. L., Toriello, P. J., & Hodgson, J. L. (2012). Implementation of a "learner-driven" curriculum: An screening, brief intervention, and referral to treatment (SBIRT) interdisciplinary primary care model. *Substance Abuse, 33*(3), 312–315.

Substance Abuse and Mental Health Services Administration. (2014). *Behavioral health trends in the United States: Results from the 2014 national survey on drug use and health.* Retrieved from   https://www.samhsa.gov/data/sites/default/files/NSDUH-FRR1-2014/NSDUH-FRR1 2014.pdf

Substance Abuse and Mental Health Services Administration. (2011) *White paper on screening, brief intervention, and referral to treatment (SBIRT) in behavioral healthcare.* Retrieved from: http://www.samhsa.gov/prevention/sbirt/

Substance Abuse and Mental Health Services Administration. (2012). *Results from the 2011 national survey on drug use and health: Summary of national findings*, NSDUH Series H-44, HHS Publication (No.) (SMA) 12–4713. Rockville, MD: Substance Abuse and Mental Health Services Administration.

Substance Abuse and Mental Health Services Administration. (2013). *Results from the 2013 national survey on drug use and health: Summary of national findings* (p. 21). Retrieved from   https://www.samhsa.gov/data/sites/default/files/NSDUHresultsPDFWHTML2013/Web/ NSDUHresults2013.pdf

Substance Abuse and Mental Health Services Administration. (2015). *SBIRT: Screening, brief intervention, and referral to treatment.* Retrieved from http://www.samhsa.gov/sbirt/about

Steenrod, S. (2014). What every social worker needs to know about screening, brief intervention, and referral to treatment (SBIRT). *The New Social Worker.* Retrieved from http://www.social-worker.com/feature-articles/practice/whatevery-social-worker-needs-to-know-about-sbirt/

Tanner, T. B., Wilhelm, S. E., Rossie, K. M., & Metcalf, M. P. (2012) Web-based SBIRT training for health professional students and primary care providers. *Substance Abuse, 33*(3), 316–320.

Thyer, B., & Wodarski, J. S. (2007). *Social work in mental health: An evidence-based approach.* New York: John Wiley & Sons, Inc..

Chapter 19
Teaching the Importance of Developing the Therapeutic Relationship

David A. Fullard

Introduction

This chapter addresses why and how to teach students the importance of developing the therapeutic relationship, also known as the therapeutic/working/helping alliance. It covers (A) the history of the development of the concept of the therapeutic relationship in general psychotherapy and mental health nursing, as well as addiction treatment and recovery, (B) the critical components of the therapeutic relationship (namely, tasks, goals, and bonds), (C) evidence-based practice showing the effectiveness of the therapeutic relationship in achieving positive outcomes, (D) the wide range of issues related to cultural competence/diversity (as well as age, gender, diagnosis, comorbidity, etc.) in developing an effective therapeutic relationship, (E) the importance of knowing the difference between a therapeutic relationship and a personal relationship and not crossing that boundary, (F) practical skills related to developing the therapeutic relationship during different stages of therapy and addiction treatment and repairing inevitable ruptures in the alliance, and (G) ways to measure and assess the effectiveness of the therapeutic alliance on client outcomes and concludes with a review of various approaches to teaching the skills needed to develop an effective therapeutic relationship with diverse clients, as well as how to improve organizational support of patients and therapists in this regard.

There is wide agreement that an effective therapeutic relationship is "the foundation of mental health care and the support for changing insight and behavior… nurtured by kindness, friendliness, objectiveness, a sense of humor, and a positive approach… where values are respected as the healthcare professional relieves distress by actively listening to concerns, improves morale through review of established outcomes, and empowers patients to participate in their own recovery" (Lecharrois, 2011, p.1).

D. A. Fullard (✉)
Empire State College/SUNY, New York, NY, USA
e-mail: David.Fullard@esc.edu

© Springer International Publishing AG 2018
T. MacMillan, A. Sisselman-Borgia (eds.), *New Directions in Treatment,
Education, and Outreach for Mental Health and Addiction*, Advances in Mental
Health and Addiction, https://doi.org/10.1007/978-3-319-72778-3_19

What Is the Therapeutic Relationship/Working Alliance?

History and Theoretical Background of the Development of the Concept of the Therapeutic Relationship

The concept of the therapeutic relationship first appeared in the twentieth century, in the early development of the field of psychoanalysis. Freud was the first to describe the rapport or positive feelings that develop between doctor and patient (Summers & Barber, 2003) based on "positive transference composed of friendly, or affectionate, feelings for the analyst" (Dykeman, 1995, p.3). Freud described various obstacles to sustaining patient engagement and commitment to treatment, including resistance to hypnosis, defenses against free association, and negative transference (of prior bad relationships to the therapist). Freud's recommendation was to "do nothing to interfere with the natural development of rapport, and listen with sympathetic understanding" (Luborsky, Barber, Siqueland, McLellan, & Woody, 1997, p. 236).

Early psychoanalytic theorists "noted the importance of the 'real' relationship between client and therapist in the therapeutic process [suggesting] that the reality-based elements of a positive bond aid in the process of therapy" (Booth, Thompson, & Campbell, 2008, p. 4). They described the therapeutic relationship as an alliance between the analyst and the patient's "conscious, uniform and rational ego against the unconscious, defending ego and its mechanisms… a stable and positive relationship [enabling] them to productively engage in the work of analysis" (Dykeman, 1995, pp. 4, 6–8).

The modern concept of the working alliance as addressing goals, tasks, and bond was developed by Bordin, who described it as a relationship between client and therapist which is common to all forms of psychotherapeutic treatment, regardless of treatment orientation or approach, *[the therapeutic alliance is] both a condition of treatment which facilitates change… as well as a change agent in and of itself* (Booth et al., 2008; Fernandez, Krause, & Perez, 2016). In contrast to Rogers, who placed most of the responsibility for creating this relationship on the therapist alone, Bordin described "the therapeutic alliance as a mutual construction of the patient and therapist" (Summers & Barber, 2003) and explained how "In a well-functioning treatment relationship, the patient and therapist come to agreement about the *goals* the patient wishes to achieve in the treatment. They also come to accept certain therapeutic *tasks* as potentially helpful for achieving those goals. The *bonds* that form between patient and therapist in the course of working on the tasks include the positive personal attachments that stimulate trust and confidence" (Luborsky et al., 1997, p. 233).

Other theorists extended the definition of the therapeutic relationship by describing the need for a spirit of collaboration or agreement between client and therapist regarding the importance of these goals, tasks, and creation of an emotional bond (Frigo, 2006). Dryden notes that the ability of health-care providers to effectively collaborate depends on their knowledge, attitudes, skills, and behaviors, and he describes this agreement (or lack thereof) as "views" of the client and therapist, regarding issues such as "the nature of clients' psychological problems… how can clients' problems best be addressed… the practical aspects of counseling [i.e., session length, frequency, cost, location, and cancellation rules, concluding that] *effective counseling occurs when the client's views are similar to the counselor's*" (Dryden, 2008, p. 6).

Components of an Effective Therapeutic Relationship

Examining the critical components of goals, tasks, and bond more closely, *goals* are the ultimate outcome or target of therapy; *tasks* are the necessary behaviors and acts required by both therapist and client to achieve those goals; and the concept of *bond* "embraces the complex network of positive attachment between client and counselor, including… mutual trust, acceptance, and confidence" (Dykeman, 1995, p. 12). A strong working alliance must establish a mutual understanding and valuation of goals, tasks, and bond to assure a positive outcome of the therapeutic process. Specifically in addiction treatment, patients "who are ready for change are more likely to have a therapeutic alliance with their therapist, are more likely to stay in treatment, and have better outcomes" (Frigo, 2006, p. 1).

   Communication is also an essential element in the development of the therapeutic relationship, since without that, therapist and client cannot come to an agreement about the importance or even the nature of goals, tasks, and bond. "[Clinicians] should therefore be competent to communicate with patients in a way that helps establish good therapeutic relationships and in achieving clinical aims" (Priebe & McCabe, 2008, p. 522). This requires specific training, supervision, assessment, and ongoing research, especially with regard to effective communication with different populations in a range of treatment settings. Effective training in communication skills instructs clinicians to introduce themselves, explain the intake procedure, get consent, and interact in a professional manner, utilizing personal characteristics and specific skills to engage with patients. The amount of time allotted for communication varies widely, of course, depending on whether the client is in open-ended talk therapy or being seen at a brief clinical visit to a community mental health-care center or even in a locked detox ward, school, or prison where they may be receiving coercive treatment.

   The three elements most strongly linked to successful outcomes are the *therapeutic alliance*, *empathy*, and *goal consensus/collaboration*, where an effective relationship fosters honesty, humility, and mutual respect. Educational programs should provide students with opportunities to learn, develop, and practice essential relationship skills: empathy, warmth, positive regard, collaboration (mutual involvement and patient engagement), agreement on goals, and management of countertransference (Perraud et al., 2006; Watson & Kalogerakos, 2010).

Evidence-Based Practice Showing the Effectiveness of the Therapeutic Relationship in Achieving Positive Outcomes

Many studies have shown that *positive therapeutic relationships improve patient results. The therapeutic alliance is a key predictor of treatment outcome, as the stronger the relationship is the more positive change that occurs for the client.* A recent study demonstrated that therapeutic alliance predicted effectiveness of cognitive behavioral treatment, interpersonal psychotherapy for depression, and medication treatment (Booth et al., 2008).

Three positive outcomes of good communication include *engagement, adherence,* and *therapeutic change of symptoms and behavior* (Hatcher, 2010). This means that when clients like and feel respected by their counselor, they are more motivated to connect with them (develop a positive *bond*), more likely to adhere to their program, show up for their appointments, attend more sessions, and follow through on treatment suggestions (agree on and perform the needed *tasks* for recovery) and thus achieve the desired change of symptoms or behavior (the ultimate *goals* of treatment). There is some question whether the third outcome, of symptom improvement, is due to the first two results (engagement and adherence) or if the relationship itself is a form of therapy that leads to recovery (Priebe & McCabe, 2008).

The centrality of the therapeutic relationship has been shown to be true regardless of therapeutic approach (psychoanalysis, role theory, systems theory, talk therapy, social psychology, social constructionism, cognitive-behaviorism, even clinical psychiatric care, and medication treatment), types of patients (adults, children, families, severely mentally ill, recovering addicts/alcoholics, members of various ethnic and cultural groups), and treatment locations (one-on-one or group therapy, formal analysis, mental hospitals, detox wards and rehab centers, schools, and prisons). Hence, the quality of the therapeutic relationship is of major importance across different kinds of psychiatric settings and treatments (Priebe & McCabe, 2008; Simpson, Frick, & Kahn, 2013).

Remarkably, this improvement is shown even in brief clinic visits or psychiatric treatment in a coercive environment, such as a locked ward or jail mental health clinic, where treatment is often open-ended, with variability in the frequency, length, and aims of meetings. Priebe et al. (2011) noted that the therapeutic relationship is at the center of the delivery of treatment, with patient noting it as the most important part of care, and is linked to fewer readmissions to hospital and more favorable changes in symptom levels and functioning measures.

Issues Related to Cultural Competence/Diversity (plus Age, Gender, Diagnosis, and Comorbidity) Regarding the Development of an Effective Therapeutic Relationship

The wider social context also affects the development of an effective therapeutic relationship, since "the patient lives within a family and/or in a community, and the nature of the various relationships with family members and other social contacts is likely to influence how a patient engages with and benefits from a therapeutic relationship with a healthcare professional" (Priebe & McCabe, 2008, p. 525). Being cognizant of and sensitive to cultural differences and family background, as well as aware of their own cultural biases, enables therapists to establish an effective working alliance with patients, regardless of cultural difference or similarity. While patients may have cognitive factors (thoughts, moods, behaviors, and reactions) that inhibit or enhance the therapeutic alliance, and there are professional variables in the skills of the therapist, it is important also to take into account the patient's environment, including "ethnicity, sexual orientation, family upbringing, socio-economic, accommodation and work status" (Grant, Mills, Mulhern, & Short, 2004, p. 15). Other issues that can impact the therapeutic alliance include stigma associated with mental health treatment (Jordan-Arthur, Romero, & Karver, 2011, p. 10).

Cultural competence is an active, not a passive quality; studies have not shown that simply having a therapist and client from similar ethnic or cultural groups improves the quality of the therapeutic alliance, nor that being from different groups lowers the effectiveness of the relationship; indeed, "client-therapist similarities and differences seem to have no effect on counseling relationships" (Erdur, Rude, Baron, Draper, & Shankar, 2000, p. 12). Rather, *engagement*, *knowledge*, *respect*, and *self-awareness* have a positive effect on therapist-client relations.

Here is an acronym to remind clinicians of the many factors that multicultural competence should be ADDRESSING:

*A*ge and generational influences
*D*evelopmental disabilities
*D*isabilities obtained in later life
*R*eligion and spiritual orientation
*E*thnic and racial identity
*S*ocioeconomic status
*S*exual orientation
*I*ndigenous heritage
*N*ational origin
*G*ender (Asnaani & Hofmann, 2012, pp.187–195)

Multicultural competence means "approaching the counseling process from the context of the personal culture of the client [and ensuring one's own] cultural values and biases do not override those of the client" (Ahmed, Wilson, Henriksen, & Jones, 2011, pp. 18–21). To achieve this, counselors must develop *cultural knowledge*, *cultural skills*, and *cultural awareness*; demonstrate that they possess the key qualities of *credibility*, *expertness*, and *trustworthiness*; and provide *validation* to their clients by confirming and respecting what they say. Being multiculturally competent also means recognizing that ethnic minority groups tend to underutilize psychotherapy services and/or drop out of treatment at a higher rate (Vasquez, 2007). Establishing a good working alliance is critical, since the success of any technique depends on patient bond with the therapist who selects and applies the various models as appropriate to each client.

Even more important to overcoming obstacles and threats to the therapeutic alliance, therapists must be aware (1) of their own biases and often unconscious microaggressions toward ethnic minority clients, (2) that they are in a position of power in relation to the client and must be careful not to abuse it, and (3) that "ethnic minority clients may be particularly sensitive to the experiences of negative judgment, rejection, and criticalness… because of a history of oppressive and rejecting experiences, [making them] easily shamed" (Vasquez, 2007, p. 881–2). Therefore, therapists should be conscious of conveying negative judgments in body language, facial expressions, voice tone, and eye contact. Personal attributes which contribute positively to the alliance include being *flexible*, *honest*, *respectful*, *trustworthy*, *confident*, *warm*, *interested*, and *open* and employing techniques such as *exploration*, *reflection*, *noting past therapy success*, *providing accurate interpretation*, *facilitating the expression of affect*, and *attending to the patient's experience*. It is also important to learn as much as possible about the various values, norms, and expectations of cultural groups with whom one works (while avoiding stereotyping) and modifying the therapeutic relationship to the client's culture, with special attention to understanding the client's voice, development of trust and credibility, and the promotion of cultural empathy, while continually maintaining a state of self-awareness regarding bias and attitudes.

An earlier focus of cultural competence was to "eliminate the cultural and linguistic barriers between health care providers and patients, which can interfere with the effective delivery of health services. Sometimes described as 'cross-cultural,' 'transcultural,' 'multicultural,' or 'culturally sensitive,' these efforts were initially targeted at immigrant or refugee populations with limited English proficiency and exposure to Western cultural norms" (Beach, Saha, & Cooper, 2006, pp.vi-vii). This approach introduced the role of interpreters and "cultural brokers," patient advocates who help individuals navigate a complicated health-care landscape. The patient-centered method notes that all aspects of the patient were important to consider, including his or her cultural background (though again, not in a uniform or stereotypical fashion), in developing the therapeutic relationship and designing effective treatment programs and, of course, "recognizing that both patients and providers brought cultural perspectives to the health care encounter… For instance, some people of color might harbor distrust of health care providers or institutions, possibly related to historical or ongoing experiences of discrimination. Providers might harbor either overt or unconscious biases about people of color that influence their interactions and decision-making" (Beach et al., 2006, pp. 6–7). Awareness of all these elements is needed for quality interpersonal communications leading to effective therapeutic relationships.

As noted above, a natural power imbalance also exists between therapist and client, with therapists having the "upper hand" due to their possessing the knowledge, experience, and expertise that the client needs; this imbalance may be further exacerbated by societal power imbalances, for instance, an older White male therapist seeing a younger Black female client in a college counseling center. Although therapists who are members of the dominant ethnic group often ignore these issues, this may impair the therapeutic relationship, because these factors affect how therapists and clients relate to others of similar or different cultural affiliation. Furthermore, the ways that different ethnic and cultural groups react to the idea and process of counseling, or the disease model of drug addiction itself, must be taken into account: "For example... research has demonstrated that Asian Americans, because of their unfamiliarity with the concept of counseling in general, have difficulty understanding the counseling process and as a consequence, tend to rate the credibility of counselors and the therapeutic alliance as low... [so it is] important to 'educate' them about... therapy from the very beginning" (Nezu, 2010, p. 172–5).

Cultural competence can improve the effectiveness of the therapeutic relationship and enable clients to feel comfortable accessing and staying with needed mental health and recovery services (Shattell, Starr, & Thomas, 2007). Specific guidance is needed about the ethnic background of the client, since some groups respond better to a more authoritative counselor, having confidence that they are experts in the field who can provide knowledgeable guidance on how to improve. Others experience more positive results with a warm, supportive, nonjudgmental therapist who listens and does not probe or question the client. Sometimes it is important to connect treatment to traditional cultural healing approaches or religious beliefs and how these general understandings are modified by individual client experience. As therapists utilize their own strengths to relate to clients in the different groups, they will create more effective therapeutic relationships which will lead to improved outcomes (Center for Substance Abuse Treatment, 2014).

The delivery of health-care services in general, and mental health-care services in particular, has long been unequal between different population groups through all phases of the counseling process, from intake and diagnosis through treatment and outcomes. Multicultural competency helps to reduce this disparity at community, organizational, and individual levels. Beyond being knowledgeable about client cultural background, therapists must also be aware of their own cultural viewpoint, personal biases, and attitudes and how this affects their service delivery, specifically relating to authenticity and transference/countertransference. Clinician self-knowledge is critical to improve the doctor-patient relationship and thus treatment outcomes.

It is also important for therapists to demonstrate *cultural insight*, by acknowledging the pain of cultural oppression experienced by clients. The multiculturally competent counselor should be sensitive to the legacies of societal racism, oppression, and discrimination; show *cultural acceptance* by maintaining a balanced perspective about one's talents, successes, and failures; demonstrate *cultural esteem* by showing respect for their client and the client's culture; express *cultural kinship* through identifying mutuality, shared experiences, and commonalities between cultures; and exposing *cultural openness* by acknowledging that clients are the "true experts" on their own lives. "Cultural attunement is an integrative construct [necessitating] self-reflection, empathy, and on-going self-development [plus the three *essential* attributes] of humility, mutuality, and transparency or openness" (Oakes, 2011, p. 51–3). An example might be a patient with chronic and multiple traumatic experiences who had a hard time seeking help due to prior experience of racial discrimination at a similar treatment setting. By adapting the treatment process, from assessment to interventions to termination, to be more culturally relevant and cultivating a strong therapeutic relationship, the patient may feel feeling respected, heard, and entrusted in contributing to her own progress leading to successful outcomes (Asnaani & Hofmann, 2012).

European-based clinicians face the challenge of treating a wide range of immigrant and ethnic minority clients from different countries, cultural backgrounds, and languages. Multicultural competency in this environment begins with the realization that although all people should have equal opportunity, there is often discrimination against minority group members. Counselors must be competent in three domains: (1) *counselor awareness of own assumptions*, values, and biases, requiring often uncomfortable self-confrontation; (2) *counselor understanding of client's worldview*, involving cultural knowledge and respect for the client's cultural perspective as well as awareness of the sociopolitical and economic factors that influence the lives of ethnic minority group members; and (3) *culturally appropriate intervention strategies* that will be effective with clients from different cultures, based in respect, flexibility, and being "responsive to the needs of the patient rather than to the philosophy of the professional" (Qureshi & Collazos, 2005, p. 309–11). Once again, the emphasis is on self-knowledge and self-awareness on the part of the therapist: *the clinician's capacity to process her or his own racial and cultural identity comprises the key to cultural competence*" (Qureshi & Collazos, 2005, p. 314).

The in-depth Treatment Improvement Protocol on *Improving Cultural Competence* notes that culturally responsive skills can improve client engagement in services, therapeutic relationships between clients and providers, and treatment retention and outcomes. Since this is the ultimate goal of all therapy, cultural competence is clearly a valuable skill for care providers. This protocol focuses on the major racial and ethnic groups identified by the US Census Bureau including African and Black Americans, Asian Americans (including Native Hawaiians and other Pacific Islanders), Hispanics and Latinos, Native Americans, and White Americans. Cultural identities are noted as including "individual traits and attributes shaped by race, ethnicity, language, life experiences, historical events, acculturation, geographic and other environmental influences… [they are] not static; they develop, evolve, and change across the life cycle" (Center for Substance Abuse Treatment, 2014, pp. xv-xvii).

RESPECT is a helpful mnemonic to remember all aspects of cultural competence:

*R*espect (understand how respect is shown within the cultural group)
*E*xplanatory model (understand how clients perceive and explain their problem)
*S*ociocultural context (recognize how race, class, ethnicity, gender, etc. affect care)
*P*ower (acknowledge power differential between client and counselor)
*E*mpathy (express genuine positive regard so client feels understood by counselor)
*C*oncerns and fears (elicit client views about seeking help and initiating treatment)
*T*herapeutic alliance/Trust (commit to behavior that enhances therapeutic relation-
    ship and realize trust is not inherent but earned by counselor)

Another "cultural identification" is the drug subculture, although in this case it is noted that treatment providers need more than just understanding the culture; they must "actively work to weaken that connection and replace it with other experiences that meet the client's social and cultural needs," such as connecting them with a "culture of recovery" (Center for Substance Abuse Treatment, 2014, pp. 159–75). While the drug culture is chosen and entered later in life versus a culture into which one is born, it nonetheless has strong influence over its members, as well as its own unique language, customs, and mores. Individuals who are deeply ingrained in the drug culture often find it difficult to reorient themselves and engage with people in "straight" society or spend time with non-using or nondrinking people. The therapeutic alliance with the counselor may be the first relationship that a recovering addict or alcoholic will have with someone outside of their subculture, making it an important milestone and waypoint in the recovery process. Also, "in general, the longer one stays in treatment, the better his or her long-term recovery. Studies show that the *quality of the therapeutic relationship* significantly influences length of stay… [and] counseling rapport… contributed explicitly to the prediction of out-come… independent of treatment retention" (Booth et al., 2008, p. 6).

Teaching the Difference Between a Therapeutic Relationship and a Personal Relationship and Not Crossing That Boundary

One of the most important things for therapists to learn is the difference between the therapeutic relationship and a personal or social relationship and how to maintain clear boundaries with clients to prevent confusion, inappropriate relations, or unin-tentional abuse of power. While building an effective working alliance, a real rela-tionship occurs based on sharing information and agreeing on treatment goals. As the therapeutic relationship develops, lines may become blurred, and the relationship could be confused with an intimate connection, by either the therapist or the client. *It is the therapist's responsibility to establish and maintain a safe space for the client and the work that needs to be done, and ensure that the boundaries remain strong.*

First and foremost, the therapist must understand the nature of the therapeutic relationship and how it differs from personal or social relationships. "A therapeutic relationship is a planned, goal-directed and contractual connection... for the purposes of providing care to the client in order to meet the client's therapeutic needs" (Professional Boundaries for Therapeutic Relationships, 2011, p. 1). The Ontario Physiotherapist Guide to Therapeutic Relationships and Professional Boundaries notes that "The therapeutic relationship differs from a personal relationship in two ways: 1) the interests of the patent always come first, and 2) there is an imbalance of power between the [therapist] and the patient... [which] means that it is not usually possible to maintain a therapeutic and personal relationship... at the same time" (2013, p. 2).

There are a number of specific relationship characteristics which are notably different between professional/therapeutic relationships and personal/social/intimate relationships. These include money (paid to the therapist by the client for care in a therapeutic relationship; shared in a personal relationship), length of the relationship (determined by treatment need vs. open-ended), location of meetings (in clinic or office vs. no boundaries), purpose (to provide client care vs. to enjoy oneself), structure (defined by care required vs. spontaneous/shared), power balance (in favor of the therapist based on skill and access to client's private information vs. equal/shared), responsibility for the relationship (with the professional vs. shared), and preparation for the relationship (the therapist is trained and the client trusts their expertise vs. equal) (Where's the line? Professional Boundaries in a Therapeutic Relationship, 2011).

Health professionals must establish clear boundaries with their clients and be aware if any boundary crossing or line blurring begins to occur, unless these are brief, intentional actions intended to meet the client's therapeutic needs, with prompt return to the appropriate professional relationship. Boundary violations occur when the client's needs are no longer the focus of the therapeutic relationship and may lead to negative outcomes. Actions that may indicate line blurring include accepting gifts from clients, therapist self-disclosure of personal or intimate information, commencing a social relationship with a former client, and/or entering a therapeutic relationship with family, friends, or colleagues. Behaviors that are unacceptable in a working alliance include abuse of any kind (physical, emotional, verbal, sexual, or financial), neglect, or exploiting information from the therapeutic process for personal gain on the part of the therapist (Professional Boundaries for Therapeutic Relationships, 2011, pp. 2–3).

Clinicians can establish a professional relationship with clear boundaries by introducing themselves to the client by name and professional title and describing their role in providing care; addressing clients by their preferred name or title; obtaining informed consent to treatment and adhering to privacy regulations; listening actively in a nonjudgmental way; developing treatment goals in a client-centered way; being aware of comments, attitudes, or behaviors that may be inappropriate in a therapeutic relationship; and reflecting on their own client interactions (Where's the line? Professional Boundaries in a Therapeutic Relationship, 2011). To avoid any confusion, misunderstanding, or unintentional triggering, clinicians should use language that is clear to the client, allow clients to have someone with them during the session, describe the assessment process, allow clients to ask questions, and revisit consent throughout the treatment process. In general, "sensitive practice should be viewed as a standard precaution, used for all client interactions" (Where's the line? Professional Boundaries in a Therapeutic Relationship, 2011, p. 14).

Two common circumstances that can produce blurring of boundaries are when the relationship slips into a social context or when the therapist's needs are met at the expense of the client's needs. This may occur when therapists are over-helping, controlling, or behaving narcissistically in relation to their clients, usually due to unrecognized transference or countertransference. Specific examples of transference include clients desiring affection or respect or experiencing and expressing hostility, jealousy, competitiveness, and love, to which normal countertransference responses include feeling flattered or important when idealized or relied upon excessively, angry when attacked, annoyed when frustrated, and so on. When the therapist experiences a strong positive or negative reaction to a client, countertransference is often the culprit and may serve as a guide to reestablish firm boundaries. A list of reactions that should inspire self-analysis include boredom or indifference, trying to "rescue" or being overinvolved with a client, overidentification, anger, and helplessness or hopelessness. A self-check index includes questions about being criticized for being overly intrusive or "too involved" with patients and their families, having difficulty setting limits, arriving early/staying late, relating to patients as one does to family members, acting on sexual feelings for a patient, deriving satisfaction from patients' praise or affection, feeling that other staff members are critical or jealous of "your" patient, or difficulties handling patients' unreasonable requests for help, verbal abuse, or sexual advances (Varcarolis, 2005, pp. 159–61).

Teaching Practical Skills Related to Development of the Therapeutic Relationship

How does the therapist go about actually developing an effective therapeutic alliance, and what happens when there are problems or lapses in the alliance which may lead to reduced outcomes for clients? There are certain interventions that the therapist can undertake to develop or enhance the therapeutic alliance at various stages in therapy, from intake and assessment, throughout the working stage, to termination. At the beginning, "role induction intervention" helps to introduce and educate clients about *"what to expect in treatment*, especially their role, the counselor's role, and common experiences which occur during treatment" (Booth et al., 2008, p. 6). This can help clients to maintain realistic expectations, and may reduce dropout rates, improve attendance and adherence to the program, as well as to continue outpatient treatment after release, such as ongoing self-directed attendance at 12-step meetings, taking prescribed behavioral medication, or keeping therapy or clinic appointments.

An in-depth session at the beginning of the program, focusing on all aspects of the therapeutic alliance by addressing the tasks and goals of treatment as well as the bond between counselor and client, may have even more positive results. Therapists can follow a script or notes to address all of these issues at one of the first meetings and ensure they display respect, positive regard, and empathy, engage in reflective listening, and praise the client's courage and effort toward behavioral change. Therapists may develop a collaborative or "team" approach with the client to agree on tasks and goals of treatment, engaging in a joint search for behavior change and recovery, so the client feels understood, listened to, and has hope and realistic expectations about successful outcome of treatment based on hard work.

Reflective listening skills are particularly important in this stage of the treatment process, involving "carefully listening to the client and communicating back what the client say, often in a slightly modified form, and sometimes including reflection of the client's stated or implied feelings. Reflection does not include advice, or the therapist's opinion" (Booth et al., 2008, p. 11). Various aspects of reflective listening include nonverbal attending, repeating, rephrasing, paraphrasing, and reflecting the emotional meaning of what was stated. The session on the therapeutic alliance should conclude with praise for the client on having positive ideas about how to use treatment, strengthening the bond and expectations, scheduling the next appointment, and further praise for any change steps which have occurred so far, "ending the session in a manner which conveys respect... a new partnership... with the next step in treatment planned" (Booth et al., 2008, p. 20).

Therapists inspire trust in their patients by demonstrating *expertise* and expressing *empathy*. Expertise is shown by therapists "who are confident, prepared, clear and logical. Empathy is not simply being kind or pleasant [but rather connotes] acceptance and understanding" (Frigo, 2006, p. 1). Beyond therapist qualities and therapeutic approaches, other factors which may affect the therapeutic alliance include patient qualities and their prior relationship experiences, with dependent, hostile, or dominant interpersonal problems indicating the likelihood of a poorer alliance (Summers & Barber, 2003). It also appears that "specific skills are required to communicate effectively with different diagnostic groups of patients... [so] one might allocate patients to different clinicians" (Priebe & McCabe, 2006, p. 71) to best match clients with therapists best able to establish a positive therapeutic relationship and thus achieve a better outcome. However, this could be difficult to achieve in practice, mostly because it could be embarrassing for a therapist who has a poor relationship with the patient, and there is no assurance that a new therapist could improve the situation.

Certain personal characteristics of therapists have been associated with better working alliance, including "less self-directed hostility, more perceived social support, and higher degree of comfort with closeness in interpersonal relationships... empathy, non-possessive warmth, and genuineness are quite likely necessary, often even sufficient, in establishing an optimal therapeutic contact in psychotherapy" (Hersoug, Høglend, Monsen & Havik, 2001, p. 206). The therapist having specific skills should not be confused with therapist and client sharing certain qualities; indeed, there are no "associations between similarity of personal characteristics and alliance, whereas similarity of *values* did influence alliance as rated by patients… [even if values are not shared explicitly they] may still have an impact on the working alliance" (Hersoug et al., 2001, p. 214). Additional clinical procedures to improve the working alliance include conveying support for the patient to achieve goals, offering understanding and acceptance, developing a liking for the patient and expressing that appropriately, helping the patient to maintain functioning, presenting a hopeful attitude that goals will be achieved and that the therapist can help the process, recognizing progress towards goals and any positive adaptive behavior change, encouraging patients to express themselves, addressing alliance ruptures directly and promptly, accurately interpreting patient issues, and providing concrete rewards when patients achieve certain goals or milestones (Luborsky et al., 1997).

It is important for therapists to develop awareness of and the ability to address any problems that arise, since "therapists tend to either ignore or miss the occurrence of therapeutic rupture events… [recognizing warning markers] can enhance therapist training and performance" (Dykeman, 1995, p.18). Ruptures in the alliance can be identified, and healing them is possible mainly by focusing on problems within the patient-therapist relationship. Troubleshooting includes responding to unexpected or negative communication calmly and with respect, utilizing reflective listening, reframing (restating the client's statement in a positive way), and rolling with resistance (rather than confronting, disputing or arguing) by accepting and respecting what the client is saying while inviting them to consider a new perspective (Booth et al., 2008, p. 21). Repairing ruptures in the alliance is especially critical so that clients do not give up on the recovery process, but are encouraged to continue treatment.

Patients with *comorbid diagnoses*, especially those with personality disorders, are especially challenging and resistant to treatment, and ruptures in the therapeutic relationship are common. To reduce the dropout rate, it is critical for therapists to address these ruptures, including attending to rupture markers and exploring the rupture experience. Indeed, the skill and attention to do so is a relationship-building activity, as "any exploration of a rupture or avoidance in and of itself can be experienced by patents as very meaningful" (Muran, Safran, & Eubanks-Carter, 2010, p. 324). An alliance-focused treatment program called *brief relational therapy* (BRT) was developed to reduce attrition in this population. Steps to the BRT approach include:

1. Establishing collaboration and agreeing on treatment tasks, demonstrating mindfulness, and clarifying goals and expectations of treatment outcomes
2. Navigating the course of treatment, observing the interpersonal field, exploring the patient's experience (with therapists monitoring their own experience), and alternating attention between self and other to increase empathic contact
3. Approaching the termination of treatment by examining separation and loss, acceptance, and being alone, helping clients to constructively work through "the paradox of our simultaneous aloneness and togetherness" (Muran et al., 2010, p. 329)

Conclusion and Next Steps/Implications for Future Practice, Research, and Education on the Importance of Developing the Therapeutic Relationship and Supportive Organizations

All of the foregoing makes it clear why *it is critical to teach the importance of the therapeutic relationship* to students across the range of behavioral treatment and helping professions: psychology, psychotherapy, psychiatry, counseling, addiction treatment and rehabilitation, mental health nursing, and physiotherapy of different types. Clinician's ability to establish and maintain positive therapeutic relationships can only be improved through continued training and supervision. While the therapeutic alliance is affected by both patient qualities and therapist qualities, specific skill acquisition and *clinical/training experience in therapeutic alliance-building skills are teachable*. Students should be exposed to the concept of therapeutic alliance development early in the course of training and specifically of the role of task, goal, and bond. The most teachable skills are discussing patient nonverbal communication, setting shared goals, identifying appropriate tasks, and addressing relationship ruptures, as the ability to create an attachment bond may be more dependent on outside variables on the part of both clinician and patient. "[Since] the degree to which clients make progress may be due in some measure to the skill with which counselors perform their tasks... skill factors need more prominent attention in counselor training and supervision... [with] concrete and detailed evidence concerning how skillfully counselors have executed their tasks [relying] less upon counselors' descriptions of what they did... and more on specific ways of appraising skills" (Dryden, 2008, p. 13).

The ability to accurately interpret patient's core conflict early in treatment and repair the inevitable ruptures in the therapeutic relationship, as well as length of clinical experience and duration of training, all positively impacted alliance scores. Therapist experience has also been shown to diminish patient dropout rate, "indicating that experience makes a difference for the therapeutic relationship. Experienced therapists... are likely to contribute positively to the quality of alliance [and those with] more than 6 years of experience had a disproportionately high percentage of patients who improved and a disproportionately low percentage... who deteriorated... supporting the importance of the therapeutic relationship" (Hersoug et al., 2001, p. 206). Therapists with confidence in their abilities based on experience are often rated more highly by patients on the alliance scale, which "may reflect patients' preference for therapists with a more structured, active involvement in therapy... more emphasis on role preparation, education, reassurance, and support might have a positive impact on the working alliance," (Hersoug et al., 2001, p. 214) as opposed to a more removed, neutral stance, which may be viewed as lack of caring or empathy.

When seeking "to integrate the essential elements of the... therapeutic relationship back into the curriculum" (Perraud et al., 2006, p. 216), the critical question is: how do we teach these skills? While patient (and therapist) personal characteristics can play a significant role in the alliance, the teachable skills that help students learn to maintain the alliance and facilitate other therapeutic work are *empathy* (including warmth and positive regard), *congruence* (being genuine), *goal collaboration* (agreement on tasks and outcomes of therapy), *clinician self-awareness*/management of countertransference, and identifying and promptly addressing relationship ruptures. *Supervision* sessions are needed to increase awareness of the importance of relationship elements, with subsequent assignments for students to practice these in a safe environment, and later *evaluation* on their progress. Tools may include a "moment map" where students describe encounters with patients, including their own reactions, which are reviewed as part of the supervision and assessment process. These approaches help to educate students in the core elements of the therapeutic relationship and to further study the correlation of the therapeutic relationship to therapy outcomes. One approach to teach these relationship skills is to have "initial supervision sessions raise awareness of the relationship elements and subsequent assignments provide opportunities to practice them in a safe environment" (Perraud et al., 2006, pp. 221–4).

Another intervention to improve routine clinical communication and thus therapeutic relationships, called *dialog*, was designed to make patient-clinician interaction more effective and improve outcomes in patients with psychotic disorders. Simply interacting on a regular basis, asking about patient satisfaction with eight life domains and three treatment aspects, as well as their wishes for help in each area, resulted in better quality of life, higher treatment satisfaction, and fewer unmet needs after 1 year. This approach is completely flexible for use in all treatment modalities (client-centered, cognitive-behavioral, solution-focused, etc.) and is simply focused on improving communication and subsequently long-term outcomes. Ultimately, individual interventions based on different patients and situations, with sensitivity to the wider social and cultural context, are needed "to enhance therapeutic relationships to optimize therapeutic effect.... This will require *better training, ongoing supervision and proper evaluation* [of] therapeutic relationships and related interventions... to systematically improve engagement, adherence and patient outcome" (Priebe & McCabe, 2008, pp. 524–5).

There are several studies showing that improved alliance between patient, therapist, and treatment organization leads to reductions in the dropout rate and improvements in patient motivation, including goal setting (Luborsky et al., 1997).

Conclusion

Given the demonstrated importance of the therapeutic relationship in patient outcomes, students should be given ample training and opportunity to practice relationship skills, as well as supervision and evaluation to determine that they are acquiring the needed ability to build, maintain, and repair effective working relationships with their patients. These skills are valuable regardless of which therapeutic method they will employ, what population they will be serving, or where they will be working. These skills include education about the importance of goals, tasks, and bond, empathy (including warmth and positive regard), congruence, active listening, self-awareness (including awareness of personal biases and patient background to ensure cultural competence), not crossing boundaries, educating the patient about what to expect from therapy, collaborating and agreeing on goals and tasks, and more. Readings, clinical work, supervision, and evaluation should focus on the central role of the therapeutic relationship, because it is through "the therapeutic relationship [that] diagnoses are made, treatment plans are negotiated and most interventions are delivered… Indeed, the relationship itself may be a curative factor in its own right" (Priebe & McCabe, 2006, p. 69).

References

Ahmed, S., Wilson, K. B., Henriksen, R. C., & Jones, J. W. (Spring 2011). What does it mean to be a culturally-competent counselor? *Journal for Social Action in Counseling and Psychology, 3*, 1.

Asnaani, A., & Hofmann, S. G. (2012). Collaboration in multicultural therapy: Establishing a strong therapeutic alliance across cultural lines. *Journal of Clinical Psychology, 68*, 187–197.

Beach, M. C., Saha, S., & Cooper, L. A. (2006). The role and relationship of cultural competence and patient-centeredness in health care quality. *The Commonwealth Fund*, pub. No. *960*, vi–vii.

Booth, R., Thompson, L., & Campbell, B. K. (2008). Developing the therapeutic alliance as a bridge to treatment. *Training Manual for the Therapeutic Alliance Intervention, National Institute on Drug Abuse (NIDA) Clinical Trials Network (CTN) 0017: HIV and HCV Risk Reduction Interventions in Drug Detoxification and Treatment Settings*. (http://ctndissemina-tionlibrary.org/display/284.htm)

Center for Substance Abuse Treatment. (2014). Chapter 5. Behavioral health treatment for major racial and ethnic groups. In *Improving cultural competence, Treatment Improvement Protocol (TIP) Series No. 59* (pp. 101–157). Rockville: Substance Abuse and Mental Health Services Administration. (https://www.ncbi.nlm.nih.gov/books/NBK248428/).

Dryden, W. (2008). Chapter 1. The therapeutic alliance as an integrating framework. In W. Dryden & A. Reeves (Eds.), *Key issues for counselling in action* (p. 6). London: Sage.

Dykeman, C. (1995). An introduction to working alliance theory for professional counselors. Information Analyses (070), ERIC Document Reproduction Service No. ED 387 755. (https://files.eric.ed.gov/fulltext/ED387755.pdf)

Erdur, O., Rude, S., Baron, A., Draper, M., & Shankar, L. (Fall 2000). Working alliance and treatment outcome in ethnically similar and dissimilar client-therapist pairings. *Research Reports of the Research Consortium of Counseling & Psychological Services in Higher Education, 1*, 12.

Fernandez, O. M., Krause, M., & Perez, J. C. (2016). Therapeutic alliance in the initial phase of psychotherapy with adolescents: Different perspectives and their association with therapeutic outcomes. *Research in Psychotherapy: Psychopathology Process and Outcome, 19*, 1–9. (http://www.researchinpsychotherapy.org/index.php/rpsy/article/view/180/156).

Frigo, D. (Oct. 2006). *Therapeutic alliance: Improving treatment outcome*. Research Update, Butler Center for Research, Hazelden Betty Ford Foundation.

Grant, A., Mills, J., Mulhern, R., & Short, N. (2004). Chapter 2: The therapeutic alliance and case formulation. In A. Grant, J. Mills, R. Mulhern, & N. Short (Eds.), *Cognitive behavioural therapy in mental health care*. London: Sage. (https://www.corwin.com/sites/default/files/upm-binaries/9667_023127ch2.pdf).

Guide to Therapeutic Relationships and Professional Boundaries. (2013). *College of Physiotherapists of Ontario*. Ontario, Canada. May 27, 2013. (https://www.collegept.org/docs/default-source/blogdocuments/therapeutic_relationships_prof_boundaries_guide130527.pdf?Status=Master&sfvrsn=0)

Hatcher, R. L. (2010). Chapter 1. Alliance theory and measurement. In J. C. Muran & J. P. Barber (Eds.), *The therapeutic alliance: An evidence-based guide to practice*. New York: The Guilford Press. (https://www.guilford.com/books/The-Therapeutic-Alliance/Muran-Barber/9781606238738).

Hersoug, A. G., Høglend, P., Monsen, J. T., & Havik, O. E. (Fall 2001). Quality of working alliance in psychotherapy: Therapist variables and patient/therapist similarity as predictors. *The Journal of Psychotherapy Practice and Research, 10*, 4.

Jordan-Arthur, B., Romero, G., & Karver, M. (Summer 2011). The importance of therapeutic alliance for transition-aged youth. *Focal Point: Youth, Young Adults & Mental Health, Healthy Relationships, 25*(1), 10.

Lecharrois, E. (2011). *Therapeutic relationships. Self-study module, information and J services.* (https://www.researchgate.net/publication/275971288_Therapeutic_Relationships)

Luborsky, L., Barber, J. P., Siqueland, L., McLellan, A. T., & Woody, G. (1997). Establishing a therapeutic alliance with substance abusers. *NIDA Research Monograph, 165*, 233–244.

Muran, J. C., Safran, J. D., & Eubanks-Carter, C. (2010). Chapter 16. Developing therapist abilities to negotiate alliance ruptures. Provo, UT. In M. J. Lambert (Ed.), *The Therapeutic Alliance: An evidence-based guide to practice*. Psychotherapy Research. https://doi.org/10.1080/10503 307.2015.1031200

Nezu, A. M. (2010). Cultural influences on the process of conducting psychotherapy: Personal reflections of an ethnic minority psychologist. *Psychotherapy Theory, Research, Practice, Training, 47*, 20.

Oakes, K. E. (Nov. 2011). Health care disparities and training in culturally competent mental health counseling: A review of the literature and implications for research. *International Journal of Humanities and Social Sciences, 1*, 17.

Perraud, S., Delaney, K. R., Carlson-Sabelli, L., Johnson, M. E., Shephard, R., & Paun, O. (Nov. 2006). Advanced practice psychiatric mental health nursing, finding our core: The therapeutic relationship in the 21st century. *Perspectives in Psychiatric Care, 42*(4), 215.

Priebe, S., & McCabe, R. (2006). The therapeutic relationship in psychiatric settings. *Acta Psychiatrica Scandinavica, 113*(*Suppl. 429*), 69.

Priebe, S. & McCabe, R. (Dec. 2008). Therapeutic relationships in psychiatry; The basis of therapy or therapy in itself?, *International Review of Psychiatry* 20 (6); 521-526.

Priebe, S., Richardson, M., Cooney, M., Adedeji, O., & McCabe, R. (2011). Does the therapeutic relationship predict outcomes of psychiatric treatment in patients with psychosis? A systematic review. *Psychotherapy and Psychosomatics, 80*, 70.

Professional Boundaries for Therapeutic Relationships. (2011). *College of Registered Nurses of Manitoba*. Manitoba, Canada. September 2011. (https://www.crnm.mb.ca/uploads/document/document_file_99.pdf?t=1438267436)

Qureshi, A., & Collazos, F. (2005). Cultural competence in the mental health treatment of immigrant and ethnic minority clients. *Diversity in Health and Social Care, 2*, 307–317.

Shattell, M. M., Starr, S. S., & Thomas, S. P. (2007). 'Take my hand, help me out': Mental health service recipients' experience of the therapeutic relationship. *International Journal of Mental Health Nursing, 16*, 275. (https://www.ncbi.nlm.nih.gov/pubmed/17635627).

Simpson, T. P., Frick, P. J., & Kahn, R. E. (2013). Therapeutic alliance in justice-involved adolescents undergoing mental health treatment: The role of callous-unemotional traits. *International Journal of Forensic Mental Health, 12*, 83–92. (https://doi.org/10.1080/14999013.2013.787559; http://psycnet.apa.org/record/2013-18818-001)

Summers, R. F., & Barber, J. P. (2003). Therapeutic alliance as a measurable psychotherapy skill. *Academic Psychiatry, 27*, 160.

Varcarolis, E. M. (Oct 7, 2005). Developing therapeutic relationships, Ch. 10. In *Foundations of Psychiatric Mental Health Nursing*. Philadelphia: Elsevier.

Vasquez, M. J. T. (Nov 2007). Cultural difference and the therapeutic alliance: An evidence-based analysis. *American Psychologist, 62*, 878.

Watson, J. C., & Kalogerakos, F. (2010). Chapter 10. The therapeutic alliance in humanistic psychotherapy. In J. C. Muran & J. P. Barber (Eds.), *The therapeutic alliance: An evidence-based guide to practice*. New York: The Guilford Press. (https://www.guilford.com/books/The-Therapeutic-Alliance/Muran-Barber/9781606238738).

Where's the line? Professional Boundaries in a Therapeutic Relationship. (2011). *College of Speech and Hearing Health Professionals of BC*. British Columbia, Canada. September 2011. (http://www.cshhpbc.org/docs/where_s_the_line_-_professional_boundaries.pdf)

Chapter 20
Teaching Students the Importance of Community Engagement and Awareness in the Areas of Mental Health and Addiction

Manoj Pardasani

Introduction

Social work is community practice (Hardcastle, Powers, & Wenocur, 2011). Although many students of social work prefer to focus on gaining direct practice knowledge and skills, the need for them to be able to engage within communities is essential to them being effective practitioners (Sather, Weitz, & Carlson, 2007). According to the Council of Social Work Education (2015), the purpose of social work is to promote human and community well-being. Social work has always emphasized the person-in-environment approach addressing individual and social problems. In the Educational Policy and Accreditation Standards (EPAS) set forth by CSWE, competencies #6 through #9 require that students learn how to engage, assess, intervene, and evaluate practice with individuals, families, groups, as well as communities (CSWE, 2015). However, many students in social work schools fail to see the importance of learning about working with communities through macro practice – community assessment, engagement, organization, advocacy, and interventions (Boehm & Cohen, 2013; Sather et al., 2007; Thomas, Netting, & O'Connor, 2011). In the field of mental health and addictions treatment, it would be very difficult for social workers to ignore the community aspect of practice when working with individuals and families.

Since the 1960s, the treatment of mental health and addictions in the field has transferred progressively from large, in-patient institutions to community-based organizations (Rosenberg & Rosenberg, 2016; Taxman & Belenko, 2012). The Community Mental Health Center Construction Act (1963) and subsequent legislations have steadily placed more emphasis on providing services to individuals within their communities (Sands, 2001). The movement toward block grants in the

M. Pardasani (✉)
Graduate School of Social Service, Fordham University, New York, NY, USA
e-mail: mpardasani@fordham.edu

© Springer International Publishing AG 2018
T. MacMillan, A. Sisselman-Borgia (eds.), *New Directions in Treatment, Education, and Outreach for Mental Health and Addiction*, Advances in Mental Health and Addiction, https://doi.org/10.1007/978-3-319-72778-3_20

1980s, the development of managed healthcare systems, and the Mental Health Parity Act of 1996 further cemented this dependence on community-based systems of care in the field of mental health and addictions (Sands, 2001; Taxman & Belenko, 2012). Integration of individuals seeking treatment within the community infrastructure is critical to success of interventions (Beasley & Jason, 2015; Cimino, Mendoza, Thieleman, Shively, & Kunz, 2015). The Affordable Care Act of 2010 further expanded access to community-based mental health and substance abuse treatment for nearly 62 million Americans (US Department for Health and Human Services, 2013). Thus, practice in this field has become synonymous with community practice in the present day. It requires social workers to adopt the systems approach to providing effective and impactful treatment for the affected population within their communities.

This chapter helps to define the evolving meaning of community, illustrate the basic concepts of community practice, and highlight the benefits of community engagement in the field of mental health and addictions. Critical skills necessarily to practice in the community context while ensuring the health and well-being of the individuals and families we serve are elucidated.

Definitions

Community

According to Hardcastle et al. (2011), communities are often the context of social work practice. According to Barker (1999), community is "a group of individuals or families that share a certain values, services, institutions, interests or geographic proximity" (p. 89). Kirst-Ashman and Hull (2011) identify three essential components that define a community – shared space, social interaction, and shared sense of identity. Communities play a critical role in supporting, nurturing, and socializing its members. Various components of a community can act as protective or risk factors for the individual needing help. The impact of social work practice can be enhanced when the various resources of a community are harnessed in favor of the client. Concurrently, barriers and risk factors identified have to be addressed as well in order to serve the client comprehensively.

Community Practice

> When a social worker engages in developing, locating, linking with, and managing community resources to help people improve their social functioning and lives, the social worker is engaging in community practice. (Hardcastle et al., 2011; p. 4).

Knowledge of community and associated practice skills are the distinguishing characteristics that separate a social worker from other professionals. Community practice skills help influence and modify behavioral patterns of the stakeholders within a community as well as change people's interactions within the community in order to promote the health and well-being of its members (Hardcastle et al., 2011; Kirst-Ashman & Hull, 2011). In recent years, the concept of *community practice* has been expanded and is referred to as *macro practice*. Macro practice is defined as "professional-directed intervention designed to bring about planned change in organizations and communities" (Netting, Kettner, & McMurtry, 1993, p. 3). According to the Association for Community Organization and Social Administration (ACOSA), the purpose of community practice, or *macro social work*, is to promote social justice by working collectively within or among community groups and nonprofit agencies to solve social problems in the community (2017). Several components of community practice have been identified such as:

- Identifying gaps and needs – and advocating for action to fulfill them
- Prevention
- Locating and connecting consumers with resources and services
- Building or enhancing social support and healthy networks
- Highlighting and fighting discrimination, oppression and injustice
- Advocating on behalf of vulnerable and marginalized populations
- Raising critical consciousness and awareness
- Organizing communities to act in their own interests

(Asamoah, Gill, Foster, & Mummery, 2016; Aubry, Flynn, Virley, & Neri, 2013; Baillie et al., 2004; Bava, Coffey, Weingarten, & Becker, 2010; Lemieux, Richards, Hunter, & Kasofsky, 2015; Ngo et al., 2016; Patel, Butler, & Wells, 2006)

Theoretical Framework

In attempting to frame community practice within a theoretical framework, systems theory, social learning theory, social exchange theory, interorganizational theory, conflict theory, or ecological theory have been widely utilized (Hardcastle et al., 2011). For the purpose of this chapter, I adapt the ecological framework that focuses on the interconnectedness of biological, social, psychological, economic, and cultural factors on the well-being of individuals (Germain & Gittelman, 1995). This framework allows us to understand the symbiotic and dynamic relationship that exists between the individual and the environment in which they reside. Within the realm of community practice, it allows individuals, families, and service providers to engage in complex relationships with one another that is based on mutual aid, interdependence, and sharing of resources (Germain & Gittelman, 1995). Community practice in the field of mental health and substance use disorders (SUDs) requires various community stakeholders to work collaboratively in order to build a comprehensive support system that enhances the health and well-being of all its members.

Benefits of Community Engagement

As mentioned earlier, the context of care in mental health and SUDs has shifted to the community. The vast majority of individuals seeking help for mental health or SUDs are directed to community-based organizations. Community-based systems of care are quite complex and comprise a mix of public and private, for-profit, and nonprofit entities. Funding sources for these services also determine access, eligibility for services, and the nature of services received. It is often hard for individuals and families to receive all the necessary services from one organization or agency. They are required to navigate a complex and complicated system to address their needs effectively. Depending on the community itself, there may be adequate or inadequate resources and services available. And it is not just essential services like treatment that individuals and families need. They may also need assistance with allied services such as housing, assistance with entitlements like food stamps and health insurance, vocational guidance, transportation, etc.

The focus of social work education for all students should be on integrating community practice into direct practice knowledge and strategies. Community practice education can prepare social workers to engage with not just the individuals seeking treatment but with the community as an entity in itself in order to access all the resources needed and create a safe and healthy environment for their consumers to thrive in (Boehm & Cohen, 2013; Sather et al., 2007; Thomas et al., 2011). The benefits of community engagement and integration can be summarized as follows:

- Enhancing service integration
- Raising awareness
- Reducing stigma
- Developing and enhancing social support systems
- Promoting treatment adherence

(DeHart, 2010; Matthew, 2017; Tippin, Maranzan, & Mountain, 2016).

Enhancing Service Integration

Since the system of care in communities is so diffuse, social workers need to understand the lay of the land. In other words, they need to understand what resources, services, and programs are available in the community and who is responsible for administering them. According to Sands and Angell (2001), service integration at the community level happens through collaboration between agencies, between professionals from various disciplines, and between consumers and professionals. In any given community, one might have to have to contend with:

- Hospitals
- In-patient detox and rehabilitation centers
- Outpatient substance abuse treatment programs

- Methadone treatment programs
- Community mental health centers
- Nonprofit or for-profit counseling agencies
- Private practice counselors
- Social service agencies that also offer mental health and addictions interventions
- Faith-based service organizations
- Legal aid services
- Volunteer or self-help organizations
- Peer-support groups like AA, NA, etc.
- Government agencies that deal with housing, food subsidies, and health insurance (Medicaid and Medicare)
- Group homes and supportive housing programs
- Day programs for people with mental illness or developmental disabilities
- Educational programs like GED completion
- Youth mentoring programs
- Vocational programs such as job readiness and placement

In order to effectively serve consumers, social workers would need to develop a record of all the programs and services available in the community and help consumers access them. This underscores the principle of a "wraparound" treatment plan. In addition, they could advocate for the consumers who may have difficulty navigating through these programs or entitlement applications. If there are gaps in services or unmet needs, they could highlight the need for fiscal support for programs that could address those needs. Connecting consumers with community-based resources and assisting them in crafting a comprehensive intervention plan would ensure that consumers and their families are served ethically and effectively (Abendstern et al., 2016; Aubry et al., 2013; Bava et al., 2010; Das, O'Neill, & Pinkerton, 2016; DeHart, 2010; Ngo et al., 2016; Patel et al., 2006).

Raising Awareness

Educating a community about mental illness and substance misuse is an important step in raising awareness about issues that may impact individuals and families (Mason & Fogel, 2013; Steiner, 2016). Frequently, people may not be aware about the various aspects of mental illness or the nature of addiction. They may also have incomplete or inaccurate information about these issues. This may prevent individuals from developing plans for prevention or seeking timely intervention when needed. Denial of the existence of mental illness or the nature of addiction may result in a community not allocating adequate resources for their redressal. Or worse, some members of the community may be denied services or access because of the very nature of their illness. Social workers play a vital role in educating affected individuals, their families, and other stakeholders (political representatives, community leaders, organizations) about these issues. Critical consciousness raising not only empowers consumers but the community at large as well and ensures that people's needs are met adequately and with dignity.

Reducing Stigma

Researchers have extensively documented the impact of stigma on individuals impacted by mental illness and addictions (Asamoah et al., 2016; Chronister, Chou, & Liao, 2013; Talebi, Matheson, & Anisman, 2016; Verhaeghe, Bracke, & Christiaens, 2010). Specifically, the fear of being treated differently, negatively judged, or discriminated against drives many to avoid admitting need for services or accessing them. The anticipated shame experienced by both the individuals suffering and the families impacted leads to denial of the problem and a distancing from community supports. This makes the problem worse for all impacted as the situation only festers and places everyone at risk of an overwhelming crisis. This withdrawal from support systems increases the likelihood of individuals dying, ending up in emergency medical care or being incarcerated, thereby increasing societal costs and criminalizing the individual. Stigma also causes community members and organizations to form preconceived notions about the affected population and erect barriers that make integration and treatment difficult. Social workers must combat this stigma through education and outreach. It is critical that they help people understand the nature and impact of stigma and make every effort to reduce or eliminate it. Reducing stigma would increase individual motivation to seek treatment and reduce systemic barriers to improving the quality of life of all members of a community. Understanding the nature of illness and SUDs would also enable families and peers to develop a strong support system for the individual.

Developing and Enhancing Social Support Systems

Researchers have established the important role support systems play in enhancing the well-being of individuals seeking help (Aubry et al., 2013; Ozbay et al., 2006; Smyth, Siriwardhana, Hotopf, & Hatch, 2015). Support systems could comprise families (both biological and ones created by choice), friends, peers, faith-based institutions, and social groups. Support systems help an individual feel valued. They help provide guidance, motivation, nurturance, and assistance for the affected individual. Support systems allow a person to feel like they are not alone and enhance their resilience in seeking help and committing to positive change. Social workers need to identify positive support systems and facilitate their involvement in the client's life. On the other hand, they also need to highlight individuals in the client's life that pose a risk to their continued health and well-being. The help-seeking individual needs to be made aware of how the various actors in their life impact them positively or negatively. A client would need assistance in navigating these relationships and developing healthy interactional behaviors. Simultaneously, various actors in the support system need to learn skills of how to support their loved one and encourage their commitment to seeking a healthier lifestyle.

Promoting Treatment Adherence

Even when an individual seeks help and engages in treatment, there is no guarantee that they will continue their participation until it is required. Relapse rates are quite high for individuals diagnosed with serious mental illness or substance abuse disorders. Adherence to treatment requires a high degree of commitment, as well as a significant investment of emotional fortitude. Various factors may jeopardize positive outcomes such as lack of support, unanticipated crises, side effects of medications, disruption of entitlements, negative perception of self-efficacy, etc. (Beasley & Jason, 2015; Cimino et al., 2015; Lemieux et al., 2015; Patel et al., 2006). Education is critical to lowering the incidences of relapse. Additionally, critical skills are needed to entice a client back into treatment even after they have relapsed or discontinued treatment. Sometimes it might be the case of a mismatch between intervention selected and the capacity of a consumer to engage with it. Social workers need to be well versed in various treatment modalities and be able to help the client select the most appropriate intervention. They also need to activate the protective factors that might assist the client in adhering to their treatment regimen. Advocacy skills are also necessary to reduce the incidence of punitive actions taken by agencies when a client relapses temporarily or is unable to comply with unrealistic expectations.

Culture and Cultural Competence

Culture is defined as the sum total of life patterns within a group of people that is passed on from generation to generation (Lum, 2010). Culture includes institutions, languages, religious beliefs, ways of living, thinking, artistic expressions, and social relationships (Hodge, Struckman, & Trost, 1975). In essence, culture is the lens through which we view the world and negotiate our existence. Culture frames how we process information and make decisions. This applies to individuals and families impacted by mental illness and SUDs. How individuals within a community view mental illness or SUDs will determine their motivation to seek help and engage in treatment. Social workers are required to be "culturally competent" in order to effectively engage and intervene with individuals from diverse backgrounds (race, ethnicity, socioeconomic status, national origin, sexual orientation, educational level, religious affiliation, etc.). According to the Substance Abuse and Mental Health Services Administration (SAMHSA, 2016), cultural competence is "the ability to interact effectively with people of different cultures." Cultural competence requires social workers to be responsive to the health beliefs and practices of diverse populations and integrate that knowledge into their outreach and intervention efforts.

As noted earlier, one of the most important steps in initiating culturally competent community practice is to raise awareness of mental illness and addictions. In some groups, these issues may be seen as something to be ashamed of or that it is caused by a lack of faith. Others might view these illnesses as a sign of moral failure or a negative reflection on parenting. This may cause individuals and families to remain in denial of the problem or shy away from seeking treatment so as not to draw attention to themselves. In other instances, inaccurate information may be shared with families in need, and this may hinder them from seeking help. Frequently, concepts and terms used in the field of mental health may not translate easily to all languages. Some groups may not even have words in their language to describe mental illness or SUDs. Social workers must raise awareness, share accurate information about mental illness and addictions, and reduce stigma in the target communities. They need to build a wide network of allies that includes community leaders, influential persons, faith-based leaders, and other institutions within the community to get the message out to the people in need – in the language that they are comfortable with. Partnering with professionals from various disciplines and peers (within the community) may allow access to those groups that may traditionally shy away from seeking information or help. When members of a community see others that look like themselves or have similar beliefs speak about their health struggles, it would reduce the feelings of isolation and internalized shame. Access to service providers who understand the cultural norms and beliefs and meaningfully integrate those in to their intervention plan will encourage more families to speak up and engage in treatment.

Practice Skills in Community Engagement

If social workers are to be effective in the field of mental health and addictions, they need to develop their capacity to engage systematically and competently within their communities (Boehm & Cohen, 2013; Sather et al., 2007; Silverman, 2001; Thomas et al., 2011). As discussed earlier, consumers need to be able to access services and resources from various sources. Additionally, they may also have unmet needs for specific resources or face barriers in accessing services. This is where social workers and other mental health or substance misuse professionals can assist their consumers within the community context. They need to develop specific skills that allow them to serve the client holistically and comprehensively within an integrated community-based service system. Some of the competencies required for community engagement are:

- Conducting an environmental scan
- Providing linkages to services and resources
- Conducting needs assessments
- Developing collaborations and partnerships
- Enhancing family support and education
- Building capacity within communities
- Organizing community and social action
- Engaging in policy practice and advocacy

Conducting an Environmental Scan

An essential first step in engaging a community is to conduct an environmental scan. Social workers need to identify the various agencies and organizations that exist within and/or serve the community. Additionally, there might be mutual aid groups, volunteer organizations, and faith-based institutions that could be potential sources of care and assistance. Foundations and centers that could serve as sources of funding or professional development for consumers and individuals working in this field would need to be engaged. A scan should include the identification of all relevant stakeholders within a community – those that could be a source of support and others who might provide resistance. Once an exhaustive search has been completed, all the data need to be compiled into a form of resource directory that could provide valuable guidance to consumers, their families, and professionals serving them. This directory could include information on specific services provided by various agencies, allied institutions (such as a church or a school) and professionals, eligibility requirements, contact information for accessing the services, and any other relevant information. The scan needs to be conducted at periodic intervals so as to ensure that the information being provided is current and relevant.

Conducting Needs Assessments

Social workers bear an ethical responsibility not just to serve consumers within their organizational context but also identify unmet needs for services and resources. They can then utilize this information to advocate for expanded services or additional resources. In order to gather accurate information on service/resource gaps, it is critical to conduct scientifically rigorous and comprehensive needs assessments. This requires social workers to be equipped with the knowledge of research methods and skills in designing and implementing community-wide assessments. Skills in designing a research study, selecting an appropriate design and methodology, recruiting respondents (all relevant stakeholders), gathering data, using analytical software for data entry and analysis, and preparing and disseminating findings are necessary to identify unmet needs and service/resource gaps in the community.

Most social workers have received some training in research methods and statistics in their educational programs. However, the content in those courses may not have been tailored to a macro or community focus. Thus, they may be able to understand and implement individual-focused, evidence-based interventions, for instance, but not know how to engage and survey a community at large. An added advantage of conducting such assessments is that it could include consumers in the planning and implementation, thereby empowering them to become more engaged and informed in the process.

Developing Collaborations and Partnerships

Once an environmental scan is completed and a resource directory developed, social workers may need to develop professional collaborations and interagency partnerships to enhance the degree of care for their consumers. Collaborations between professionals from various disciplines would ensure integrated care through enhanced communication and planning between providers and a systematic implementation of the intervention plan. Formal and informal agreements between agencies would enable consumers to access a greater number of resources through expedited application procedures. Such collaborations also limit the possibility of service overlaps and duplication, while increasing the judicious use of precious resources within a community. Integrated interventions prevent the possibility of consumers falling through the cracks in transition from one form of care to another – such as when an individual is discharged from a hospital back to an outpatient setting. Social workers need to know how to negotiate and prepare effective linkage agreements that benefit the individuals and families they serve. This process also increases an understanding of the practices of various disciplines and how they contribute to the overall well-being of the consumers.

Enhancing Family Support and Education

Although the primary focus and responsibility of a social worker is toward the individual consumer, families become the secondary client in the process. Families can be biological or naturally occurring and are critical to the health and well-being of the consumer. They may serve as sources of strength, support, and assistance. They enable the individual to seek out help and stay committed and motivated through the process. On the other hand, they may pose as risk factors. If families lack knowledge about mental illness or SUDs, they may increase denial on part of the consumer, and this may limit help seeking on their part. Additionally, the family may lack the resources and capacity (both financial and emotional) to support the consumer adequately. Family members are also directly impacted by the illness or addiction. They may experience emotional distress, trauma, financial hardships, social isolation, and discrimination. Thus, social workers need be able to provide education to families, link them to needed services and resources, and provide guidance on how to support their family member in treatment.

Building Capacity Within Communities

Once a comprehensive needs assessment is conducted, service gaps, unmet needs, and inadequate resources can be identified. Social workers can then utilize this data to modify existing programs, create new programs or services, or redirect underutilized resources to serve the consumer more effectively. Relying on the linkages and partnerships created, they can encourage other agencies, organizations, and professionals to expand their services to address unmet needs. Social workers can also build capacity by raising awareness and knowledge about critical issues in mental health within the community. Such education reduces stigma, incidences of social ostracism, and barriers. It also builds the capacity of a community to address its members' needs in a competent, sensitive, and comprehensive manner. An informed consumer is an empowered consumer. Furthermore, professionals and service providers within the community may need specialized knowledge and skills in order to work with the target population. Social workers can conduct these trainings themselves or link the providers to the necessary training resources.

Organizing Community and Social Action

Frequently, community members, especially consumers and their supporters, need to be rallied to raise awareness about unmet needs or inadequate resources. A community may need to bring attention to issues that impact its members' lives. Communities usually have limited experience with organizing for action. People may need guidance and training in order to create an effective and impactful plan for social action. Social workers can be very helpful in this arena. Working with their consumers and families, they can prepare and support organizing efforts. They can help address their fears of being "exposed" in the community or of losing their current benefits for speaking up. These efforts require skills in persuasion, planning, coordination, communication, drafting effective arguments, etc. When it comes to communication, the creative use of multiple media outlets such as newspapers, radio, television, and social media would be critical to successful efforts. It is also important, in social action endeavors, to build and activate provider networks. These networks comprise professionals and experts who can develop plans to influence legislators, funders, and other major decision-makers. Experts could come from various professional disciplines, consumer advocacy groups, scholars in the field of mental health and addictions, and government. Social workers can help coordinate the work of these collaborative networks and establish synchronicity between the consumer efforts and that of these professional networks. Social workers need to be exposed to exemplars of successful social action ventures and be able to practice these skills in their educational programs.

Engaging in Policy Practice and Advocacy

The vast majority of social work and healthcare (physical, mental, and SUD) services are funded through government contracts and grants. Agencies and organizations rely heavily on this public source of funding while also raising resources from other sources to supplement their budgets. This public funding stream is reliant on social policies that determine the type of services and assistance offered, as well as eligibility requirements. Thus, it is imperative that social workers develop skills to analyze public policies and highlight their costs and benefits to consumers. Additionally, they would also need to engage in systematic and strategic advocacy efforts to influence change. Knowledge of how government functions and how policies can be enhanced is important information for social workers. Students are exposed to social welfare policy and advocacy courses while preparing to become social workers. However, their preparation for actually carrying out these tasks in practice may be limited.

Conclusion

The Council on Social Work Education (CSWE) prescribes the nature and direction of social work education through its EPAS (2015). Both BSW and MSW programs are governed by the competencies laid out in them. Schools of social work are then assigned the task of designing courses that meet those competencies. While many courses are common across schools – such as human behavior in the social environment, social policy, research and statistics, generalist practice, etc. – each school may place emphasis on different content and specializations depending on their organizational mission and focus. Schools also strive to offer choices that are popular with students. As mentioned earlier in this chapter, when students express interest in working in the fields of mental health or addictions, they think mainly of practice with individuals and families. Students struggle to see a connect with, and relevance of, community engagement and macro practice in this field. So it is up to faculty and administrators to integrate this content into their practice courses in order to better prepare students to work holistically within a community context. Generalist and advanced practice courses should be revised to help students understand the importance of community engagement in direct practice. Field placements must also be reimagined to give students an opportunity to see the integration between individuals seeing help and the community in which they reside. At a minimum, students should learn how to:

(i) Engage in holistic and multifaceted practice in mental health and addictions
(ii) Implement models of integrated care that provide comprehensive and effective interventions
(iii) Strategically raise community awareness, organize consumers and stakeholders, and build resource capacity
(iv) Systematically identify service and resource gaps, as well as unmet needs
(v) Advocate successfully for consumers and their families

It has always been an ethical imperative for social workers to preserve human dignity and promote social justice. The person-in-environment lens through which they serve requires them to integrate the individual within the community and engage the community at large for the betterment of the individual. The field of mental health and addictions has always reflected interdisciplinary practice. Given these practice realities and our mission as social workers, it is critical to learn how to practice within communities. Engagement and integration are vital to securing effective and sustainable outcomes for our clients. Preparing social workers to do this work would not only benefit the target population but also serve to underscore the importance of social work as a profession.

References

Abendstern, M., Tucker, S., Wilbeforce, M., Jasper, R., Brand, C., & Challis, D. (2016). Social workers as members of community mental health teams for older people: What is the added value? *British Journal of Social Work, 46*, 63–80.

Asamoah, P., Gill, S., Foster, E., & Mummery, C. (2016). Receive information. Reduce stigma. Reflect on strategies: The caregiver series. *Canadian Journal of Community Mental Health, 35*(3), 119–123.

Association for Community Organization and Social Administration (2017). *Macro social work practice: MSW*. Retrieved from http://www.acosa.org/joomla/mswstudents

Aubry, T., Flynn, R., Virley, B., & Neri, J. (2013). Social role valorization in community mental health housing: Does it continue to the community integration and life satisfaction of people with psychiatric disabilities. *Journal of Community Psychology, 41*(2), 218–235.

Baillie, L., Broughton, S., Bassett-Smith, J., Aasen, W., Oostrinde, M., Marino, B. A., et al. (2004). Community health, community involvement and community empowerment: Too much to expect? *Journal of Community Psychology, 32*(2), 217–228.

Barker, R. L. (1999). *The social work dictionary* (4th ed.). Washington, DC: NASW Press.

Bava, S., Coffey, E., Weingarten, K., & Becker, C. (2010). Lessons in collaboration, four years post-Katrina. *Family Process, 49*(4), 543–558.

Beasley, C., & Jason, L. (2015). Engagement and disengagement in mutual-help addiction recovery housing: A test of affective events theory. *American Journal of Community Psychology, 55*, 347–358.

Boehm, A., & Cohen, A. (2013). Commitment to community practice among social work students: Contributing factors. *Journal of Social Work Education, 49*, 601–618.

Chronister, J., Chou, C., & Liaso, H. (2013). The role of stigma, coping and social support in mediating the effect of societal stigma on internalized stigma, mental health recovery and quality of life among people with serious mental illness. *Journal of Community Psychology, 41*(5), 582–600.

Cimino, A., Mendoza, N., Thieleman, K., Shively, R., & Kunz, K. (2015). Women reentering community: Understanding addiction and trauma-related characteristics of recidivism. *Journal of Human Behavior in the Social Environment, 25*, 468–476.

Council on Social Work Education. (2015). *Educational policy and accreditation standards for baccalaureate and master's social work programs.* Washington, DC: CSWE.

Das, C., O'Neill, M., & Pinkerton, J. (2016). Re-engaging with community work as a method of practice in social work: A view from Northern Ireland. *Journal of Social Work, 16*(2), 196–215.

DeHart, D. D. (2010). Collaboration between victim services and faith organizations: Benefits, challenges and recommendations. *Journal of Religion & Spirituality in Social Work, 29*(4), 349–371.

Germain, C., & Gitterman, A. (1995). Ecological perspective. In R. L. Edwards (Ed.), *Encyclopedia of social work* (19th ed.). Washington, DC: NASW.

Hardcastle, D., Powers, P., & Wenocur, S. (2011). *Community practice: Theories, and skills for social workers* (3rd ed.). London: Oxford University Press.

Hodge, J., Struckmann, D., & Trost, L. (1975). Spirituality and people with mental illness: Developing spiritual competence in assessment and intervention. *Families in Society, 85*, 36–44.

Kirst-Ashman, K., & Hull, G., Jr. (2011). *Generalist practice with organizations and communities* (4th ed.). Toronto, Canada: Brooks/Cole.

Lemieux, C., Richards, K., Hunter, D., & Kasofsky, J. (2015). Interrelationships among physical health, health-related and psychosocial characteristics of persons receiving integrated care in community mental health settings. *Journal of Social Service Research, 41*(5), 561–583.

Lum, D. (2010). *Culturally competent practice: A framework for understanding diverse groups and justice issues* (4th ed.). New York: Thompson.

Mason, S., & Fogel, S. (2013). Prevention, community engagement and social work. *Families in Society, 94*(3), 139–140.

Matthew, R. (2017). Community engagement: Behavior strategies to enhance the quality of participatory partnerships. *Journal of Community Psychology, 45*(1), 117–127.

Netting, F., Kettner, P., & McMurtry, S. (1993). *Social work macro practice.* New York: Longman.

Ngo, V., Sherbourne, C., Chung, B., Wright, A., Whittington, Y., Wells, K., et al. (2016). Community engagement compared with technical assistance to disseminate depression care among low-income, minority women: A randomized controlled effectiveness study. *American Journal of Public Health, 106*, 1833–1841.

Ozbay, F., Johnson, D., Dimoulas, E., Morgan, C., III, Charney, D., & Southwick, S. (2006). Social support and resilience to stress. *Psychiatry (Edgmont), 4*(5), 35–40.

Patel, K., Butler, B., & Wells, K. (2006). What is necessary to transform the quality of mental health care? *Health Affairs, 25*(3), 681–693.

Rosenberg, J., & Rosenberg, S. (2016). *Community mental health: Challenges for the 21st century.* New York: Routledge.

Sands, R. (2001). *Clinical social work practice in behavioral mental health: A postmodern approach to practice with adults* (2nd ed.). Boston: Allyn & Bacon.

Sands, R. G., & Angell, B. (2001). Social workers as collaborators on interagency and interdisciplinary teams. In K. J. Bentley (Ed.), *Social work practice in mental health* (pp. 254–280). Pacific Grove, CA: Brooks/Cole.

Sather, P., Weitz, B., & Carlson, P. (2007). Engaging students in macro issues through community-based learning: The policy, practice and research sequence. *Journal of Teaching in Social Work, 27*(3/4), 61–79.

Silverman, S. (2001). Social workers as advocates and community organizers. In K. J. Bentley (Ed.), *Social work practice in mental health* (pp. 281–296). Pacific Grove, CA: Brooks/Cole.

Smyth, N., Siriwardhana, C., Hotopf, M., & Hatch, S. (2015). Social networks, social support and psychiatric symptoms: Social determinants and associations within a multicultural community population. *Social Psychiatry, 50*(7), 1111–1120.

Steiner, A. (2016). Assessing the effectiveness of a capacity building intervention in empowering hard-to-reach communities. *Journal of Community Practice, 24*(3), 235–263.

Substance Abuse and Mental Health Services Administration. (2016). *Cultural competence*. Retrieved from https://www.samhsa.gov/capt/applying-strategic-prevention/cultural-competence

Talebi, M., Matheson, K., & Anisman, H. (2016). The stigma of seeking help for mental health issues: Mediating roles of support and coping and the moderating role of symptom profile. *Journal of Applied Social Psychology, 46*, 470–482.

Taxman, F., & Belenko, S. (2012). *Implementing evidence-based practices in community corrections and addiction treatment*. New York: Springer.

Thomas, M. L., Netting, F. E., & O'Connor, M. K. (2011). A framework for teaching community practice. *Journal of Social Work Education, 47*(2), 337–355.

Tippin, G., Maranzan, K., & Mountain, M. A. (2016). Client outcomes associated with interprofessional care in a community mental health outpatient program. *Canadian Journal of Community Mental Health, 30*(3), 83–96.

U.S. Department for Health and Human Services. (2013). *Affordable care act expands mental health and substance use disorder benefits*. February 20, 2013. Retrieved from https://aspe.hhs.gov/report/affordable-care-act-expands-mental-health-and-substance-use-disorder-benefits-and-federal-parity-protections-62-million-americans

Verhaeghe, M., Bracke, P., & Christiaens, W. (2010). Stigma and client satisfaction in mental health services. *Journal of Applied Social Psychology, 40*, 2295–2318.

Index

GPSR Compliance
The European Union's (EU) General Product Safety Regulation (GPSR) is a set
of rules that requires consumer products to be safe and our obligations to
ensure this.

If you have any concerns about our products, you can contact us on

ProductSafety@springernature.com

In case Publisher is established outside the EU, the EU authorized
representative is:

Springer Nature Customer Service Center GmbH
Europaplatz 3
69115 Heidelberg, Germany

www.ingramcontent.com/pod-product-compliance
Ingram Content Group UK Ltd.
Pitfield, Milton Keynes, MK11 3LW, UK
UKHW021327230425
5596UKWH00003B/5

* 9 7 8 3 3 1 9 7 2 7 7 7 6 *